Getting Back On Track

Using Megapotency Homeopathy

JILL R TURLAND
Dip Hom, Dip Herb Med, Dip Hol Massage

Getting Back on Track - Using Megapotency Homeopathy
© Jill R. Turland 2003
Second Edition 2014
Revised and Reprinted 2019

Getting Back on Track - Using Megapotency Homeopathy is copyright under the
Berne Convention. All rights reserved. Apart from any fair dealing for the purpose
of private study, research, criticism or review, no part of this publication may be
reproduced, stored or transmitted without prior permission of the copyright owner.
Enquiries should be addressed to Jill R. Turland at the Publisher's email address
below. (She does not bite!)

*Disclaimer: This book is not intended to replace the services of a qualified health practitioner. While the book
describes well proven research, any application of the recommendations outlined within is at the reader's
qualified discretion. The author and publisher take no responsibility for the outcomes of such application.
Untrained users of homeopathy are requested and advised to seek skilled assessment by a professional
homeopath before taking any of the remedies as described herein, and to maintain close communication with
that practitioner. Only through professional clinical record-keeping can this new knowledge be expanded
and results confirmed for the greater benefit of humanity.*

ISBN 978-1-951670-00-9 - Paperback
ISBN 978-1-951670-01-6 - Hardback
ISBN 978-1-951670-02-3 - eBook
National Library of Australia
State Library of New South Wales

Published by Author's Note 360
info@authorsnote360.com

Typeset in Palatino 10 using QuarkXpress Vers7
Cover and cover photograph Comfrey in Flower ©Jill R. Turland 2003

First printed 2003 by Southwood Press

AUSTRALIAN HOMEOPATHY RESEARCH

AUSTRALIAN HOMEOPATHY RESEARCH was founded for the purposes of

- research into the treatment of chronic and degenerative conditions through the resolution of their psychosomatic origins
- research into commonly used homeopathic trauma remedies to gain greater understanding of their specific psychological attributes, which understanding can then be applied to the treatment of a wider range of conditions than previously thought possible for these remedies
- research into the relationship between the emotions and attitudes and corresponding muscle tensions and structural changes
- research into identifying specific muscle tensions and spinal patterns visually and by palpation in relation to specific homeopathic remedies
- research into the usefulness of megapotencies of homeopathic trauma remedies in chronic conditions
- through such research, simplifying the application of homeopathy in clinical practice while expanding the usefulness of trauma remedies
- the publication of such findings

AUSTRALIAN HOMEOPATHY RESEARCH is the research and clinical practice division of *QUALITY OF LIFE* Products. The research work was begun in 1990 by Jill Turland, homeopath, and Bryan Barrass, osteopath and chiropractor. To date, more than a dozen trauma remedies have been investigated through personal provings of megapotencies and through analysis of Clinical Practice. We present our findings relating to twelve of these remedies in this book for the benefit of all seekers of true healing through personal responsibility.

AUSTRALIAN HOMEOPATHY RESEARCH
A Division of *QUALITY OF LIFE* Products
P.O. Box 91
Barraba NSW 2347
AUSTRALIA
Ph. 61 2 6782 1085
turland.jill@gmail.com

Truth, like the infinitely wise and gracious God, is eternal. Men may disregard it for a time, until the period arrives when its rays, in accordance with the dictates of Heaven, shall irresistibly break through the mists of prejudice and, like Aurora and the opening day, shed a beneficent light, clear and inextinguishable, over the generations of men.

- Dr Samuel Hahnemann, founder of Homeopathy

We should be ready to change our views at any time, and slough off prejudices, and live with an open and receptive mind. A sailor who sets the same sails all the time, without making adjustments when the wind changes, will never reach his harbour.

- George

It is now high time that all who call themselves physicians should at length cease to deceive suffering mankind with mere talk, and begin now, instead, for once to act, that is, to really help and to cure.

- Dr Samuel Hahnemann

ACKNOWLEDGEMENTS

My sincere thanks go out to the following people for the creation of this book:

The late Alan C. Jones, my homeopathy teacher, to whom I owe my somewhat radical, unconventional attitudes and methods. Alan always taught us to think, to analyze what was happening in the body when a certain process was in train, or a certain effect was being seen. It was not enough for him, and is not enough for me, to rely on the symptom picture alone in the selection of the remedy, or to follow blindly all who went before us. Discovery must continue beyond the foundations of the past.

George Vithoulkas, world renowned homeopath, who first realized the necessity of finding the psychological 'essence' of each remedy in order to see more clearly the similarity to the patient. George has revolutionised the practice of homeopathy in the Western world with his insights, upon which my own research was initially modelled.

Bryan W. Barrass, osteopath and chiropractor, my much loved partner, who has shared with me the trials and tribulations of proving and benefiting from remedies in megapotencies, and added his own insights and chiropractic knowledge into the melting pot of ideas.

The late David Tansley, D.C., who taught me the principles and art of dowsing, the importance of considering the subtle anatomy of man in the science of healing and, through his extensive writings, the foundations of radionics, the science of vibrational energy.

All our patients, family and friends, who have, wittingly or unwittingly, been part of the learning, and who have been an endless source of enthusiasm and excitement by receiving and reporting on the amazing effects and benefits of the new treatments - in particular, my ever-supportive mother, the late Jean Hopper, my great friends Helena Bushell and the late Donie Scott, and long-suffering, ever persistent patients/friends Helen Lorraine, Barbara Leeson, Anna Flesselles and Lynda Mary Gorman-Burrows, and many others who stayed with me, participating in the research, long enough to find their health answers.

Dr Candace Pert, Ph.D., research neuroscientist, a forerunner in the new science of psychoneuro-immunology, whose excellent book 'Molecules of Emotion' first alerted me that science was at last catching up with two-hundred-year-old homeopathy and finally proving its truths, that emotions and health are linked at the molecular level.

Dr Bruce Lipton, M.D., Ph.D., research cellular biologist, whose insightful studies confirm that quantum physics, quantum mechanics, provides understanding of the communication channels that link the mind and body; that vibrational patterns and resonances impact molecular communication within the body; in short, that our thoughts, attitudes and beliefs create the conditions of our body and the external world.

The many homeopaths who have gone before us, who are still studying homeopathy in the greater Halls of Learning, and who pass on their insights to all homeopaths who will listen, for our experimentation on the physical plane. Without their inspiration, hints and clues, imparted to me through my Inner Tutor (intuition), my personal guide, Gonjesil, I would still be floundering.

CONTENTS

CHAPTER 1

Discovery consists of seeing what everybody has seen and thinking
what nobody has thought
- Albert Szent-Gyorgi von Nagyrapolt

HOW IT ALL BEGAN

At a seminar given by the Australian Institute of Homœopathy in Sydney in 1988, there was some discussion about the need for standardised procedures to be defined and implemented for the proving of new homeopathic remedies. Some suggestions were also made of substances that could be proven.

After about ten minutes of such talk, one man arose from his seat in mid-hall and declared that he could not understand why we would want to find new remedies, when we have already thousands. Surely, what we need is to learn more about those that we already have, many of which have not been proven adequately and are therefore not being used to their greatest potential, even though in common use. This man was the late Wallace McLintock.

I was impressed by this line of thought and Wallace's words still stick in my mind. In my research work, I have focused on understanding the thought pattern, attitude or emotion underlying the problems that the common first-aid kit remedies can affect for the better. It seemed to me that if chronic disease develops out of insufficiently healed acute problems, as it does, then perhaps the remedies needed for the acute conditions could be the same ones we still need once those conditions, denied the appropriate remedy at the acute level, develop into chronic ill-health. And surely, if a small range of remedies is helpful to a large, even enormous number of people for first aid, surely an enormous number of people who never received their remedies at the acute level, need these remedies for their chronic conditions?

There is some evidence for this in general homeopathic practice. We have long used, for instance, Aconite for acute heart attack, to allay fear of dying and thus relax the patient and restore order to the blood vessels. Yet a heart attack is an acute sign of insidious ill-health - it never strikes the truly healthy. What I discovered was that the reason Aconite becomes needed for heart attack is that the underlying condition of the person is also Aconite by nature - the person has had previous events in life where there has been fear for survival or fear of great harm, either for himself or a loved one, and this fear has traumatised the heart on a sub-clinical level.

Ever since the beginnings of homeopathy two hundred years ago, the mental and emotional characteristics of the patient have been of primary importance in the selection of the remedy, whether in acute or chronic conditions. I came to discover that social attitudes and beliefs have also a prominent part to play, and that remedies can remove unhealthy social conditioning and allow greater insights and understanding of life to develop.

That is the subject of this book - the use of ten common homeopathic remedies in the treatment of chronic disease, through the application of very high (mega) potencies, which enable the release of commonly held, stored emotions, attitudes and false beliefs from the body, mind and spirit of the individual, and thus allow the body to heal itself.

This is a book that is going to rock you back on your heels and get you thinking along new lines. It is time to tell you about the discoveries our research has unearthed, which will enable you to lift up your lives and get free of social conditioning that has been crippling, not only individuals, but the nations of the world for thousands of years. In addition, where necessary, the book will show you how many of the complications to health brought about by medical procedures and drugs over the last century, based on false beliefs, can be resolved.

My aim is to explain to all of you what these crippling beliefs are, how they have allowed us to be led along, like lambs to the slaughter, into a cul-de-sac of personal, social and medical ignorance - and what you can do to get back on track.

The book also deals with internal chronic disease resulting from all kinds of injuries, and demonstrates how even accidents relate directly to specific attitudes and emotions. Through the new understandings we have been able to piece together the mechanisms by which, say, bowel cancer can develop both from lifting heavy weights and carrying everyone else's loads, or breast cancer can develop out of injury to the lymph nodes or a sense of dependency, and surgery and dental work cause hormonal imbalances - and we show you what can be done about them.

Homeopathy has long been used to counteract the harmful effects of surgery, puncture wounds (injections) and pharmaceutical drugs. My research has given me some exceptionally valuable insights into the adverse effects of common drugs being over-prescribed, how to recognize patterns of ill-health to understand their source and deal with that, and how to counteract and prevent the downward spiral into degenerative disease.

It all relates to who we think we are, our attitudes and false beliefs that are ingrained in childhood, coming down from many generations of forebears, combined with unhealthy emotions such as fear, guilt, shame, grief, bitterness and anger, which have shaped the way we live our lives.

Unhealthy, that is, for our bodies, which are created into destruction by destructive thoughts and feelings.

Every adult, and particularly every parent of children has the right to this understanding, to be able to take responsibility for getting back to mental, physical and/or emotional health. Reclaim your personal power and take charge of your thoughts, your feelings and your circumstances! It's easier than you think, once you take advantage of the new knowledge. Let the miracles happen for you.

The book is the culmination of over ten years of research that suddenly thrust itself upon me. I had no such plans. I found it quite astounding when remarkable events led me to piecing many facts together that provided new insights into how the remedies release stored emotions and where, in the body, these emotions have been stored.

I had learned in 1988 from Roger Morrison, a Californian homeopath, about the sweet, helplessly indignant, anger-suppressing nature of many people needing Staphisagria. Roger was giving a seminar in Sydney, demonstrating his case studies with video presentations of consultations. One of these was of a woman, quietly indignant over injustices in her husband's treatment of her. 'Look how sweet she is,' Roger said. 'You can always tell Staphisagria by that sweet smile.' I laughed and laughed when this point was brought out, as only a week before, my husband, Maurie Turland, had looked amusedly at me and said, 'You're a sweet little thing, aren't you.' Well! Red rag to a bull, that was. 'Sweet! Sweet! How dare you call me sweet! That's the last thing on earth I want to be called!' Sure enough, it was a smile similar to mine, and although I had not suppressed my indignation on that occasion, I knew I often did, as this woman had done.

I went home and took Staphisagria. I had a blood disorder at the time, of very few, very inactive leucocytes, an immune disorder, and this was the first remedy to begin to show improvement in it. (The situation resolved fully after I discovered the megapotencies in 1991, and how Staphisagria frees up the pituitary gland to boost the thymus and the immune system.)

Later, I recognised this helplessly indignant feature in Bryan in 1991, and Staphisagria enabled him to take a stand for himself to save his life. But my first insight into the amazing guilt-clearing action of the higher potencies came with an experience that Bryan and I had with Hydrastis in January 1992, and this incident also gave us far more knowledge of Hydrastis than I have been able to find in any of the Materia Medica at my disposal.

Bryan had had a problem, all his life, with obstinate constipation, and this had been complicated in more recent times by diverticuli and haemorrhoids, which often bled. He had not had a normal bowel motion for over twenty five years, he said. He also suffered from discomfort in his lower back, which forced him to walk around to relieve the ache after standing too long in one place.

His lumbar spine was visibly out of correct alignment - the fifth lumbar vertebra was anterior to the curve, a spondylolisthesis, and twenty-one years of chiropractic adjustments had failed to make a lasting correction. Six months prior to this I had given him Staphisagria CM, which had made lots of improvements in him but had failed to touch the bowel problem or the lumbar spine. I decided on Hydrastis, and by some intuition made it up in MM, a potency I had never used before. He took the remedy over three consecutive nightly doses.

The results were immediate. Next morning I gaped in amazement - the lumbar vertebra was visibly back in perfect alignment with its fellows! Bryan began to feel stiffness in the lumbars, and a lot of pain in his pelvis that day.

He had had a silly injury at age 15 on the soccer field, when his left foot stuck in the mud and he crashed down heavily, fracturing the pelvis in three places. Now he could painfully trace those break lines along the left pelvis. (I thought we might need Symphytum to clear these symptoms.) He did not relate these symptoms to the remedy at first, thinking he must have strained himself pumping up the car tyres. I knew this would not have corrected the vertebral misalignment, and watched keenly for further developments. We agreed that there would have to be some muscular adjustments to be made as a result of the spinal correction, which could account for the soreness in the back, but this did not account for the pelvic injury pain.

After the second dose the aching continued. After the third, Bryan experienced an interesting sequence of symptoms: on attempting to urinate, though the bladder was full, he could only get out a dribble at a time. It took ten minutes of wait/trickle, wait/trickle before he felt comfortable. It reminded him instantly that the same thing had occurred on the day of the pelvic break, when he had been in hospital all day without being asked if he need to relieve himself. Being a Staphisagria type, he had been too embarrassed to mention it to anyone (not nice, you know), and was barely able to pass water by the end of the day. Old symptoms recurring, which, to a homeopath, always indicates healing is taking place, of very old damage.

Then he began to limp. The only time in his life he had ever limped was when getting back on to his feet after this accident. This new limp came on after the pelvic pain had subsided, and lasted a couple of hours. Two weeks after all these effects relating to the pelvic break had gone, a severe pain arose in the right hand. It lasted for half an hour, and surprisingly, did not in any way impair the function of the hand. Bryan uses his hands all day, massaging backs and limbs and making joint adjustments - this work was not compromised, although the pain remained strong while working. It was a real mystery, but he knew enough by now to blame me! I just kept saying, 'You've hit someone, I bet you've hit someone in the past', and he would reply jokingly, 'Not me, I don't hit, I run.'

4

It took him a week to understand where this pain had originated. At this stage there was still no improvement in bowel function.

We now had the job of working out why all this had happened after taking Hydrastis. I remembered that Hydrastis had been a favourite amongst the North American natives for the healing of injuries, particularly battle wounds. Bryan had had many injuries through his life - why did only these ones surface? Having been involved in guilt research for some time I felt it had to be a guilt-related reaction. If so, what kind of guilt? What would be the guilt connection between war wounds and Bryan's hurts?

Well, we came to the conclusion that the guilt was of harm caused by oneself. 'It was my fault' was the over-riding thought that had stopped complete healing of Bryan's injuries of so long ago. Consider this: the soccer-field injury had been a most frustrating and guilty experience, as it was the first and only time his father ever had the chance to go and watch Bryan play. Bryan, whose whole life revolved around soccer, was Captain of the team and had led the team on to start play for the second half a few minutes ahead of the scheduled time, and his father had not yet returned to his seat in the stand. Only a few minutes had elapsed before the injury occurred.

To perpetuate the guilt of this, his father died suddenly within a year, and never had been able to see his son play again. As we understand it, the fifth lumbar anteriority was part and parcel of the whole injury, and was 'locked in' by the irresolvable guilt-regret.

In respect to the hand incident, the story is quite amusing. After a week of searching his memory, Bryan came up with the recollection of a story his mother used to tell him. Apparently, at the age of about four years, Bryan had been put into a Day Care centre when his mother, a nursing sister, was unexpectedly called to work. A rather large, fat child at the centre had taken control of the slippery-slide and was not allowing other children, including Bryan, to use it. When it came time for food, the fat boy came down from the slide - food being even more important - and Bryan, infuriated, gave him such a powerful fistful that the boy was knocked unconscious. Guilt was cast very heavily on to Bryan, he was made to sit quietly and guiltily until his mother came to get him, no doubt had a sore hand for a while, and was made to feel he had brought it on himself. The guilt factor held the pain in until now, forty five years later, it was released by Hydrastis MM.

Later Xrays (January 03) showed his lumbar spine to be still free of spondylolisthesis.

We hit on the Hydrastis revelation in January 1992, worked with this for some time and really came to know it well. Hydrastis releases the weight of responsibility from the lower spine and realigns it as it lifts you free of the need to be responsible for other people, or the guilt over harm you have caused yourself or others.

The other thing to happen in 1992, was that for a few months, I kept getting the mental instruction, 'Look at the sphenoid. Look at the sphenoid.' After a while I said to Bryan, 'What is so great about the sphenoid? Where is it, exactly?' 'It is a bone in the head,' he said. 'Look it up.' So I consulted the anatomy textbook and saw where the sphenoid bone fits into the cranial structure. It runs across the front part of the head behind the eyes, from temple to temple, below the frontal cortex of the brain. So what? I looked again for anything that might make this bone of more significance than we knew, and saw that it has a cavity in the centre in which the pituitary gland sits. It must be that. Neither of us understood why this information was of special importance, but I kept trying to work it out. All I knew was that if you get hit on the temple area you could be badly damaged or die, as boxers know well.

Then, later in the same year, we received word of a chiropractic seminar to be held in Sydney, on Sacro-Occipital Technique Cranial work. There was to be a seminar for chiropractors and one for chiropractors' assistants running concurrently. We booked in, he to the professional course and I to the assistants' course.

It was an absolute revelation. On the first morning, my speaker began his talk with discussion of the bones of the head, describing each one separately, and beginning with the sphenoid bone. 'And this sphenoid,' he said, 'which is in perpetual motion....' 'What?' I interrupted. 'Say that again?' 'Yes,' he said, 'it is in perpetual motion caused by several different influences of pressure all happening at once in the head,' and went on to describe these pulsing forces. Phew! Now I knew why I was there. If this bone is in perpetual microscopic motion, this must be important for the healthy function of the pituitary gland, and anything that compromised that normal motion would compromise the normal output of pituitary hormones.

This was the answer to my puzzlement. I hurried excitedly out at morning coffee break to tell Bryan, only to find that Bryan was racing excitedly towards me. 'You must see this video we've just been shown,' he said, 'I asked the tutor if we could replay it at lunchtime for you. You'll be amazed!'

At lunchtime we ignored food and raced into the other room to play the video, and it was really amazing. Dr Marc Pick, an American chiropractor and anatomist, in order to teach cranial movement and the different forces that generate this movement, had created latex models of each of the skull bones.

In the video, he describes each bone separately, showing how the sphenoid is the keystone of the cranial structure. It is the one bone that cannot be removed from the skull before other bones have been removed, the bone on which all the structure of the head is built. His latex models could be clicked together. He demonstrated how each bone influenced its neighbours, and how important is the flexibility of the cranial sutures, those mysterious joints between each bone.

When all the bones had been clicked into place, he then demonstrated, through the flexibility of the latex, an exaggerated interpretation of how different forces or pulses influence the cranium to be constantly moving, and how these (known to be three but believed to be possibly four) influences have differing rates, causing this movement to be in a gyratory manner. The three known forces were respiration, circulatory pulse and cerebro-spinal fluid flow, each of which have an alternating active and passive stage.

We laughed with great joy and delight to see how the wonderful little latex bones were moving first one way, then another, distorting the shape of the head amusingly as these different influences were demonstrated. What a revelation! No wonder many people's heads change shape to some degree as they progress through life.

I had been drawn already to the study of Staphisagria, long known to be a remedy for conditions following indignation. We had both gained a lot from Staphisagria in high potencies ourselves and found a widespread need for this remedy in the community. This is the remedy for the effects of indignation and suppressed anger and also the trauma effects of surgery and wounds from knife blades, when the body has 'taken offense' painfully and is not healing easily. When we learned about the sphenoid bone and how its free movement influences pituitary function, we were able to work out how pituitary function can be impaired by suppressing anger, locking anger tension into the muscles of the face which attach to the sphenoid and neighbouring bones, thus preventing full movement of these bones, and how this pituitary function could be restored to order by releasing the stored anger with Staphisagria, freeing up the muscles and thus allowing full mobility of the bones.

We continued working with Staphisagria with this new understanding, finding great numbers of people were getting benefits we would never have given them, before this knowledge was given us. My current estimate is that eighty per cent of British and those of British descent need Staphisagria in megapotencies to free them of their cultural, socially imposed guilts. You will read why, later in the book.

Later in 1992, I began to notice a lot of Arnica cases, and realized this was another powerful guilt release remedy, for the guilt of not feeling tough enough to take all that life throws at you. Arnica was not a remedy with which we had personal guilt-release experiences, but we knew that Arnica is a great remedy for muscles and therefore the heart muscle and we had numerous people coming in for muscle treatment who needed Arnica. All we had to do here was observe what their spinal subluxations and muscle tensions were, to see what all the Arnica people had in common. On the mental side, they all felt that they were perfectly OK if only they did not have this physical problem! They could not admit that they had any weakness or soft-heartedness. The majority of Arnica people were truck drivers, footballers, farmers and mothers of young children, and they all had subluxations anteriorly of the 2nd and 4th thoracic vertebrae.

Conium was the next remedy to come to light in the guilt release work. We already knew that Conium people have a lot of pre-occupation with money and worried over where the next dollar was coming from. We began to observe that some people would get very panicky at the thought of relying on their own wits and skill to attract enough money in, and would go on the dole at the first sign that their income was not going to be steadily sufficient. We also found that this belief encouraged people to expect that they would always be reliant on someone else to pay their way for them. We noticed, for instance, that women of middle age and older, whose husband had been the provider, were shocked into developing cancers of the Conium kind when the husband died. They could not imagine how they could ever provide for themselves. (The Conium person, we found, craves independence yet cannot believe it is truly possible.)

It was not a great leap in thinking to realize that dependency on financial support was also of similar impact on the consciousness to dependency on drugs, doctors, surgeons, wheelchairs, walking sticks and crutches, and that some Conium people followed through in this direction, encouraged by our over-protective society. Big Brother wants us all dependent.

We continued, meanwhile, to learn about Ruta (ligament remedy, for guilt of not pulling together for strength) and Ledum (tendon tension - inability to let go or forgive the past). The most staggering revelations came in 1993 when I began to look into Hypericum.

My mind still boggles at the import of this remedy. When you read about it, yours will, too. I still shake my head in wonder at how this commonly used remedy has been so partially known for so many years, and how much so many people need it. It was this remedy that taught us so much about the killing power of an injection, a simple puncture wound. When I first realized what Hypericum in megapotencies could achieve and saw what it was achieving, I was dumbfounded for two years, in that I could not talk about it to any other practitioner, I could not believe they would ever believe me, the implications to society were so confronting. The funny thing was, I was handing out articles to my Hypericum patients to read about themselves and the remedy, they would happily pass them around amongst their friends and family and I would have a steady stream of Hypericum sufferers coming in to get free of their needle-shock complaints.

The realization of Hypericum was a discovery of the profoundest importance and awe-inspiring in its far-ranging implications. It had taken me over two years of puzzling over a handful of people with similar characteristics to realize that their similarities of personality pertained to this one remedy, and to see their common factor, spinal injuries. It took another major leap in concepts to grasp the other side of Hypericum, the puncture wound/tetanus/injection connection, and to realize that this was also relating to the same deeply-held belief.

8

We worked this remedy to death for two years before letting the information out to practitioners. During this time I proved the remedy on myself, and this is documented in the Hypericum chapter. After thinking for the previous three years that everyone in the world must need Staphisagria (nearly everyone did who was coming to us), we found ourselves besieged by people in need of Hypericum, for an amazingly wide range of problems.

Not all my group under study had the full range of characteristics as we finally understood them - the one most significant factor that all had in common was *low self-value* buried under an overlay mantle of ego, and a desire to be seen to be the greatest, the winner; and it was only after using Hypericum, or recognising the potential need for it for the resolution of old, violent injuries in these people, that the realization came that I was seeing a clear personality picture for this remedy. Our textbooks are surprisingly devoid of any indications of a particular mind-set or attitude, and Hypericum's full usefulness has never been imagined before now.

The most astounding insight into Hypericum, though, related to the adverse effects of injections on the central nervous system. We found that many people who had had frequent injections early in life were hyped up, never able to slow down and concentrate for long enough to read a book or listen to what others had to say. The Hypericum chapter is astounding, and you will see lots of people you know, described there. [We later realised that other puncture wounds - stings and rusty nail injuries (Ledum) and mosquitoes (Staphisagria) - shocked the body in different ways according to what the inherent attitudes and beliefs were.]

The early insights into Hypericum were accompanied by some insights into Symphytum, the remedy, we found, for guilt if not working - a workaholic's remedy, also for those who felt denied a trade or profession; the primary remedy for all who feel they are not earning their existence if they are not working, and for the common complaints of many retirees.

In order to find out more about Symphytum, in 1994, Bryan and I both took Symphytum MM. Next morning we awoke with white-coated tongue and a sensation as though the dentine had been removed from our teeth. This dry, chalky feeling lasted all that day but was gone by the next, as was the white coating on the tongue. I also had, that day, white, powdery skin on the soles of my feet, as though I had stood in talcum powder. We had no other changes from our normal selves, but I wondered about the mineral loss.

We are still learning about this amazing Symphytum and its benefits in degenerative complaints and dementia. Care must be used, with such powerful remedies, that the person matches the remedy and the miasm that it relates to, lest mistakes be made - for what can be corrected in one person could be created in another of the opposite constitutional type. You will read in the Symphytum chapter how we learned this, from Bryan's painful experience.

We lived with and learned from Symphytum, Hypericum and the other remedies for four years before the next big remedy surfaced - Ignatia, in 1997, which deals with the guilt/grief of things not working out the way you had planned or expected, causing a stymied, stagnating feeling of not knowing how to get back to the plan.

This time, it was my own symptoms of Ignatia that prompted the discovery. I had developed a problem of a lump in the throat and a tight, weighted chest, sighing, having to take a deep breath now and then to expand the ribcage enough to get a good amount of air in. I also began to get a rather sad look around the mouth, the opposite to my lifetime's smiley look. ('Smiler Jill', I was called years ago.) This was quite inexplicable. I had nothing to be sad about, life was as good as it had ever been, I thought. How could I be needing Ignatia? After months of resisting, I finally gave myself a dose of CM.

I awoke next day knowing exactly why. The grief-like symptoms related to an on-going sense of grief that, because of the death of my late husband Maurie, my plans for the land we had bought - plans to develop a healing retreat in the bush where people could come, stay a few weeks if necessary and go away improved by homeopathy and osteopathy - had never eventuated. His death, and my taking a new direction subsequently, had left the whole scheme still on the backburner. The new insight was that it was not up to me to create this, that my job was to do the research that would enable many others all over the world to create such miracle healing centres. I sold the land and put the money into this research, Ignatia lifting the weighty feeling off my chest.

Many people need to get weight off their chest, or a lump from their throat. Ignatia is a communication remedy, it releases people from the belief they need to keep quiet about their feelings and allows them to express their griefs in words. The benefit of this is that the person is not trying hypocritically to convince the world that he is unaffected by grief and sadness, and again, emotional energy is not locked into the muscles, and the cranial bones and pituitary gland are not affected by muscle tensions. We found that the benefits from Ignatia pertained to the posterior pituitary hormones and conditions relating to these, with the same facial muscles as Staphisagria being affected in an opposite way.

Ignatia was followed by further insights into Ledum in the following year - it proved to be amazing in prolonged grieving and resentment situations, allowing the past to be let go and forgiveness to set in, instead. Many people who had needed Ignatia also needed Ledum to help them let go of the past, forgive and move on into today and tomorrow. Ledum people have a fear of moving into the future, unlike Hypericum who cannot wait to get ahead. Ledum helps people at critical changeover points in their lives, to shift out of their (no longer) comfort zones and embark on new beginnings. We saw a great deal of Ledum in George W. Bush, whose lack of forgiveness extended into vengeance towards the Taliban and determination to control

Iraq - two separate issues that he wanted us to think were only one. Bush's inability to let go and take a different stance could only lead to big trouble. Who will disarm the USA? The Ledum person allows his loyal heart to be controlled by his inability to let go and move on, and even his inability to forgive or allow. (Our own Prime Minister Julia Gillard is also a Ledum personality.)

Only recently have I begun to see the extended understanding of Ruta. Ruta is the remedy for those who believe in combining forces for greater strength, in the need for takeovers, creating conglomerates and multinational companies, and on a more personal scale, for those who have guilt over lack of unity in a family or community, a grief/guilt that they are not pulling together for greater strength against the adversities of life. 'We must be strong', they think, 'We must all pull together.' A great remedy for our times, applying as it does to government bodies, defense forces, unions and associations, clubs and even the local football team. Australia's former Prime Minister, John Howard, is a Ruta type. He likes to 'get with the strength.'

By 2003 the knowledge we had gained had been well consolidated by clinical practice involving both the homeopathic and osteopathic patients, and this book was first published. We had only just begun to see the full understanding of Aconite, and many patients from the past (who needed Aconite and I never considered it) were coming back to get free of deepseated, suppressed fear, the result of long-ago frights. The patients do not know it is fear causing their problems. Suppressed fear manifests in the intellectual, logical person and enough of it can cause brain spin-outs similar to the destructive effects of marijuana, resulting in mental disorders. We found Aconite to be the major remedy for mental illnesses like depression, bi-polar disorder and schizophrenia associated with brain faults after frights, terror and prolonged fear, as well as marijuana damage.

All of these are shock/trauma remedies and social attitude remedies, freeing people of injury and illness patterns they have had, in some cases, all their lives or through many generations of forebears, and allowing them - when we give them the remedies in megapotencies - to take charge of their lives and their relationships and get their act together. Some of the remedies carry immense power to offload the guilt of harm done by medical drugs and procedures of all types. You will, as I say, be amazed.

I am particularly keen to see these remedies in use in our aboriginal communities and other ethnic groups in Australia who have suffered so much of man's inhumanity to man. The benefit to all social groups is cleansing and empowering, enlightening and freeing people from the handicaps of social injustices, domestic violence, political outrage, war trauma, terrorism, personal violence, criminality, drug dependency and abuse, family breakup, depression and mental derangements. Prisons and correction centres, institutions of all kinds, support groups, everywhere where there are people in need of big help, are places where these remedies should be put in use.

There is still much to learn about the mechanisms by which remedies effect change, and about the origin of the initial derangements - how a symptom picture develops, and what it tells us about the thinking and feelings of the patient prior to and at the time of the development of symptoms. My research is along these lines. I seek to know what is really happening in the body, in the structure and the various functions on all levels, when a remedy is working, and why it is doing what it is doing. I also search out the particular belief, attitude or emotion associated with the event, as this is critically important in the choice of remedy, and specifically relevant to the particular physical pattern that develops after the event. Each type of shock, whether physical or psychological, has its own specific way of registering in the body, and in the face. Often the face indicates the remedy needed, often the spine and muscles shout it out.

My research has been done along the lines of Francis Bacon, whose writings and experiments inspired the formation in 1663 of the Royal Society, one of the most prestigious scientific societies in the world. Bacon proposed that a discovery is only scientific if it is guided by facts and not misguided by theory. When studying the hidden mysteries of nature and science, the natural philosopher should both observe and experiment *before* proposing a theory. He said that a scientific mind is a *tabula rasa*, a blank page devoid of all content, so that it can receive the imprint of nature without distortion. I have tried, at all times, to avoid the prejudices and misinformation of prior knowledge and rely only on what I was observing, confirming the discoveries through repeated experimentation in order to fine-tune and give specificity to to what seemed initially to be generalisations.

Undoubtedly, there will be more knowledge coming forward, and we are learning all the time. We have enough here, though, to get started on cleaning up our society, our planet. If you are in a position where you regularly encounter people who need the kind of help offered in this book, take action. Either start trialling them in your practice, if you are qualified to do so, or impress on your local homeopaths the need to do so. I hope this extended knowledge will be incorporated into homeopathy curriculi as teachers become sufficiently familiarised themselves.

Without a spirit of exploration and enquiry, no progress can be made. I offer you this book as a trigger for your own investigations and observations, and wish you all the excitement and relief the discoveries have brought us.

CHAPTER 2

The greatest discovery of any generation is that human beings can alter their
lives by altering the attitudes of their minds
- Albert Schweitzer

HOW DID WE GET OFF TRACK?

Certain untrue beliefs and attitudes prevail throughout the world.
Because of the 'helplessness' effects of some of these attitudes and beliefs, we
have allowed the development of an insidious, destructive curse that is
crippling the western world and destroying the mental and physical strength
of the individuals of whole nations. Chapter Three deals with this second,
more recent divergence from sense. Here, let us talk about our ingrained
beliefs.

BELIEFS AND EMOTIONS

We are trained in childhood to a lot of false beliefs, which alter our view
of life and change our enjoyment of it. We all have different backgrounds and
life experiences. Many attitudes are based on ingrained false beliefs held by
whole societies, whole groups or subgroups of people, and it is very difficult,
from within the group, to see that everyone may be wrong.

Psychiatrists call this phenomenon 'consensus reality' - a framework of
values and judgements in which religion, science, culture and education all
contribute to a coherent world-view. Consensus reality varies from society to
society.

Certain very strongly held, community taught, unhealthy ideas are
actually causing considerable deterioration, not only in the health of
individuals but also in the state of health of the planet. These attitudes and
beliefs are taught by emotional manipulation - fear-mongering, blackmail,
controlling by guilt; many also arise out of attitudes to death and fear of life
and death; all inhibit joy and love, and invite the presence of anger, hate,
greed, vengeance, fear and grief. Ignorance is the major reason.

Among the most powerfully destructive beliefs in the western world are:

- *God is judgemental and will punish you if you are bad.*

When you look around you it is obvious that God does not judge, only man judges. Universal Intelligence simply allows everything to happen, allows us all to use our free will and suffer the consequences of such use, whether good or bad, until we learn the laws of life. This mistaken belief accounts for half the world's guilts, fears and untrue beliefs.

- *Emotions cloud good judgement. Emotions are a sign of weakness and must be suppressed.*

Emotions are powerful creative energies that must be used to our advantage if we are to create a better world. Destructive emotions can be converted into creatively constructive energies for good. Without emotions nothing would ever be created or achieved, even we ourselves would not exist. We must get free of this misunderstanding in all its forms.

- *Men are naturally aggressive.*

This is a cop-out attitude that men have, to hide their guilt over being so keen to go to war rather than learn to use their physical energy and emotions more creatively. They can get free of this guilt. The desire to kill an adversary is confused with early man's need to corner and kill his prey, as animals do, and to protect his kill from others. Men play competitive sports that replicate the hunt, like football, where the ball is the weapon and the goal is the prey - this is evidence of hunting memories, but not of a desire to kill or harm each other, which is a symptom of unnecessary distrust and frustration.

- *Men's (logical) word is important, women's (intuitive) word is not worth listening to. Women are men's slaves and chattels.*

This stems from the teaching that Eve was made out of Adam's rib, therefore men are the leaders and more important. It all falls apart when you find that science knows that all men start off as female embryos and develop their male characteristics further down the track. (Many cultures through time have recognised the importance of women and particularly the Earth Mother, Mother Nature, from whom we all arise.) There is also the mistaken belief that the intellectual functions of the brain are superior to the intuitive. True intelligence, as I will show later, requires an equal balance of both, and this can be achieved.

- *Work is the only honourable way to earn your place in society.*

This insidious brainwashing has been accentuated by the industrial revolution, when it became necessary to find many labourers to man the factories. And the industrial revolution was a creation of bankers and industrialists, who saw unbounded ways of increasing their wealth. Never before in history have people been obliged to earn money in order to eat. Our dependence on money for our very existence has now spread to all countries of the world and almost all populations. We desperately need to get free of this destructive belief, and we can. It is still slavery, based on bankers' greed.

- *We have a duty to others.*

Shakespeare had it right - 'To thine own self be true, and it must follow, as the night the day, Thou canst not then be false to any man.'[1] Learn what healthful attitudes and beliefs are in your own best interests, towards your own personal growth and spiritual consciousness, and follow them, and you can do no harm to anyone. Try to live for others and you only suffer frustration that kills you.

- *I am responsible for all you weaker people.*

You are not. Mind your own business and let others mind theirs. By all means show kindness, but don't weaken others by carrying their burdens for them. It ends up weakening you as well. This is not in anyone's best interests.

- *An eye for an eye, a tooth for a tooth.*

The belief in justice is another big killer. We can get free of this aggressive belief. Whether you want vengence of this kind or simply to see justice done legally, this is another of those long-held teachings that need to be thrown out the window. God has been created in the image of Man, with all his failings. The universe does not judge, seeks no justice. There is no such thing, it is a man-made belief like the law of karma, that one must always pay a price. The only price you need to pay is to learn from your experiences, forgive yourself (you 'miserable sinner') and others and keep on progressing in your understanding of the laws that do govern life, which are pretty basic - Do unto others only those things that you would not mind being done to you - Respect all others - Respect the planet, the universe and the Creative Intelligence behind it all; and do not confuse respect with fear. Homeopathy helps you to allow that all are in their right space at all times.

- *I am alone, no-one can be trusted to have my interests at heart.*

This is such a widespread feeling in western society that it has lead to the breakdown of the community as a com (together) -unity (as one). The old extended family groups have become the nuclear family, now these are splitting up and leaving fractions of families all over the place, all feeling separated and isolated from people they ought to be loving and living with. The degree of distrust is both created by and contributes to a lot of the emotional pain and distress in the western world. But it is all an illusion, this belief in separatism, opposition, competition, enemies - and it falls away once you get the remedy that clears the fog from your vision.

Rejoice! There are powerful homeopathic remedies that can release all these ideas and lift people out of this bog the world is in. Once enough people experience the benefits the world will become a place headed for peace; without the release of these stored emotional energies resulting from destructive beliefs, no such peace will ever be possible. Civilization will remain barbaric.

THE GUILT OF EMOTIONS

It is our beliefs that generate unhealthy emotions, i.e. any emotion that is not adding life and vitality to your cells but instead, has the power to undermine your vitality. False beliefs about the true nature of life create our fears, griefs, anger and indeed, all our guilts. It surprises me that so little attention has been paid to this widespread and insidious aspect of dis-ease, considering that there is hardly a soul alive on the planet who is not afflicted with guilts in one way or another. Perhaps it is our very guilt itself that stops us from seeing the magnitude of the scourge, and creates a veil through which enlightenment and insight are slow to penetrate. Yet within the standard range of well-proven homeopathic Materia Medica we have some very powerful tools for the release of guilt.

Guilt overlies many attitudes and emotions. When I talk of guilt I mean bad conscience, in many different ways - a sense of having sinned, a sense of shame, of embarrassment, of grievance, even of grief; we suffer from guilt over not doing what is expected of us, over doing what others expected of us against our own instincts, over things done and things undone, feelings felt and feelings left unfelt, over 'right' and 'wrong', even over pleasure at our own successes, or joy in loving relationships; for many even being alive and daring to breathe brings its own guilt.

Some are guilty over eating too well, too often, too little, or over not giving proper respect to their bodies' requirements; leading to guilt over being too fat, too thin, having poor skin, body odour, and many forms of elimination problems. Some are guilty over grief issues (if only I had - or hadn't - done...) thinking to have averted some death or suffering. Some suffer a lifetime of grief and guilt over a parent, over parent or self not having come up to expectations.

On a broader scale, those in responsible positions suffer many guilts over having, in the course of their jobs, to make decisions or take actions that disadvantage or upset others. Medical practitioners know all about it! Many a drug has been guiltily removed from the market after destructive effects have been discovered. Many a judge has had to live with having made judgements that, although technically legally correct, he has felt were morally unjust or harsh. Social reforms begun in the eighteenth and nineteenth centuries are still bringing changes in the laws of the land, the old laws being guiltily replaced.

One of the most fascinating things about guilt is the way we can be made to feel guilty about not feeling guilt. Guilt benefits only the one who wants power over others, never the guilt-sufferer. So power-seekers, for many centuries, have succeeded in keeping their power over people through the relentless application of guilt and fear. Churches have, to the present day, been the most guilty of this: through the use of the dogma of hellfire and eternal damnation, fear dominates a large percentage of the world's social customs, and guilt is its inevitable accompaniment.

We will have to pay, we have been told for centuries, with damnation, if we take pleasure in such things as fine food, good company, fun, music and dancing, prosperity, loving relationships, good sex (the most sinful thing of all) and work.

Serious business, work! - often used to offset the guilt of enjoyment, so therefore acceptable as part payment for our sins, and scarcely something to have fun at. The enthusiast in his work is regarded as something of a crackpot, and a danger to his mates who, guilty, might be expected to work harder! We must also always take good note of what others (church, government, gods, family, neighbours or simply 'they') think is best for us.

'Do unto others as you would have them do unto you' is interpreted as 'I've done you a favour so you now owe me one'. 'It is better to give than to receive' is another common teaching. How can it be, if you deny the recipient the pleasure of receiving, thinking he must immediately give back in order to regain some level of grace? And why is self-denial better than deserving as much as the next?

If we take a stand at any time and start acting outside of guilt, especially if it appears to disadvantage someone else, we are immediately judged, and judged harshly, and the guilt flak starts flying thick and fast. By this means, then, we see that guilt is self-perpetuating, feeding on itself like a virus in the mind. Having started the ball rolling, many centuries ago, modern man has succeeded in creating himself guiltier and guiltier. We have even come to accept it as a normal state of living.

Why has this state of being become the norm? Why do we place so much emphasis on what others think, inevitably to our own detriment? By what right does anyone else know what is best for me? How can he possibly know, when only I know the fullness of my own experiences, my own hopes and intentions for myself, the range of experiences I need for my own development? Who else can judge, and find me wanting in any respect, not being in possession of full knowledge of these things? And therefore, by what right do I hand over my personal power to others, and allow their judgements and opinions to take control of my life?

How did we ever come to lose the intuitive sense of knowing what is best for us, what is right for ourselves in what we do and how we do it, and the courage to stand by this knowingness, no matter what?

I believe that guilt is at the basis of all loss of Self-value, Self-esteem, personal power, Self-trust, Self-love, Self-honour, and our loss of faith in the God Within, and that this loss has resulted in our creation of the world as it is today. Recurring patterns of war, famine, financial greed and imbalance in the distribution of the world's resources, insularity of nations, tribes and families,

17

isolation even within these groups leading to breakdown of love and forgiveness in relationships - all these would not exist were it not for the guilt that each one feels, of one kind or another.

By guilt, I do not mean remorse. Remorse is an acknowledgement that some harm has been done, a sense of guilty sorrow. The guilts that are perpetuating strife in the world are, for the most part, not registering in the conscious thinking of man, which is why they are so difficult to alter without enlightened help.

For it is strange but true, that once we release the guilt from participation, we cease to participate in war. Remove the guilt of ill-treatment, we cease to ill-treat; remove the guilt from apathy and loss of love, and the love returns; remove the guilt from grief, and the grieving one can put the past behind and get on with the game in hand; remove the guilt from poverty, and the impoverished begin to take charge of themselves; remove the guilt from the controllers and they will cease to need to control; remove the guilt over ceaseless argument, and conflict dissolves; remove the guilt over feeling hopeless, and hope is rekindled; remove the guilt of being afraid or terrified, and a healthy confidence in oneself and the processes of life replaces it.

THE SUBTLE ANATOMY OF MAN

Let us have a look at who we really are, in our totality of mind, body and soul.

Our non-physical self attaches to our physical body as an enveloping force field, a mass of colourful, swirling energies entering and activating the body at various vortices, known to the Indian mystics as chakras. This is pure light.

In a state of poor health, mental or physical, the colours of the force field or aura can be seen (by those with such psychic clarity) to be in a state of murkiness. The areas most in trouble are the muddiest. As healing takes place, brighter, clear colours return to these areas. It is emotions that first muddy the energies, the physical areas depleted of energy or vitality then must deteriorate. These polluted energies transfer to the physical level of the body and cause poor communication between cells.

The seven major chakras are located along the spine, energising the endocrine glands which are the interface between our physical and non-physical forms, and which are the emotion centres of the body. Each of the seven major chakras resonates to one of the seven colours of the rainbow. Red is the colour of the Base (of the spine) chakra, the survival centre; this is the slowest resonating colour, activating the adrenal glands' fight and flight responses. Orange relates to the Sacral chakra and the reproductive glands, and affects our socialisation and the continuation of our species. Yellow energises the Solar Plexus chakra and activates the pancreas, influencing all the digestive processes, the 'yellow systems' of the body.

Each of these three chakras is inextricably linked to the emotions attached to survival - fear of death, fear of the elements, of non-survival of the species, fear of not finding food (or, in modern western countries, of not having enough money), and all sexual power emotions. The emphasis is on fear for one's life and wellbeing, very self-oriented.

The chakras centred above the Solar Plexus chakra - the Heart chakra (green, thymus gland), the Throat (blue, thyroid gland), the Brow (indigo, pineal gland) and the Crown chakra at the vertex of the head (violet, pituitary gland) are only partially active when thoughts and emotions are focused in the lower body. Green, the colour for the heart chakra and thymus gland, is the colour most needed to lift people operating from the lower energy centres of fearfulness into the light of love. For remember, fear is only the absence of love. Only then can they begin to develop the potential of the higher chakras in their journey towards the great wisdom of the Crown energy. We need to become personal Greenies.

Long ago, I believe, the Crown chakra used to energise, directly, the pineal gland and the pituitary. Over time and adaptation, these have become separated in their activities, mainly owing to our suppression away from full usage of the energies of the Crown. Activation of the Crown chakra will see these pulled back into unity, opening the pineal to lost consciousness of our god qualities, and not only shall we begin to reverse all manner of ill-health but if continued far enough, we shall cease to age.

The pituitary gland is the Master Gland of the endocrine system, which is the interface between your physical body and your non-physical energy centres. Clairvoyants see these energy centres as vortices, funnel-shaped gateways through which universal energy - as life-sustaining cosmic rays - enters the body, maintaining the vitality of each gland, which then distributes this energy through the body in the form of hormones. False beliefs and guilts impair the distribution.

Megapotency homeopathic trauma remedies cleanse the lower chakras and purify the heart. They enable the heart energy, pure love, to work with mind/will in creating our perfect desires. An unpurified heart chakra is held back by the powerful destructive energies of our guilts, griefs, angers, resentments, fears, doubts, jealousy, lust, envy, hatred and greed - these are the Devil Incarnate that we all need to dissolve, before we can become our best selves. In doing so, we reactivate our thymus gland, the source of our immunity and the residence of our soul, to strengthen our life force.

This is why I say we need to re-green the planet and the people. For until people can begin to feel love for and confidence in themselves instead of fear for their survival, there can be no world healing. Inner love brings a sense of well-being, of confidence and faith that one's inner tutor (intuition) is always on hand to guide one out of harm's way. One lives with a totally new outlook and thence a new experience of the same outward circumstances. It brings

19

one the opportunity to love others, fearlessly and seeking no rewards. How can one ever hope or expect to follow the injunction to 'love thy neighbour as thyself' without first loving oneself?

One of my favourite exercises that I give my patients is to look into a mirror and repeat aloud to the image, 'I love you' - seventy times seven times! In other words, seventy times a day for seven days. It is amazing how many people cannot complete this number. They fall in a screaming heap of tears, as it becomes clear to them how untrue the statement is. Perseverence and repetition, however, retrain the subconscious body-mind to the new belief, and this is really worth doing.

Why is this so hard? I came to realize that most people have a very impaired concept of who they are, really are. We live with an image of ourselves that is shaped by so many emotionally coloured beliefs and experiences that the real identity has been shrouded. The overlay of acquired guilts, griefs and fears shapes the way we understand ourselves and our world, and imparts a sense of hopelessness, of helplessness and, in many cases, worthlessness. With such beliefs, it is impossible for some to feel love for themselves. Yet until they can, it is impossible for them to truly love all others.

Victim-consciousness is an inevitable accompaniment of helplessness. It ranges from the sense of powerlessness of one dominated by a stronger personality to those fearful of the infinitely small - viruses and bacteria; those frustrated and helpless under threat of violence, whether domestic, social or war; those affected by the frustrations of stymied plans and lost hopes through circumstances not of their own making, or of ill-conceived laws and regulations; and those whose inability to face responsibility causes them to blame anything and anyone for whatever happens to them.

The combined guilts of old fears and helplessness can open the person to a belief that they are the hapless victims of entity attack. Entities from the unseen dimensions are thought to be the cause of all manner of ill-health and psychic attack, feeding on and depleting vitality or controlling the mind and actions of the sufferer. In medicine this is called schizophrenia. It is merely caused by emotional shock trauma fragmenting the energy field or aura of the sufferer. Many people believe that the aura normally forms a protective barrier around us, so that if damaged, undesirable energies from the lower unseen dimensions are able to enter the body's fractured force field and disrupt the life of the sufferer. Heal the shock/fright trauma and you heal the aura so that such disruption ceases to be possible. Quantum physics shows us a scientific explanation for schizophrenia, which I shall detail in the Aconite chapter, and which also allows the possibility of an opening to another dimension of reality.

In every victim of whatever circumstance, we find lack of confidence, lack of awareness of the infinite power we all have to control and create our own lives exactly as we would wish. Once we get free of victim-consciousness we are able to unleash the mind-power lying dormant, just awaiting the chance to be brought into our service. Answers come to our dilemmas and we are able to shake free and fly into greatness.

MAN THE CREATOR

Fred Alan Wolf, who has described quantum physics for the layman in his easy-to-read book *Parallel Universes*[2], says 'Quantum physics appears to be telling us that what we choose to observe alters, and even creates, what we observe. Thus in a quantum world view, we have choice - something I see as synonymous with consciousness. In other words, to have consciousness, there must be choice.

'But how can choice manifest? There must be mind. In other words, it is self-consistent to have choice if there is mind, and choice then exists in the mind. Mind, I believe, exists as fleeting energy in parallel universes. The universe we perceive consists of the overlap of these fleeting flashes of energy. The patterns create mind as surely as they create matter. Both the existence of matter and the perception of it are the same thing.

'Thus it is that the mind of any sentient being that is capable of perceiving a reality is capable of reaching into parallel universes and performing the task of choosing that reality.' However much it may seem otherwise, we always have choice, though our available choices may be inaccessible owing to our psychological blocks.

Let us consider the reason, or the mechanism, by which mind and emotions create your physical problems. In essence, the universal law under which all sentient life operates is as follows:

Conscious *thought* plus the *energy* of emotions creates the nature of our reality, our physical form and all our environmental circumstances. We are the totality of our thinking, our ideas and imaginings, acted upon by our emotional energy to give them manifestation.

Einstein is credited with having said, 'Imagination is more important than knowledge.' Through imagination we can envisage and this is the first step towards altering our reality.

No thought or idea is of any value without the application of an emotion to activate it. All the great geniuses of all time would have gone unnoticed if their emotions had not been brought into use: enthusiasm, joy, excitement, courage, confidence, love have all been employed to bring the thoughts into reality.

In the same way, thoughts can be of undesirable happenings, destruction and devastation, accidents, misfortunes of any conceivable kind. These thoughts also pass out of the mind without changing anything unless an emotion is attached to them. Whether the emotion is excitement (joy at the idea of war is common enough), horror or fear makes no difference - the thought begins the process of manifesting on the physical plane.

Imagine the chaos if every thought you ever had became a reality! Thank God, we have an inner censor that can choose whether or not to be fired up by an idea. Most of our thoughts are fairly emotionless. But some are coloured by experiences and beliefs that stir up feelings - fear, envy, grief, resentment, anger and so on - which have no option but to result in a physical event. It is a law of life - mind plus emotion creates your reality on the physical plane.

And what does this really mean? It means that most of the time, most of us (if not all) are sparking from emotions relating to a whole range of false ideas, old guilts, griefs and fears, social programming and conditioning, and we are living in a false concept of life. We have had so much wool pulled over our eyes by our experiences and social influences that we cannot see the truth that would set us free, so we create and perpetuate physical ill health.

The fact is that life is seen as a duality of light and dark, good and evil, black and white, love and fear, joy and depression, God and the Devil, positive and negative. But the reality is that these are concepts devised by man, without knowledge of the Law.

The Law is of universal unity. Black and white are but two faces of the same coin; fear is the dark side of love, evil is the dark side of good. Dark cannot exist in the presence of light. Darkness is only the absence of light; black is the absence of colour, while white is the blending of all colours; fear is the absence of love, anger is the absence of an allowing, loving tolerance. We need to fill ourselves with the brilliance of pure light to expel all the fears and guilts and griefs and other self-destructive emotions that are causing deterioration in our physical form.

Once we allow this light into our lives, the release of these undermining emotions is immediate, as fast as switching on a light switch. We are then freed up to experience the previously suppressed joy of living. Some people achieve this healed state in a religious experience, a sudden dawning of enlightenment. These people are rare. But this same healing is available to all through the wonders of megapotency homeopathy, and the enlightenment is just as great. Nothing compares with the totality of healing available through homeopathy. This is the most powerful form of colour healing, specific enough to apply accurately to the different types of emotional healing.

Everything is actually one energy; it just appears to be broken up. This is true of the universe, the human body and the microcosm of the atom. Life in the material world requires a condensing of this energy into denser form - matter - but it is still pure energy.

In physics, we have recognised a natural law of magnetic attraction and repulsion. It relates to the other law we all learned at school, that every action has an equal and opposite reaction. Because thoughts activated by emotion are energy forms, they come under these laws, which we describe in more philosophical terms as the law of cause and effect, or the law of Karma, which means, basically, that 'as ye sow, so will ye reap,' life ensures that you get what you deserve, or, 'what goes around, comes around.' We have these sayings in even the oldest cultures, they are ideas that were recognised as facts of life thousands of years ago. However, thoughts sent out by fear, grief or guilt energies can be neutralised by self-forgiveness and release of the stored guilts and fears, thus neutralising the Karmic retribution and putting you instead, into a 'state of grace', debt-free.

'We have completely lost sight of the Self, our divine consciousness residing in our crown chakra, the centre of our greatest wisdom and our access to all-knowing, the universal totality of knowledge. We have become engrossed in the material world of phenomena, trapped in the ego as surely as if we were caught in a web. Our Self-knowledge is shrouded in this limiting web, we wander around in fear and ignorance of who we really are, the Supreme Lord of our Being.'[3]

The Supreme Self is omnipotent, there is nothing it cannot do. Faith can literally move mountains. The human body is actually a vast storehouse of power, lying latent and always ready and waiting to be brought into activation. Indian mystics call it Kundalini, Christianity calls it the Christ, the Chinese *chi*, the Japanese *ki*, the Kalahari tribemen know it as *ngum*. The Aztecs called it Quetzalcoatl, ancient Egyptians worshipped it as the Serpent of Wisdom. When Christians talk of 'letting Christ into your heart', they are simply advising you to open up your consciousness to the already existing power of love lying waiting in the Heart chakra. It is a power that has been known of by the early priests, the passers-on of knowledge, since time began, though they kept it shrouded in mystery lest it be misused by the uninitiated, irresponsible in their ignorance.

The Self is always in communication with all of life, always conscious of the unity of all things. All information is always available to it, all truths on tap. But instead of identifying ourselves with our great Self, we identify with our body, the vehicle we have created to carry us through our material life, and our ego, the limited view of ourselves as separate, individual, alone in our passage through life and learning. The illusion is perpetuated by our misunderstandings of how to handle daily life's interactions and vicissitudes, which continue to feed us false information on which to base our lives.

Our ability to receive enlightenment or become consciously aware of the creative principle and the creative energy within us is limited by our perceptions of life, which in turn are beliefs and attitudes based on eons of experiences and our emotional reactions to, and interpretations of, these experiences. We need to expand our understandings, to cleanse and free ourselves of misunderstandings and the limiting emotions they carry that are continuing to inhibit our progress towards All-knowing.

We have to retrace our steps and return to our source, reclaim our personal power, accept responsibility for who and where we are, and get back on to our original path, the track to knowledge of who we are, where we came from and where we are heading.

It is our denial of the Love principle, the creative energy lying dormant in our hearts, and our refusal to allow this great power to activate and transform our lives and our world, that keeps our planet in a state of war and destruction, on a personal level as well as global. And it is only this way because all our destructive emotions are preventing us from even knowing that there is a light waiting to be switched on.

Let us throw off these shackles and free ourselves to get moving along the pathway to peace and harmony, health and happiness. All our physical problems stem from this ignorance, even the most grossly physical, cancer. The new biology proves that toxins created by our destructive emotions cause irritations in the blood vessels and organs, leading to erosion, tumours, congestion and coagulation of the blood.

Who needs this? It's high time to get back on track.

THE MIND-BODY CONNECTION

The idea of the mind having power over the body has to be changed in the light of modern research, to the view that body and mind are one, that the body is the outward manifestation of the mind. Dr Candace Pert, PhD, who describes her research into neuropeptides as carriers of emotional energy through the body in *Molecules of Emotion*[4], says 'it could be said that intelligence is located not only in the brain but in cells that are distributed throughout the body, and that the traditional separation of mental processes, including emotions, from the body is no longer valid.

'If the mind is defined by brain-cell communication, as it has been in contemporary science, then this model of the mind can now be seen as extending naturally to the entire body. Since neuropeptides and their receptors are in the body as well, we may conclude that the *mind* is in the body, in the same sense that the mind is in the brain, with all that that implies.

'We can no longer think of the emotions as having less validity than physical, material substance, but instead must see them as cellular signals that are involved in the process of translating information into physical reality, literally transforming mind into matter. Emotions are at the nexus between matter and mind, going back and forth between the two and influencing both.

'The mind, then, is that which holds the information network together, often acting below our consciousness, linking and co-ordinating the major systems and their organs and cells in an intelligently orchestrated symphony of life. Thus, we might refer to the whole system as a psychosomatic information network, linking *psyche*, which comprises all that is of an ostensibly non-material nature, to *soma*, which is the material world of molecules, cells and organs. Mind and body, psyche and soma.'

Dr Pert's groundbreaking work on the neurotransmitters of the brain took her firstly from realizing that certain neurotransmitters created emotions that were predictable, to later realizing that emotions alter the numbers and activity of neurotransmitters - a two-way street. The longer Pert studied neurotransmitters, the more she realized that man is firstly a non-physical being of mind and emotions, and secondarily, a physical entity. She moved from being a factual analyst to an enlightened scientist. That is how it is - the more you study the body, the more you realize that emotions are the prime movers, mind is the master.

Dr Bruce Lipton, PhD, research biologist, states in his lecture *The Biology of Belief*: 'Cells work together in a community. When the community falls apart, that's when you get disease. The cell always is intelligent and can adjust to its environment. It reads it through the brain, whose *perceptions* cause it to send messages to the cell, telling it about the environment as perceived by the brain. Perception gets between the environment and the cells - your beliefs adjust your physiology. Beliefs select your genes. You are controlled by your beliefs. Your biology adjusts to prove your beliefs right. Aging is a belief that kills, as is cancer. Only 5% of cancer victims have a predisposition to cancer genetically. Genes may correlate to an expression of life, but are not a cause. Without the cause, the gene can do nothing.

'Belief is a filter between the environment and the cell. You can only see what you were trained to see, through the filters. BUT you can change your beliefs, substitute new ones, and thereby change the way your cells are informed from your brain's output.'

Perceptions about our life and what is going on in it are determined by programming early in life. Lipton points out that in the early years of childhood, our brains are operating in delta wavelength, where all information comes to us as truth and is absorbed without rationalisation. We are like sponges, soaking up everything we encounter without discernment or judgement. This is why perceptive societies have always sought to protect young children from exposure to potentially harmful, emotionally upsetting events and circumstances. It also explains why the Roman Catholic Church is relentless in its determination to indoctrinate children before the age of seven years.

Much of this book describes the ways in which many programmed ideas and beliefs about life have influenced the development of our lives and our descent into ill-health, and gives you tools by which these ingrained untruths may be dissolved away, allowing new patterns of thought to be substituted.

CREATIVE VISUALISATION

Much has been re-discovered over the last century about the ways we can create what we want from the creative power of our mind and heart. One critically important factor seems to be the lack of a disbelief. As long as you don't believe something is impossible, it is possible. If you believe with your mind you can do something, you can, provided you put enough heart energy into it.

The Melbourne psychiatrist, the late Dr Ainslie Meares[6], pioneered the teaching of creative visualisation in healing in Australia. Dr Meares taught his patients how to meditate, and while in meditation, how to look into the body's problem areas, see what was going wrong and apply the power of creative imagination to restoring order to the cells and tissues.

Many patients were successful in ridding themselves of conditions as difficult to shake off as cancer by using his methods. One, Ian Gawler, who had lost a leg to cancer, was inspired to continue the teachings and began to run meditation groups in his own home. The popularity and success of this regular meeting in Melbourne led to the formation of the Gawler Foundation, which disseminates information and runs classes to educate cancer sufferers in the methods.

Success depends on the quality of the emotion put into daily life - if fear for your life, guilt or grief predominates, you will not do as well as those in whom confidence and positive determination prevail. Even then, some unrecognised, subconscious destructive belief may undermine the effort.

Children are particularly clever at creative visualisation, because they have not yet accepted the teaching that it is impossible. In many parts of the world now, children in cancer wards are being taught to imagine their bloodstream carrying hosts of little PacMan-style white blood cells seeking out and gobbling up, thus destroying, the cancer cells. Of course, cancer is not the only disease condition susceptible to the power of creative thought. The fact that it is believed and feared to be one of our most intractable diseases only shows how much could be done if the methods were applied across the board.

We can all use our mind power to create anything we want, and many people do, even without knowing how they are doing it. Uri Geller[7], famed for his spoon-bending abilities, began bending spoons, quite unintentionally, at a very early age. For years this happened quite spontaneously, which did not please his parents much and did little to endear him to households they were visiting socially. As time went on, he developed the ability to control the happenings, and was able to make a living demonstrating this strange ability, along with other equally strange skills. However, there are times when he fails to bend spoons at will, and he interprets this as the result of others' antagonistic mind power out-performing his own.

Many people tell me how they willed themselves well, and we have all read stories of heroic achievements of survival against all odds. Mastery of the body and mastery of the elements are possible. Isn't there a story about Jesus standing up in the stern of a boat caught in a fierce storm, and didn't he wave his fist at the clouds and demand, Cease! and the storm abated? He knew these things. And didn't he also say, 'All that I do, you also can do'?

When I first learned about creative visualisation, life provided me with an opportunity to give it a try. We lived on a bush property which had dairy farms on two sides. Every winter the farmers would set fire to their grasses and treed areas with the idea of preventing summer bushfire infernos. Eucalypts drop a lot of dead branches and leaves which become hazards in the summer heat, and as the trees regenerate quickly after fire, it is a good idea to burn sometimes to clean up the undergrowth. The habit is to wait for a good wind so the fire is carried as far as possible, it prevents them from having to re-light areas where it might have fizzled out. It is called 'controlled burning', but this year there was no control given.

I could see from our home near the top of a hill, that fire was beginning to rise up the adjoining slope on my land. This slope was all bushland, and presented no risk to our home, being separated by a gully that I did not expect the slow-moving fire to leap. However, we did have a little shelter on that hill that we'd built to house various tools and equipment. We removed everything of value to our home hill and waited. The little shed was very flimsy, made only of pliable, re-inforced plastic sheeting wrapped around some trees, roofed with the same material, and it sat smack in the centre of a clump of dense underbrush and scrub to three metres high amongst tall eucalypts.

The men went off to work and I was left there, expecting the fire to consume our little shelter. I suddenly remembered about the power of thought and decided to put it to the test, see if I could do what others claimed they could. So I sat at my desk, closed my eyes and focused my thoughts on the little shed. I visualised it as emitting a powerful opposing force - in my mind, I saw the flames rise up the hill, try to attack and consume the structure, but the forcefield emanating from it caused the flames to be forced back, leaving the building intact. I watched as all around was burned to the ground and saw the fire move on up the hill, leaving my shed behind. I spent about ten minutes doing this, after that I could not visualise it any more so I went on with my day's activities and hoped for the best.

The fire reached the top of the slope and burned out, and it was not until the next day that the ground was cool enough to walk on, to go and see what had survived. Imagine our great amazement to see our little structure, certainly not flame resistant generally but now not even sooty, standing alone in the middle of a sea of black, all scrub burned to the ground right up to within half a metre, yet only a few tiny spark holes in the fabric of the roof where cinders had landed afterwards. The things we had left inside - plastic plant pots and ice-cream buckets - had also been unscathed by the heat.

In the same way as thought can be used to create what you wish to happen, undisciplined thought - imagination, imaging - combined with fear-emotion energy can also, indeed will, always, result in creating the very undesired event you are envisaging. If you fear cancer or some other destructive condition, allowing your thoughts to dwell on it fearfully gives that idea the power to become a physical reality. If you are fearful while driving, and envisage that truck coming towards you suddenly on your side of the road, sooner or later that is exactly what will happen. You will have set the scene on the astral plane and it will manifest itself physically sooner or later, unless you deliberately take steps to annihilate it.

Wipe that image from the blackboard of your mind as soon as it appears, substituting a more preferable one, and continually discipline yourself to do this every time destructive thoughts are envisaged. Fill your heart with confidence that it was only a passing thought that has not the fear energy to manifest itself. If this seems impossible, use the remedies in this book to clear out your accumulations of guilts and fears and it will be a lot easier.

BASIC PRINCIPLES OF GUILT RELEASE

'Jill's Law' states: *The key to healing is the release of muscle tension.* This was something that became clear to me when I studied Holistic Massage in Bryan's diploma course, the year before we began our research work together. I had already a fair idea of this since studying osteopathy way back in 1968-70, when Bryan and I were students together, and the massage school reminded me and reinforced this understanding.

Whether this release of muscle tension is done by manual methods like massage, osteopathy or chiropractic, by self-realization, yoga, hypnotism, autosuggestion, meditation, energy healing methods such as Reiki or laying on of hands, through herbs, nutrition, flower essences or homeopathy, matters little. Without release of the related muscle tensions there can be no full healing.

Muscles are the primary storage areas for tensions stemming from emotions, attitudes and beliefs. Any muscle in the body can become affected by emotions, including the emotions associated with attitudes and beliefs.

Each end of a muscle attaches to a bone. Muscles in prolonged tension pull bones out of their normal positioning. This can impair the flow of nerve and blood supply to the related organs, causing depletion of tissue integrity, or in other words, disease. Thus the muddy colours seen in the aura, the colours of unhealthy emotions, manifest on the physical plane.

Each strongly held belief or emotion creates a specific pattern of muscle tensions unique to itself. Muscles work in groups to effect particular reactions to emotions. It is possible, through observing patterns in muscle tension and structural (skeletal) misalignments, to know which emotion is being stored, and which homeopathic remedy is going to release it, and relate this specifically to the internal disease the person has been suffering.

THE SPHENOID - PITUITARY CONNECTION

The positioning of the sphenoid bone in the cranium has a critical influence on the correct functioning of the pituitary gland. The sphenoid is known as the keystone of the skull, it cannot be removed from the skull before other cranial bones have been removed, and by far the greater part of its body is within the skull, only a small area meeting the outside world at the temples. Well within the head, it is protected from many bumps and blows, a safeguard for its precious cargo: for, in the centre of the sphenoid, in a cavity called the sella turcica, is the pituitary gland.

Known to osteopathy since its founder, Andrew Taylor Still (1828-1917) first inspired his student, William Garner Sutherland to study the design for motion of the cranial sutures is the fact that the sphenoid bone, along with all the cranial bones, is in perpetual motion, vibrating microscopically under the influence of pulses created by the flow of cerebrospinal fluid, blood flow, respiration and a mysterious, slow cranial rhythm. These pulses are of differing rates or frequencies, their combined forces generating a gyroscopic motion of the cranium which is essential for healthy functioning of the organism.

Dr Sutherland devoted thirty years of research to this discovery, and called the process the Primary Respiratory Mechanism, deeming it the basic ordering and healing principle of the human body.

Strong emotions such as anger, grief, joy and courage are registered first by the hypothalamus (in the top of the brain) and then responses are transferred to the hypophysis or pituitary gland for appropriate action to be taken, by releasing hormones that initiate certain muscle responses to express (or *press out* of the body) the emotion. Other emotions are registered in different parts of the brain, e.g. fear is felt by the hippocampus, and is overridden, it is believed, by the major part of the cerebral cortex. This ex-pressing may take the form of clapping, cheering, laughter, tears and lamenting, rage or flight, depending on the emotion felt. Each reaction releases the emotional energy from the body through the action of the muscles involved. There is no residual effect and good health is maintained.

However, thanks to social conditioning, we suppress the activity of these muscles and withhold all that emotional energy, which, from being a self-healing energy release, becomes a powerful internal energy for suppression of body functions leading, in the long run, to degenerative and destructive diseases.

A belief that anger and offenses must be swallowed or ignored in order to keep the peace, avoid offense, avoid unpopularity or simply because 'nice people don't get angry' causes the angry one to clench his jaw, bite back his words and contain the energy of the emotion within the body. The jaw is the first place to suffer - muscles of the temporo-mandibular joint and the whole of both sides of the face become filled with this emotion and begin to store tension. These muscles include those that attach on to and around the lateral aspects of the sphenoid bone, which then becomes locked and pressurised by the tensions, unable to perform all its microscopic vibrations. Similar effects occur from the suppression of grief, disappointment and sadness.

Changes in the positioning and range of motion of the sphenoid occur as a result of such muscle tension, which may arise from psychological shocks, sport or work postures, accidents, dental work, surgery but most particularly, from suppression of emotions. This partial or total immobilisation or minute shift in the positioning of the sphenoid restricts the delicate nerve and blood vessels within the sella turcica surrounding and feeding the pituitary gland, which then becomes compromised in its ability to give optimum performance. I suspect that the normal microscopic, vibrational movement of the bone has a stimulatory effect on the pituitary, as well, and this stimulation also becomes reduced. A wide range of endocrine problems are the results of such restriction.

The pituitary gland, then, is being acted upon from two aspects: via the signals being sent out from the hypothalamus as it registers emotions, and via the physical pressure applied by a misaligned, stalled sphenoid bone. In truth, the hypothalamus is telling the person to adopt a certain behaviour in response to emotion, while guilt is causing the person to override this message and suppress action or speech. The pituitary is caught between two powerful, opposing energies.

Prolonged or repeated suppression of emotion causes prolonged muscle tensions affecting the sphenoid in a permanent way. One grief, fear, frustration or indignation builds upon the previous, causing the body to become somewhat fixed in its holding of these tensions, and allowing serious endocrine deficiencies to develop.

Freeing the guilt of feeling such emotions by use of the megapotencies allows these muscle tensions to relax and the sphenoid is enabled to return to its normal position and freedom of motion. Similarly, the jaw that has been pulled out of alignment by these muscle tensions returns to its correct position, and the pituitary begins, often instantly, to function at its best again, thus sending adequate hormones to all the endocrine glands and all organs throughout the body, to restore their normal functioning.

30

Anywhere in the body, muscle tension causes a drawing or pulling force to be applied to the bones to which those muscles attach, leading to restricted motion of those bones. Such muscle tension can be caused by the full range of human emotions.

Shock, fright, terror and panic, even if only once experienced, can cause chronic effects through muscle tensions unresolved, the effects of which some people never overcome without powerful help. These experiences cause sudden changes in the positioning of the parietal bones, albeit sometimes microscopic, which cause these bones then to impinge upon the internal tissues and this impairs the flow of fluids and puts pressure on the brain and any or all its component parts. Malfunction is the result.

Other suppressed emotions also affect the muscles of the face and head. Grief occurs not only as a result of death or partings, but can be an on-going sense of disappointment that things did not turn out as previously expected, planned or hoped. This is often put to the back of the mind, but the storage of that grief energy, unexpressed, tightens certain muscles of the face and has an effect on many body functions by impeding the sphenoid and the posterior pituitary.

Many attitudes and beliefs are not harmonious with life and health. The majority of our social conditioning is based on false understandings which are perpetuated through many generations. Religious and political dogma have also led us away from the truth and generated unnecessary fears, guilts and griefs. Even when we feel intuitively that such beliefs may be wrong, we suppress such feelings in order to conform. We are afraid to be honest, in case we are reprimanded or not loved. Because our intuition, our Inner Self or God-Within knows the real truth, a state of disharmony is created.

Social attitudes teach us it is bad to show emotions, that only the intellectual mind can be allowed expression. This imbalance between our respect for intellect and our respect for feelings is causing inappropriate reactions in the body when feelings are felt. Suppression has become the order of the day, the acceptable way to behave. How often were you told, as a child, 'only babies cry,' 'there's nothing to be afraid of,' 'stop that fighting,' without any real help given as to how to resolve the feelings? Emotions - energy forces - are held back and get locked within the body, in the muscles, waiting to be set free, stored as prolonged tension.

Stress is the product of wrong beliefs and attitudes - work guilt, duty guilt, fun guilt, fear guilt, grief guilt, guilt guilt - combined with held-in detrimental emotions. Stress kills because of the accumulation of these stored emotions in the physical body, and their subsequent effects on the structure. It is quite amazing to see how health is regained once the relevant emotion or shock is released.

We need to know what type of fear is in the mind of the sufferer, and which remedy deals with that particular fear. For example, great benefits

31

came from using Conium once it was revealed by Vithoulkas that Conium people are materialistic.[8] I further discovered that the people needing Conium always had a sense of financial helplessness, a belief of not being able to provide enough for their perceived needs or ambitions, a fear of lack of supply from outside themselves. This specific information has opened up the uses of Conium, a lymphatic system and cancer remedy, to a much wider degree, and the prevalence of such people in our money-oriented society makes it a very important remedy.

You really need to understand that healing your emotions, freeing yourself of your accumulated emotional baggage and getting your life on track, is not traumatic, not a slow process, does not require intense investigation into your childhood nor the re-experiencing of harrowing traumas. It does not require hours or years of counselling, psychology, hypnosis, auto-suggestion, religious conversion, past-life therapy, meditation, vegetarianism, self-analysis, relationship analysis, praying, New Year resolutions, will-power, months in the wilderness or sailing singlehanded around the world. Using the guilt-releasing remedies, it is as easy as ABC, and as rapidly freeing, energising and joyful as you could wish.

In subsequent chapters I will show you the ways to get back on track. Not the way to unrestrained, detrimental emotions, not the way to violent outbursts of anger or floods of tears of grief, not the way to guilt-free irresponsibility. None of these is healthy, either. What you will get is personal growth, so that new insight gives you freedom from anger, freedom from grief, freedom from guilt, freedom from fear, and with this freedom, a new strength to take positive steps in planetary healing.

I will show you also the relationship between our attitudes and why we have handed over our personal power to so-called experts, authorities vested in a little importance who cannot possibly know as well as we do, what is good for us, and can only act from what they think is good for themselves, from the perspective of the lower energy centres of fear and greed. And you will find knowledge that will enable you to reclaim that power and take charge of your life again. I aim to empower you to overcome these guilts, shake off the overlays and find your true, powerful, magnificent self. The world needs you as your best self.

CHAPTER 3

Entrenched belief is never altered by the facts
- Dick Francis, 'Hot Money"

MODERN WESTERN MEDICINE - ON SHAKY FOUNDATIONS

In 1981, a study evaluating the reasons for admission to a respected university hospital in Boston, Massachusetts revealed that an astonishing 36% of the patients were admitted for iatrogenic (doctor-induced) conditions.

Using statistics from a 1984 Harvard Study, the National Safety Council and other sources, the Campaign to Protect Consumer Rights said that more people die from medical negligence than any other accidental cause. If these (USA) statistics are valid, medical errors kill more people than the combined total of accidents involving automobiles, falls, drownings, fires, choking, guns and poisons. This group's study found that anyone admitted to a hospital faces a 1 in 400 chance of dying as a result of medical negligence or malpractice: one every six minutes.

That was many years ago. Do you think it is any better here in Australia, today? A decade ago, the (Australian) AMA was quoted as claiming that 85% of Australians entering hospital do so as a result of doctors' treatments.

Did you know that the World Health Organisation lists homeopathy as the second most widely used system of medicine in the world, after Traditional Chinese Medicine? Western medicine is only fourth on the list. Homeopathy is *more widely used* than the system Australians think of as 'proper medicine'. More people in the world use 'alternative medicine' than that which you thought was conventional medicine.

Why is it, then, that Australia and America lag behind in our recognition of the great benefits of homeopathy? There can only be one answer, and you know it already - vested interests continue to promote drug therapy, because they cannot patent homeopathy. Vested interests own and control drug companies, fertilizer and pesticide companies and the petroleum industry from which they make their products. They control their own drug research and train our doctors to be their salesmen, their pushers, ignoring all the genuine research that proves how far off the truth they are, in order to keep their power and wealth; despising us all as silly sheep, mindlessly following their propaganda, even if it kills us, like lambs to the slaughter.

Evidence that western medicine kills is shown in the huge increase in litigation in recent years. People are, at last, trying to show their intolerance of the failings of the medical world by trying to seek compensation from drug companies, from doctors, surgeons and from hospitals, with the result, since cases are often very successful, that insurance has become an absolute essential in the minds of these pillars of integrity. So panicky have they become, in fact, that when the largest medical insurers in Australia went bust, the medical profession demanded that the government guarantee to cover them against litigation, or they would have no alternative but to close their doors. They know full well that what they do is a public liability, that they cannot practice their profession without risk to the patients - well may they panic! Let them close their doors, those who work so dangerously, wolves in sheeps' clothing. Their insurance premiums are incredibly high - but not high enough, evidently, to keep the insurance company's head above water.

Meanwhile, those of us in the harmless professions are very rarely sued. Many of us do not even carry insurance, though our professional associations now have swayed to pressure from the health insurance companies who require us to be insured if we want our clients to be able to claim rebates. When is the government going to wake up that they are being conned to the back teeth by the medical profession and their suppliers, and that health does not have to be expensive?

The plain and terrible truth is that one of the major causes of the diseases prevalent in our society is the medical drug profession itself, since it works from a false standpoint without respect for the innate super-intelligence of the human totality of body-mind-spirit. And it does so despite the growing mass of scientific knowledge within its own research establishments, whose evidence demands that attitudes, beliefs and methods must change.

Complications in health arise from:

- the failure of 'modern' medicine to have grasped the most basic understanding of the body's inherent self-healing ability, known for centuries by many cultures; and the relationship between thought and form;

- the failure, owing to this ignorance, to perceive that symptoms of illness are actually signs of unhealthy attitudes and beliefs condensing into matter - 'coagulated thought' - signs that tell us that a change needs to be made, that something is throwing our bodily order into disorder, and our inherent self-healer is working on this correction to the best of its ability;

- the failure, because of such ignorance, to apply treatments that support the body's attempts at self-healing, but instead, applying forceful treatments that suppress these self-healing efforts, purely to eliminate the

34

signs of such efforts, and without regard for the mind-creator of the patient;

- the failure to understand that such suppression merely drives the problem into deeper organs and tissues, to break out later as an apparently new and more serious disease condition, while the patient's body becomes ever more congested and depleted of its inherent self-healing energy, and the mental and emotional aspects remain unhealed and continue to maintain and fuel the problem;

- the misconception that bacteria and viruses are always invasive micro-organisms of evil and sinister intent that must be fought and killed out at every opportunity, which is not the case.

In his excellent article *'Pleomorphism of Germs'*, Horst Poehlmann[9] puts germs and viruses into proper perspective. According to Poehlmann, current bacteriology is based on a fundamental error: the Germ Theory of Louis Pasteur (1882-1895). Louis Pasteur was a French inorganic chemist (untrained in physiology) who became the god of bacteriology. In his theory, disease is the result of germs entering the body and multiplying. Various chemicals and vaccines are thought to prevent the germ from doing this. What is conveniently ignored is that Pasteur denounced his own theory from his deathbed, and acknowledged the superiority of the rival theory of Claude Bernard: 'Bernard is right. The microbe is nothing. The environment is all-important.'

Claude Bernard (1813-1878), a French physiologist, had claimed that the germs or microbes, the seeds of disease, would not grow, and therefore would not cause disease, unless the environment in the body ('terrain' in French) was favourable for their metabolisms. Most established researchers in our time base their research on an artificially-created environment in their laboratories, so their conclusions cannot be safely carried through to apply to the human body, which has defense mechanisms for keeping bacteria under control, cleansing mechanisms for keeping the inner environment clean, and the ability to respond to healing factors intrinsic in our fruit and vegetables, the most notable of which is Vitamin C.

Antoine Bechamp[10] (1816-1908), an extremely well-educated French microbiologist, found that disease can originate from within the body, and his findings were confirmed many times over by dedicated researchers in each succeeding generation. Bechamp continually emphasised that pathogenic microorganisms are not the cause of disease but rather the secondary manifestation of a state of toxicity in the body. His experiments showed that he could, by changing the environment of the cell, convert a healthy cell into a virus, and with further alteration to its environment, from a virus into a bacteria.

You know how a common cold starts out with a watery mucous discharge indicating a viral 'infection' which becomes, after a few days, a thicker, yellow mucus indicating a bacterial 'infection'. As the cold clears up (of its own accord, no help from medicine needed) this reverts to clear discharge (viral) and back to none. Exactly the same process occurred in Bechamp's experiments - by altering the environment of the bacterial cells back to the original nutrition he was able to see the bacteria revert to viruses and then back to normal cells.

Another great microbiologist, Royal Rife, followed on from Bechamp and found that there are only ten different types of germs. All varieties are different forms of these ten basic germs. Any organism within its group can be readily changed to any other within the ten groups depending on the medium with which it is fed or grown. For example, if we take a pure culture of bacillus E coli, and alter the medium by as little as two parts per million by volume, we can change that organism within thirty six hours to a bacillus typhosis according to every known laboratory test. Further controlled alterations of the medium will produce the virus of poliomyelitis or mycobacterium tuberculosum or the cancer-producing virus discovered by Rife which he called the BX virus. And then, if you please, you can alter the medium again and change the micro-organism back to a bacillus coli.

So the appearance of so many viruses, so prevalent nowadays where they were quite uncommon when I was young, can be directly attributed to environment. Viruses are simply cell replication going wrong.

Faulty cell replication can occur in any life form dependent on soil. Unhealthy farming practices are creating faulty cell replication to occur in grains, fruits and vegetables and particularly, food animals and birds. Wild animals are also affected, as their habitats are impinged upon by chemically polluted air and water and by degradation and deafforestation. Little wonder that insects like mosquitoes, fleas and ticks can transfer viruses - rogue cells - from one animal to another and to people, and that animal proteins used in immunisation serums are carrying viruses from those animal tissues into the human body.

Chemicals used in agriculture and the home garden are being linked to the increasing prevalence of some diseases. The Sydney Morning Herald of Nov. 6, 2000 ran an article 'Gardening pesticide linked to Parkinson's disease', describing how researchers in Atlanta GA fed steady amounts of a 'non-toxic' pesticide, Rotenone (or derris dust to Australians) into the bloodstreams of rats and they developed all the symptoms of Parkinson's. The scientists said that the finding was the best evidence so far that chemicals in the environment may be factors in parkinsonism. (We know from clinical experience and from the evidence of the many Drug Compendiums available that many drugs have 'side' effects of tremor.)

We need to continue to push for modernised natural, organic, biodynamic and permacultural methods of sustainable agriculture to become mainstream. Chemical pesticides, herbicides, fertilizers and broadacre pastures are destroying our internal and external environment, not to mention our farmers' financial stability. Annual ryegrass and wild oat control costs Australian cereal farmers at least $120m a year to control[11]. Alternative methods are still in the minority.

Royal Rife also found that the cancer-growth-inducing BX virus became absolutely violent when it was exposed to X-rays, and tumour growth was severely sped up; an observation that can be regularly made after cancer patients receive their death sentence in the form of radiotherapy. Statistics show that untreated cancer patients live up to four times longer than the conventionally treated patient. Insiders also know that practically no cancer cell is sensitive to radiation; only the body's defense wall around the tumour gets destroyed.

For the last century and more, those who have debunked the Germ Theory have been crucified. Pasteur, wealthy and politically powerful, was able to bring about the less well situated but honest Bechamp's exile from scientific circles; Royal Rife, who also discovered a totally harmless and extremely effective cure for cancer using radio frequencies (shades of homeopathy and radionics) to destroy the cancer cells, refused a rip-off offer from the US AMA who wanted to suppress his information, which led to his laboratories' being burned down and Rife's being driven to alcoholism after several staged court cases. Supporters of Rife were threatened with loss of their license to practice medicine if they continued to support him.

The same happened to Hoxsey who discovered the famous herbal cure for cancer. The Hoxsey Clinic is still alive and thriving in Mexico, proving the success of Hoxsey's methods. More recently in Canada, Gaston Naessens[12], another post-Rife researcher who even had video film of the germ transmorphology, was taken to court by the Canadian Medical Association with the aim of gaoling him for life, but this attempt was not successful. Others, too numerous to mention, have been defamed, ridiculed and exiled from various countries including Australia for their successes in treating cancer. (e.g. Google Jenny Barlow Foundation)

There is big money to be won from the preservation of the cancer industry, for some. Strange that trillions of dollars, much of it raised by well meaning individuals and groups, have been spent over the last hundred years in the pursuit of a cure that never appears; strange to what lengths some will go, to keep you, the public, in ignorance of the great hoax being perpetrated against you. Notice how they behave like cornered wild beasts when faced with the potential loss of their powerbase. A multitrillion dollar business (the cancer industry is the second largest industry in the world after petroleum) employing millions of people has been built on the foundation of Louis Pasteur's disproven theory that invading germs are the cause of diseases.

Abandoning that theory and embracing the proven truths of cell biology would make the pharmaceutical industry, that also produces insecticides, pesticides, food colourings, preservatives and many other harmful chemicals, teeter towards collapse unless it could find ways of patenting life-force enhancing treatments instead of powerful, bullying, often deadly chemicals. Could this ever happen? Not in my opinion, as the whole mind-set requires a total turnaround from fear-based greed and self interest to loving, genuine concern. They keep telling us that healthful, safe practices are not financially viable so we cannot be encouraged to pursue them. If I were religious, I would say this sounds like the voice of the Devil.

FAITH, HOPE AND LOVE - LOST FROM MEDICAL PRACTICE

Have you ever stood back from today's medical practice and taken a look at the big picture? Have you noticed that medical procedures are all aggressive, invasive assaults on the human body? Have you noticed that the philosophy governing the prescription of drugs is one that believes the body must be coerced into certain actions or reactions by forceful or controlling methods?

The latter half of the twentieth century will be looked upon, in centuries to come, as the darkest age in medical history. Faith, hope and love, the primary creative energies required for healing, have been abandoned by technology and 'science' to the point where it is difficult to find any medical procedure or drug that incorporates even one of these. Indeed, doctors are so far removed from them that they have come to regard it as a dangerous practice to give a patient hope, to have faith in the patient's innate self-healing abilities, or to apply methods of healing based on a loving standpoint rather than cruelty. Why?

Modern medicine claims to have its foundations in the Hippocratic oath, the Hippocratic writings (c. 400BC, Greece) and the writings of Galen (130-c.200AD, Rome).

Let us have a look at these venerable sources.

We find that the Hippocratic oath, as used nowadays, is more modern in its English language form,[13] but here it is, in its original translation, in full:

THE OATH

'I swear by Apollo the physician, and Aesculapius, and Health, and All-heal, and all the gods and goddesses, that, according to my ability and judgment, I will keep this Oath and this stipulation - to reckon him who taught me this Art equally dear to me as my parents, to share my substance with him, and relieve his necessities if required; to look upon his offspring in the same footing as my own brothers, and to teach them

this art, if they shall wish to learn it, without fee or stipulation; and that by precept, lecture and every other mode of instruction, I shall impart a knowledge of the Art to my own sons, and those of my teachers, and to disciples bound by a stipulation and oath according to the law of medicine, but to none others. I will follow that system of regimen which, according to my ability and judgment, I consider for the benefit of my patients, and abstain from whatever is deleterious and mischievous. I will give no deadly medicine to anyone if asked, nor suggest any such counsel; and in like manner I will not give to a woman a pessary to produce abortion. With purity and with holiness I will pass my life and practice my Art. I will not cut persons labouring under the stone (i.e. gallstone) but will leave this to be done by men who are practitioners of this work. Into whatever houses I enter, I will go into them for the benefit of the sick, and will abstain from every voluntary act of mischief and corruption; and, further, from the seduction of females or males, of freemen and slaves. Whatever, in connection with my professional practice or not in connection with it, I see or hear, in the life of men, that which ought not to be spoken of abroad, I will not divulge, as reckoning that all such should be kept secret. While I continue to keep this Oath unviolated, may it be granted to me to enjoy life and the practice of the art, respected by all men, in all times! But should I trespass and violate this oath, may the reverse be my lot!'[14]

Well, the reverse is fast becoming the lot of many, nowadays, as orthodoxy loses credibility and many doctors face or fear litigation owing to the riskiness of their medications.

According to Professor Lloyd, there is no evidence that Hippocrates ever wrote anything down. However, he travelled and taught, and numerous others wrote volumes claiming to be his teachings. It is not known now how much of these writings were actually pure Hippocrates. No matter. The part most quoted as coming from the Hippocratic Oath is the injunction that says 'First, do no harm', which is actually expressed as 'abstain from whatever is deleterious and mischievous'. The original phrase, *prima non nocere*, is Latin, not Greek, and probably was written by Galen.

Galen left over 500 treatises, some eighty or ninety believed genuine are still surviving. He was a great philosopher and believed a physician must be also a philosopher. He was an incessant critic of the contemporary medical sects then flourishing in Rome. He opposed all fads and cults, and every doctor who lost sight of what he held to be the Hippocratic teaching on the unity of the living organism and the forces of nature.

Galen believed that 'animals are governed at once by their soul and by their nature, and plants by their nature alone, and that growth and nutrition (which are common to both plants and animal) must therefore be the effects of nature, not of soul'. He nevertheless believed that nature was smarter than the mind of man - 'They cannot do what Nature does, for to imitate this is beyond the power not only of children, but of anyonesoever; it is a property of Nature alone' - referring to the intricacies of the growth processes. Contrast this with the arrogance of modern medicine.

Man's inhumanity to man reaches its peak in today's medical methods. There is hardly a procedure used in orthodox medicine that does not involve force, manipulation, aggression or violence; and the same can be said of pharmaceutical drugs. The whole mind-set seems to be 'If it can't harm you, how can it help you?' or even worse, 'If it can't kill you, how can it help you?' And the killer mentality is accepted as normal.

Drugs are manufactured with the intention of forcing the body to produce more or less of hormones, enzymes or amino acids; or of replacing these with synthetic chemical hormones that encourage the body to shut down on its own natural production of them; and of forcing chemical reactions to take place that are not the choice of the innate cellular intelligence and therefore not in line with healing. Despite the fact that the body is the grandest problem-solver there is, quietly and perpetually overcoming billions of obstacles without our conscious instruction, doctors don't trust it. They turn to chemical drugs. Confusion and congestion result, the body's elimination channels become clogged up with chemicals it has no programming for neutralising or cleaning out. It is a dangerous practice requiring critical doses that make scant allowance for variations in human tolerance and carry high risk factors, even when considered 'safe' enough to be prescribed over the counter, in pharmacies and in supermarkets.

It is no wonder that some doctors suffer guilt. How terrible it must be, to work in a practice where you know, at the end of the day, that you have not made one prescription that offers real healing; not one person has been given gentle, non-invasive treatment chosen to co-operate with the body's intentions and stimulate the person's natural self-healing capabilities.

Many medical practitioners are doing post-graduate study in a wide range of alternative or complementary modalities. A survey in Perth (W.A.) recently suggested that more than fifty per cent of GPs had done some such course. However, there is a massive shift required to leap from orthodox allopathy to homeopathy. As medical disciplines, they are poles apart, as dark is to light, as ignorance is to enlightenment. Most medical doctors cannot jump this gulf. It requires first that they recognize that their methods are dangerous, then forgive themselves for the years of harmful practice; the guilt is often too great, and some refuse to face its existence. By denying guilt and suppressing it, they entrench themselves even more firmly in the darkness of their limited understanding.

The English homeopath, Dr Dorothy Shepherd, wrote in the 1940s:[15] 'As I read in a medical paper some time ago, a doctor spoke of himself to a coroner thus: his first duty, he considered, was to relieve pain. Not to cure the patient, mind you. Medical Science has forgotten when and where to look for a cure; it sees in a drug, only a way of obliterating suffering and drowning pain. And to an already weakened constitution, weakened by disease, is added the unnecessary cumulative effect of a drug disease; a disease caused by the action of a drug or drugs.'

There is a concerted attempt on the part of drug companies to jump on the 'natural' bandwaggon lately. Have you noticed the increasing number of pharmaceutical products coming out now that claim to be herbal 'extracts'? Just be careful. What the drug companies mean by extract is something extracted from the plant, that is now being isolated and given to you in concentrated form, and even as a synthetic copy, in a patented drug form.

Some of these so-called 'herbal' drugs on offer have no relationship to the known uses of the plants as used in herbal medicine or homeopathy. They are still trying to offer a suit-everyone treatment without regard for your individuality, and it is put to you as natural. Nature does not work that way, and healing is not found from these methods.

In herbal medicine, a plant extract is made by simmering the plant material in water for some length of time, until *all* its readily available components are extracted into the water and the water is reduced in volume. This is also known as a decoction, and it can be preserved by adding a little alcohol. It contains many minerals, plant hormones, enzymes, vitamins, chlorophyll and many other substances which are in the perfect balance to provide you with the kind of healing that that plant is capable of offering.

Well, you might say, they're heading in the right direction, they're trying, aren't they? No, they are trying to bring herbal medicine into the control of drug companies, by turning naturally occurring plants into patented drugs, just as they have always done. The whole baseline is wrong. Don't get any warm, fuzzy feelings when you see such things, it is not a sign of awakening.

In Australia, many small herbal and vitamin manufacturers have been bought up by drug companies, who continue to use the old brand names while altering the quality and content of the original formulae. Is this a deliberate ploy to bring discredit on natural products? I believe so.

One doctor I know studied acupuncture and herbal medicine after finishing his medical degree. He told me, 'From the first week of acupuncture, I saw a whole new world unfolding. I had no idea that healing existed like this.' He still practises medicine as well but has reduced this to a minimum by becoming a Patch Adams-style clown, creating laughter and joy in children's hospitals and in war-torn parts of the world. He has found the healing and soul-restoring power of laughter.

Those doctors who take up homeopathy - a rare few are willing to do the study involved, de-program themselves from their medical training and spend the greater time required to find the appropriate remedy - enter a wonderful world that allows them to offer hope and love in their prescriptions, with the certainty that their well-chosen remedy will effect healing without harmful side-effects or complications.

The experience of homeopathy in one's own life is the stimulus - no-one who has done so cannot wish to pass on his joy and excitement to others. To find suddenly that there are healing, even curative treatments for conditions he had previously believed incurable - such as the after-effects of injuries, asthma, arthritis, heart disease, endometriosis, prolapses, fatigue, depression and a thousand other named conditions - is a great joy that uplifts and inspires him to further study and practice.

To find that there are homeopathic remedies that will even antidote the adverse effects of drugs, surgery, anaesthetics, X-ray, injections of any kind, chemotherapy and other traumatic offenses to the body is an even greater joy, as his guilt can then be released by their use. Wouldn't you think a genuine medico would want this? Yet it is a risky business in Australia, I know of several doctors who turned away from drugs into safer practice and were subsequently struck off the medical register for not practising according to the standard practice of their peers. Furthermore, they were then not covered for Medicare subsidisation and their patients had to pay full consultation fees, as mine do. It reduces the clientele, but integrity counts.

Unfortunately, most don't have time to see past the end of their nose, they are so overloaded with waiting rooms full of people requiring help. Take it from me, you will not find true healing there for any condition you may have, no matter how many drugs you try. You will simply be drugging yourself into such a poor state that there will be no alternative but to cut out the diseased organ - or so your doctor will lead you to believe - or die of side-effects.

In both America and Australia it has been left to individual enthusiasts to maintain the true and genuine knowledge. Truth will not be suppressed forever, and the time has arrived for greater public education. Armed with knowledge, you will be able to demand better medical care.

SIDE EFFECTS AND AFTER EFFECTS

Still feeling sceptical about what I'm saying? Think I'm being a bit hard on all those well-meaning doctors with their lovely bedside manners? Have a look at the ways that commonly used drugs and procedures are affecting our children and ourselves, and then see if you don't think I have a strong case against these white coats who terrify many children with their cruel methods.

ANTIBIOTICS

The first antibiotics were the sulfa drugs developed in the 1930s. These were followed by Penicillin in 1941, a drug derived from penicillium, a mould. Curiously, this was found to be effective against fungal infections of the mucous linings of the airways (homeopathic action!). Used in the micro-doses of homeopathy, this is a powerful remedy for the same kinds of bacterial and fungal infections it is used for in Medicine. The big difference is that in microdoses, there are no adverse effects, no side effects and no resistant strains develop - the medicine is simply stimulating the body to overcome in its normal way, energising its immune system to conquer the problems similar to those that penicillin can itself cause.

Antibiotic means anti life. Antibiotics kill indiscriminately, not concerned about which organisms they are killing, and that means you and your kids. And what antibiotics, whether herbal or pharmaceutical, can cause, if used too frequently or for too long, is one or more of the following:

- Sore throats that recur, sometimes within two weeks of the last course of antibiotics; with mucous congestion that quickly becomes thick, yellow, greenish, causing coughing, often going to the chest; mouth breathing; blocked eustachian tubes, causing deafness; in children this is 'treated' by putting grommets (pieces of plastic hose) in the ears, which fall out as the child grows, by which time he will have grown out of the problem by himself, hopefully.

- Depleted immune functions, rendering us more susceptible to infections. As years go on, it is common to see mononucleosis, known as Glandular Fever or Epstein-Barr Virus, set in. This is usually triggered off by stress such as the workload of higher education - high school and university students are the most common sufferers, and almost invariably they have had lots of antibiotics in childhood.

- Depleted friendly bowel bacteria. Antibiotics kill out the friendly as well as the unfriendly microbes. Depleting helpful bowel microorganisms like lactobacilli means that unfriendly microorganisms are given a greater opportunity to thrive and multiply.

One of the worst of these is candida albicans, the thrush yeast, which feeds on sugars in your digestive tract. When candida is encouraged to multiply by your killing out of its enemies, it devours all your food sugars and demands more, causing cravings for sweet foods and fermentation in the stomach and bowel, and you become a bubbling beer-factory - indeed, alcohol can be produced, making you feel intoxicated. It also gets prolific enough to change from a yeast into a fungus that sends root-like filaments through the bowel walls and into the bloodstream, into the pelvic cavity, through the uterine wall or the bladder, and conditions like endometriosis set in.

These processes develop over a good number of years. The immune system has initially been compromised by antibiotics given years before, sometimes also by Glandular Fever, then, often, the use of The Pill and generally a lifestyle stress situation creates the final trigger. The range of symptoms arising out of and concurrent with a Candida problem is vast, and includes inability to keep the mind focused, short-term memory loss, mental spaciness, food intolerances, asthma, arthritic aches and pains, fibromyalgia, uterine aberrations, constipation and/or diarrhoea, panic attacks, acute sensitivity to the environmental chemicals in, for example, a supermarket, rashes, acute energy loss and chronic fatigue.

The breakdown of immunity eventually leads to malignancy in one form or another. But antibiotics are only one of the killer forms of medicine.

IMMUNISATION

World wide, medical research and statistics show indisputable correlation between immunisations and brain damage, death, arrested development, autism, mental and physical hyperactivity (ADHD), social violence and criminality. Our society is mystified by the massive, continuing increase in children's and teenagers' instability over the last few decades. A massive increase has also been noted in the number of children being born with defective brains and/or bodies. Researchers have provided a phenomenal amount of evidence correlating these with immunisations, particularly with the pertussin vaccine. To ignore them is to bury your head in the sands of determined ignorance.

Despite vaccinating babies several times in their very early months, pertussis is still increasing. The resurgence is especially found in infants, where it is most dangerous. According to Infection and Immunity[16], vaccination has apparently changed the age at which children get infectious diseases, from childhood to infancy (when they are most vulnerable). When countries stop vaccinations in infancy, the age of occurrence returns to older children who have greater coping ability.

I am often given the argument, 'How is it that vaccination is claimed to be so dangerous, if it has succeeded in eliminating smallpox from the world?' Smallpox vaccination was developed because of the supposed immunity to smallpox given to milkmaids by the cowpox virus, which is harmless to humans but causes a similar complaint in cows. It was introduced to the human body after being cultured in the lymphatic systems of cows. This was risky enough in itself, because of the possible presence of other viruses in the lymph, but it worked remarkably well - homeopathic to the problem, according to the Law of Similars (see Chapter 4).

However, it is not the cowpox virus culture that causes today's problems. Vaccination (from *vaccus*, Latin for cow) was discontinued in 1980 after the World Health Organisation declared that the world had seen its last case of smallpox in 1978. Laboratories became the growth centres for smallpox, and the virus has been perpetuated and used in various experimental treatments for desensitising to allergies and cancer, and - how sick is it, that at present, decades since the last smallpox case in the world, stores of the smallpox virus are still kept in the USA and in Russia, for the stated purpose of developing new weapons of germ warfare? (Who will disarm the USA?)

The serums used for the cultures for all the immunisations nowadays contain formaldehyde, aluminium phosphate, thiomersal (a mercury compound lately said to be being phased out - after half a century! - because of its damaging effects), foreign proteins (antigens) and contaminating animal proteins and viruses from the tissues used as the growth medium on which the viral and bacterial components of the serums are cultured.

Far from being safer, more controlled, these serums develop, alongside the desired culture, many other viruses. Some scientists admit to as many as twenty extra viruses being present in the DPT serums commonly stuck into babies. They know this, but have no way of filtering out these very tiny rogue cells, so they simply say, 'Hopefully, the benefits will outweigh the risks.' The benefits go to the drug companies, while the parents take the risks with their children's health.

And what are the risks? Aside from death, there have been thousands of cases of encephalitis and other crippling diseases, but most widespread of all is the astounding increase in childhood asthma and diabetes - a terrible money-making scam for drug companies. First, they fill your children with filthy pollutants, then they fill them with more chemicals to try and force the body to cope, with nothing being offered to help eliminate the toxicity or stimulate vitality. And this drugging becomes an expectation for the whole of life, unless the individual somehow, mysteriously, 'grows out of it'.

And that is only the half of it. Vast numbers of children are also suffering brain and nervous system shock effects simply from being stabbed with a pointed instrument, which can overstimulate the brain causing hyper-sensitivity, hyperactivity (ADHD) and loss of functional balance in the systems of the body, and at the other extreme, tetanus-like encephalitis causing shut-down of some functions of the brain and leading to cot-death, autism, paralyses of various kinds and loss of intelligence. *The very act of stabbing a child* causes, in many, the loss of self-value that we find so prevalent in today's youth, leading to social violence, loss of respect, criminality, drug abuse and suicide. It makes no difference what was in the injection, all kinds can have these effects on some children, simply from the hypodermic stabbing. What is a kid to think, after all? Either he thinks he deserves better than this and suffers mental and physical indignation at the offense, which causes its own range of problems, or he thinks he can't be worth much if even his own mother is not protecting him from this assault, she doesn't value him very highly. And if he grows up thinking he is not worth much, how can you expect him to value or respect other people?

According to the US Center for Disease Control and Prevention's national survey[17], seven per cent of US children aged 6 to 11 have been diagnosed with attention-deficit/hyperactivity disorder (ADHD), and half of them have a learning disability as well. This is plague proportions (2.6 million children) and directly attributable to needle shock, which, perversely, is being increased each year, children are receiving more injections and skin-piercing procedures from their day of birth than ever before.

A relationship between cot-death, immunisation and vitamin C deficiency was recognised as long ago as the early 1970s. Dr Archie Kalokorinos[18], a NSW country doctor treating both aboriginal and caucasian children, found that sudden infant deaths were caused by a form of infant scurvy, or vitamin C deficiency. He found that he could prevent these deaths if contacted swiftly, by injecting them with 200mg of liquid ascorbic acid, intramuscularly, sometimes in conjunction with a million units of penicillin, and the result was a dramatic recovery in thirty minutes of infants who were on the verge of death. Autopsies had shown him that the livers of such infants showed liver change. Sick infants displayed symptoms of liver tenderness with remarkable frequency, as well as irritability of temperament.

Factors that contributed to sudden, unexpected infant death also included mild infections (burning up vitamin C) and any routine immunisation, which quickly used up increased amounts of the vitamin, making it absolutely vital for immunised children to be supplemented with ascorbic acid after their injections.

Dr Kalokorinos found that administration by the mothers of oral ascorbic acid failed to give the benefits of the injected vitamin, if the child showed signs of an infection. (I have observed that an injection often counteracts the adverse effects of a previous injection, i.e. the effects of a puncture wound can be counteracted by another puncture wound - this is a homeopathic action, much the same principle as cauterising a burn to counter the painful destruction of the previous burn.) He found that irritability was a sure sign of infantile scurvy, and found that such children, if then immunised, could and would die from 'this lethal combination.' Dr Kalokorinos found that the best cared-for and best-fed babies in the district - whether aboriginal or white - were dying, and that the risk was even greater if they were given sedatives because of their irritability.

Needless to say, orthodox medicine and government refused then and still refuses to take responsibility for such deaths, despite an enormous amount of literature supporting his findings, even then. When Dr Kalokorinos took his findings to Canberra, he got nowhere. When he wrote an article for the Medical Journal of Australia on the subject, the article was refused and the editor called the subject 'irrelevant'. As Archie Kalokorinos angrily said, 'Since when does the subject of infant deaths become irrelevant?'

Sparked by the US government's potential program of inoculation against hypothetical germ warfare, the (US) Foundation for Health Choice[19] on January 13, 2003, issued a press release that 'two health groups are launching a challenge to the very constitutionality of subjecting infants and children to mandatory vaccinations for a variety of diseases.

'The joint effort by the Washington, DC-based non-profit consumer groups Foundation for Health Choice and Citizens for Health is based on the fact that such 'preventive measures' can be expected to kill a certain number of children and substantially harm others.'

'The two health organisations have already begun to utilize this approach in a 'friend of the court' brief filed in a case now in federal court, citing both a recent opinion by a US district court judge that federal capital punishment law is unconstitutional based on findings that some people facing execution were actually innocent and the argument used by the 2nd Circuit Court of Appeals in reversing that ruling.

'In overturning the lower court decision, the appeals court affirmed the need for due process for the taking of a life by government but, contrary to the district court's opinion, held that a criminal trial provides all necessary due process to support the death penalty. It is the citizens groups' contention that children deserve at least as much due process as a convicted killer before being subjected to a possibly lethal injection.'

'"The lives that are lost by this program are lost without even a pretense of due process," noted James S. Turner, a lawyer, consumer advocate and spokesman for the groups, who pointed out that those for whom vaccination may prove to be a lethal injection are not even granted the legal recourse open to defendants facing the death penalty.' Go to the Koren Publications[20] website to view a poster now available called "Do You Know What's In a Vaccine?" The list of vaccine ingredients is one of the most important pieces of information for parents to consider, if they are to make an informed choice - what role these ingredients play, how they interact with each other and how they affect their child's health. As parents you need to know the answers to these questions.

A nurse writes in Tedd Koren's newsletter, 'I worked in a care centre for children. Most of the kids were extreme cases from car accidents, child abuse and the end results of childhood vaccinations. Most of the "shot" kids were suffering from side effects from their intro shots under three months of age. I read files (wasn't supposed to) but I had to find out why children unrelated in any way, looked similar but were not diagnosed with the usual diagnosis. It read in their files that there were complications from such and such an inoculation. It was horrible. All the children came into this world healthy, normal reflexes, breathing, Apgar .... until the shots. This is why, even at the age of 17, barely educated, I decided my babies would never get a shot! Three years later I had my first child, and the decision was upheld.'

There is much that can be done in homeopathy for many victims of immunisation, and much better preventive health measures. While the concept of immunisation is OK, the methods being used are destroying our societies. There are other ways, inexpensive, effective and harmless, but they do not make money for drug companies, so you are protected from knowing about them. Instead, you are fed the foolish propaganda that harmless treatments can only be ineffectual. We deal with these methods later.

VACCINATION ASTHMA

Asthma is now one of the most prevalent childhood conditions. When I was young, it was rare, only a small handful of children (less than 1%) suffered it. Nowadays, teachers tell me that there are only a few children in their classes who do not have a puffer of Ventolin. No-one used to die of asthma. Nowadays, they do. I read once that the manufacturers of Ventolin acknowledged that used indiscriminately, Ventolin could cause death by heart attack. Rybacki and Long[21] give as its possible risks, 'Increased blood pressure, fine hand tremor, irregular heart rhythm and fatalities (with excessive use).'

We have seen how immunisation pollutes the body with chemicals and viruses that challenge its organs of elimination. A first line of elimination is via the airways. A temperature is the first evidence of this, as the body chooses heat to kill out invading organisms. It then brings out mucus to flush away the residues of the battle. A runny nose, hoarseness, cough and wheezing follow. Huge amounts of antioxidants are required to help the immune system at this time. In the absence of extra Vitamin C, the fever symptoms may abate without finishing the cleansing process; or the child may die. Vitamin A is also needed to maintain the functional integrity of the mucosal linings of the airways. The self-healing mechanism having exhausted its available supplies, the mucus congestion becomes a set-in condition.

We have created a world full of people who cannot breathe well because the processes the body normally uses to keep foreign matter out are being bypassed, deliberately and indiscriminately (one day this will be called 'criminally') at every stage.

Skin's main function is to protect the body from the outside world. Most of the properties of skin are qualities of elimination and defense against attack from the environment. When you assault this intelligent, ingenious organ by penetrating it with a syringeful of foreign, filthy serum, you are bypassing the normal functions of the immune system. The pollutants go straight into the lymphatics and the bloodstream. The body is designed in such a way that it expects its intake of nutrients and medicines to come via the mouth and digestive tract, which has the ability to deal with and extract toxic elements and either destroy or eliminate them. It has no way of dealing with chemical toxins and viruses when they come through the skin. No wonder, then, that many children suffer brain fevers as these viruses and toxic chemicals go straight into the blood that is going to the brain.

Medical scientists tell us that the immunising must be done by needle because otherwise, it is rendered ineffectual by the stomach and its surrounding lymphatic glands. Yet the Sabin polio vaccine, the only one not implicated in cases of vaccine damage, is given orally. Is this ineffectual, or is the other claim a lie? If they can make one successful vaccine for oral administration, why not the others?

Either way, no-one needs to be put at risk of years of asthma by this method. It is far more risky than the risk of death or after-effects from childhood diseases, which only occur in a very small number of cases and even more rarely in those treated homeopathically. Vaccination asthma is only the beginning of a lifetime of problems that move gradually into deeper tissues: muscles (heart and circulatory disorders), joints (arthritis), chronic lymphatic congestion (lymphomas), liver congestion, tumours, not to mention the potential for a lifetime of allergies and sensitivities, hyperactivity and chronic fatigue. We are now seeing the age for deaths from these most serious and deadly conditions coming down to include people under thirty, even teenagers.

PAINKILLERS

Research now tells us that taking pain-deadening drugs after an injury (this also means surgery) appears to interfere with healing. Researchers at the University of Medicine and Dentistry of New Jersey[22] found that using NSAIDs (non-steroidal anti-inflammatory drugs) appeared to slow or modify bone healing after a fracture. These drugs apparently blocked the cox-2 enzyme associated with pain and inflammation. Researchers may be beginning to realize that the enzyme and perhaps the pain and inflammation itself, plays an important role in healing.

Pain is an indicator of something going on, a healing process in action, in the body. Its purpose is to warn you of this process, to protect you from taking the body beyond its limits of tolerance at that time. To suppress pain, therefore, is to take away the warning signal, the indicator, and allow you to pretend there is no need for care. Drug companies want you to do this so that your healing process can develop into a problem that requires long term, even lifetime treatment. It makes sense, businesswise, to have the whole population on lifetime treatments. That is the only sense there is in using a painkiller. If you seek out healing practitioners, find out why the pain is there and take steps to treat and heal the source of the problem, bad luck, you don't have to take constant medications! That means you will not develop complications and need more drugs to counteract the effects of the first ones. You have just reduced the national ill-health bill by half.

You thought paracetamol was harmless? In the Sydney Morning Herald, Aug 10-11, 2002, we read that 'a coroner is expected to recommend that paracetamol be removed from supermarket shelves and sold only in pharmacies, after a teenage boy died from an overdose of the drug.' The coroner issued a draft recommendation to this effect, despite the fact that 31 gms of the drug was administered over 14 days to the boy, not at home but while hospitalised following a hip operation, for the purpose of relieving pain. (That is two grams a day, a common enough dosage.)

After four days he developed a fever, and more paracetamol was given to relieve his rising temperature and nausea. He eventually died of end-stage liver failure seventeen days after the operation. It is estimated that as many as 30% of liver transplants occur as a result of paracetamol damage. It really amazes me how many people take it almost like confectionery, and even feed it to their babies. No doubt this teenager had had plenty before reaching the stage of needing his operation (it would not have stopped his condition from worsening), and the trauma of the operation plus the anaesthetic and the extra drug was more than his liver could handle.

A decade later, paracetamol has been found to put people at risk of heart attack.

Still think I make mountains out of molehills?

ANTIDEPRESSANTS

Depression is a huge social problem, and no wonder. There are far too many hopeless, helpless, mystified, worried and frightened people, and this is a direct result of the insidious brainwashing we are fed daily. Noticed? Our TV films and news are full of violence, war, frightening images of destruction, smashing, blasting, gunfire, body image improvers (you are ugly!) and wonderful cars and holidays you will never afford, not to mention the bombardment of political hoo-haa, news and views of horrendous motor accidents, kids' cartoons of evil wizards and terrifyingly realistic space wars events. The media seem to feel obligated to present only the most horrendous images they can find.

On top of this, we are constantly at risk of losing jobs or financial investments, companies going to the wall, family breakups, teenagers getting on to drugs, kids breaking into homes and mugging the elderly, cars stolen and trashed ... enough to depress everyone in the country.

Read the rest of this book and take appropriate action and you will never need to suffer again.

My patients, when trying to unhook themselves from addictive anti-depressants, tell me they make them hyped up, racy, nervous, give heart palpitations and thumping headaches and make them extremely quick-tempered, alternating with great teariness. These are also the withdrawal effects. Thank God, our remedies clear this quickly and solve the problems at their source.

Psychiatrist Dr Andrew Powell[23], former Oxford academic and founder Chair of the Spirituality and Psychiatry Special Interest Group of the Royal

College of Psychiatrists, UK, blames the Newtonian world-view for the current increase in depression.

'Our scientific model of the psyche has no place for the soul; there is nothing before birth and nothing after death. Everything has to be understood as arising from within this temporary, physical existence, with the human self the only source of consciousness. We are all separate beings, bounded by the envelopes of our skin and moving around in a fixed, impersonal, three-dimensional universe utterly indifferent to our comings and goings. Little wonder that depression is the ailment of the modern world. In the first five years of Prozac's coming on to the market, over 10 million prescriptions were handed out.'

Drug companies still work from the old, limited Newtonian physics rather than moving with the times. Science shifted beyond this outlook eighty years ago.

STEROIDS

The most commonly used steroids are the cortisone-like drugs such as prednisone and prednisolone, anti-inflammatories used for allergic disorders such as arthritis and skin complaints and to create immune system suppression; and the sex hormones oestrogen and progesterone, used in the various forms of The (contraceptive) Pill and HRT.

From The Essential Guide to Prescription Drugs, we learn that possible risks associated with corticosteroids include altered mood and personality, cataracts, glaucoma, hypertension, osteoporosis, aseptic bone necrosis and increased susceptibility to infections. They are thought to work by *inhibiting the normal defensive functions of lymphocytes and antibodies.* How can anyone believe this is OK, or without destructive effects?

Also, from the same source, possible risks associated with the use of The Pill include serious, life-threatening thromboembolic disorders (e.g. deep vein thrombosis, so don't fly), hypertension, fluid retention, intensification of other problems like migraines, fibrocystic breast changes, accelerated uterine fibroid tumours, drug-induced hepatitis with jaundice, and less commonly, liver tumours.

HRT (Hormone Replacement Therapy) is given to replace oestrogen loss when this occurs from ovarian failure or removal in a young woman, or from menopause, and is used to treat post-menopausal conditions of osteoporosis and genital atrophy. What is ignored is that the whole of the body is producing oestrogen in virtually every cell - it does not just come from the ovaries, otherwise where would men be getting theirs? (All human organisms depend on oestrogen.) It also ignores that 30% of osteoporosis sufferers are men. The problems of low oestrogen have to be addressed at the level of the thyroid gland and most importantly, at the pituitary, which is the master of the endocrines and can replace the hormones of all the endocrine glands below it, given half a chance.

As I was first writing this book, we had just been given The Big HRT Scare. As with almost every drug in widespread use, the adverse effects eventually come to light. Curious that the very conditions found in the US Women's Health Initiative investigation, a ten-year study, to be adverse outcomes of HRT (causing death) were already known years ago from previous research. I wrote the same list of conditions - breast cancer, coronary artery disease, stroke and pulmonary embolism - in 1996 in my Flower Essence Handbook, in describing the essence Wisteria (which deals with fearful compliance with 'authority' figures, or doing as the 'experts' tell you, such as taking HRT).

In one of the trials done, more women than expected stopped taking the drug - two fifths of the starters had opted out by the sixth year. The researchers ruefully noted that if all these women had stayed on the medication, the adverse outcome would have been more pronounced. How nobly compliant of the stayers to hang in and, perhaps, to die for the cause. How much better if killer drugs were never released, and the healing modalities were in vogue instead.

Steroids are synthetic or animal-sourced forms of hormones the body generally produces naturally. Western medicine takes the view that once your body is deficient in its production it will always be so. Not true. It also presumes to know exactly how much hormone to add, which only the body can know, so production becomes even further deranged by forcing the body to accept amounts that are rarely spot on. The result is often that the endocrine glands, particularly the pituitary which is easily deranged by bodily indignation at forceful things done to you, get into a state of numbness and apathy and begin to go on strike. You will read later how the pituitary responds very rapidly to the friendly energy of Staphisagria, which leads to normalisation of all the endocrines and steroids can be avoided, reduced or discontinued; and also how we normalise bone calcium levels, ease off menopausal effects, regulate thyroid and a host of other hormone benefits.

And did you know that the form of oestrogen most commonly supplied comes from the urine of pregnant mares, who are kept in tiny stalls day and night without exercise so their urine can be collected easily? How healthy can this product be? And how does a waste product of a horse come to belong in a human body?

Possible risks of hormone (oestrogen) replacement therapy include increased risk of uterine cancer in as little as three years use, increased risk of breast cancer even if combined with progesterone, increased frequency of gallstones, accelerated growth of uterine fibroid tumours, fluid retention, post-menopausal bleeding, deep vein thrombophlebitis and thrombo-embolism, increased blood pressure and decreased sugar tolerance, with increased likelihood of Candida infections[24].

DEBUNKING SOME COMMON MYTHS

SCIENCE AND SPIRITUALITY CAN'T MIX?

Since the beginning of time the priests were the holders and teachers of all knowledge. Science, mathematics, medicine, music, astronomy and theology were all known to the priesthood of the earlier civilisations and their secrets were carefully protected from the unwise and the uninitiated. Knowledge and insights into the healing powers of Nature were gained through meditation and intuition, and the priests were reverentially respected and bowed to by the common man, as doctors are today.

Habits die hard, this worship of knowledge not available to the uninitiated has been deeply ingrained into our culture for thousands of years, though few doctors go beyond their arrogant intellects to find truth, these days. They have sold out to ego and materialism, and the ancient skills taught to the early priestly initiates have been all but lost.

There was no separation between knowledge (science) and spiritual truths until the philosopher René Descartes, in the seventeenth century, declared body and soul to be separate entities totally unrelated to each other. This notion was taken up by Isaac Newton, whose discoveries laid the foundation of a mechanical universe where time is absolute and space is structured according to the laws of motion. Medical 'science', henceforth, has always seen the body's functions and development as being separate from the soul of man.

Science and Medicine even developed the belief that there is no such thing as a soul, which then created the mighty rift between science and theology that we saw throughout the twentieth century. Knowledge of how the 'miracles' of early Christianity happened, once taught in the Mystery Schools, had been suppressed long ago by the Church of Rome, in favour of keeping the populace awe-inspired but ignorant, and with the loss of science from the Church, such spiritual understandings of the laws of physics have waited until more recently to be rediscovered.

With every year that passes, more and more research into the microcosm of the human body and into the mind is proving its spiritual nature. Science and spiritual knowledge are merging again, as they must. Truth cannot be antipathetic to truth. Both medical science and Christianity are undergoing cataclysmic revolutions, and not before time.

DRUG RESEARCH MONEY IS USED FOR HUMANITY?

The popular belief is that the medical profession and drug companies in particular, are spending all that wonderful money we hear about on research into diseases that are rampant in the world. Fact is, they have given up on trying to find drugs for diseases like malaria and tuberculosis, so prevalent in third world countries, where five billion of the world's six billion people live. It is simply not profitable enough, the poor cannot pay the premium costs levied against the richer countries. These diseases, once thought defeated or at least controlled, are back with a vengeance and have developed resistance to the drugs once thought to have vanquished them.

One drug research centre alone has more than 600,000 natural product samples in its library in Melbourne, housing extracts of plant, microbial and marine macro-organism samples. The plants are discovered by global positioning satellite trackers that pinpoint their locations in various parts of Australia, New Guinea and Borneo. Once each plant is collected, it is crushed and mixed with organic solvents to produce extracts containing the compounds present in the raw tissue, much the same way as a herbal extract is prepared.

From here, the scientists have no way of determining whether they are going to find a new, magical compound from which to create a new drug, except by doing literally millions of screenings and random testings of various components of the plants. There is no attempt to discover what the whole plant can offer - plants cannot be patented, so only the products made or synthesised from one or a few components can be considered profitable.

Millions have been spent on all the wonderful technology and computerisation of this laboratory - to discover less than homeopaths could discover at virtually no cost, with only a handful of volunteers working on each plant extract over quite a relatively short time, with a resultant very inexpensive medication (see Chapter 4). Keep your hands in your pockets or look carefully, next time you feel urged to contribute to drug research.

In order to establish itself as a necessary and valuable part of society, the medical profession has seriously exaggerated what it can do, pushing the 'miracle' cures and sophisticated gadgetry which cost more and more to achieve less and less. There is no doubt that medical technology is awesome - but the knowledge of what to do with the findings is still pre-historic.

People are now also seeking drug treatment for all the emotional problems of their lives, as if medical drugs are going to solve their family relationships, addictions, bad temper, kids' behaviour and learning difficulties and lots more. Whether it is absenteeism, self-harm, mood disorders or sheer panic, there is usually a medication out there to deal with the condition, to keep you in your slot. (There *are* answers for these, but they lie in the direction of getting to the causes rather than drugging the results.)

New Australian research has raised some concerns regarding drug companies and scientific research. The Medical Journal of Australia published a report which indicates that both researchers and GPs are influenced in their clinical decisions by their (financial) relationships with drug companies. A man came to see me once, whose best mate worked for a drug company as a travelling sales rep. This friend had been to a seminar put on by the company to educate doctors and sales reps. In the course of the seminar, the young man nearly fell off his chair when the speaker announced, 'Whenever you get patients whose diagnosis is unclear, always tell them they have cancer, because we'll give you $x for every patient you put on this drug.'

HOSPITALS ARE SAFE, YOU ARE IN GOOD HANDS?

In the western world, we find that staphylococcus strains are resistant to antibiotics. In the 1990s, between 100,000 and 150,000 people died of infections they contracted in US hospitals. The same happens in Australia. So much for modern hygiene and sterility methods - they strengthen the bugs and weaken our immunity. Our hospitals are hotbeds of infection, and staphylococcus kills, frequently.

A senior professor of surgery in England recently came out with his assessment that half the operations for breast cancer were a complete waste of time[25] (and that coming from a conservative country where the hysterectomy rate is only one tenth per capita of that in Australia). A long-standing statistic has been the acknowledgment that rates of operation - in any western society and for a wide range of conditions - vary only according to how many surgeons are living and working locally. They have little relationship to the actual prevalence of particular diseases, or the success of the surgical procedures.

WE WILL ALWAYS NEED SURGERY?

Of course, some will have a need for skilled surgeons for some time to come. Surgery and medicine are quite separate fields. Homeopathy is a good complement to surgery, having such excellent, normalising trauma remedies. All we lack is an anaesthetic, which plants, hypnosis and acupuncture can supply. Homeopathic remedies allay fear, prevent and treat shock, speed up recovery after anaesthetic, resolve pain (without the hallucinations of morphine), prevent complications, prevent and treat infections, prevent scarring and adhesions and heal cuts, prevent and treat haemorrhage and generally make surgery less hazardous than with drug therapy.

The more important point, though, is that much surgery can be avoided if the healing remedies are employed before you get beyond the point of no return. Vast numbers of operations would not eventuate, and do not eventuate, where conditions are treated homeopathically and the organs or tissues are stimulated to heal themselves.

Many people are panicking in Australia at present because there is an increasingly long waiting list for elective surgery for public patients, historically those least able to afford to pay their own way. Our public hospital system is so overloaded because no attempt is ever made to heal problems before they get to requiring surgery. It is a case of 'Take these drugs until you are bad enough to be operated on, then we'll cut the whole problem out. Too bad if it is an organ you cannot live without, but perhaps you may get a transplant.'

If this is your case, seek true healing, do not sit back and wait for your surgeon-god to put you on his sacrificial slab. There is so much offering in the healing professions. Sure, it will cost you, but only in terms of a few consultations, no cost to your body.

If there is one kind of surgery above all others that is a gross offense against the patient, it is the currently worshipped organ transplant surgery. True, there are some people walking around who are happy to have been given someone else's organ. But the day will come when it will fade out of fashion as did almost every other medical and surgical practice of the past. Most transplant recipients are people who have been reduced to their unenviable state through drug poisoning and the failure of medicine to resolve fears, guilts and griefs. They must be kept on immunosuppressant drugs forever more, destroying their liver, because if they regain an efficient immune system, the transplanted organ is rejected. It is a Catch-22 situation, buying time without quality of life. Harvesting of spare parts is a really sick social attitude problem that has grown out of failure and ignorance.

If you are on the wrong track, the further you continue down that track, the denser the jungle of ignorance becomes. Try climbing a tall tree, to get a perspective of how far you have come from that clear, straight track over in the distance, then head for it, however hard the journey.

BLOOD TESTS REVEAL ALL - WE NEED BLOOD TESTS FOR DIAGNOSIS?

Do we? If you are dependent on the logical brain that can only deduce from what it can see, perhaps yes. If you open up your mind to other ways of knowing that defy logic, you may find that there are many skilled practitioners around who can heal you without ever knowing the name of the bug associated with your problem.

Indicators in the blood are often misunderstood. For example, it used to be the case that when an antigen for say, rubella, was found in the blood, it meant that the patient had previously been exposed to that disease and had gained immunity. It often seems, today, to be a good sign that this person is in need of a rubella immunisation injection.

This kind of misrepresentation is really common with many viruses and bacteria. Is it deliberate? Or have they really lost the plot?

Blood tests of any kind are only of limited value. They are like looking at several disjointed pieces of a jigsaw. Even when you line them up it is not possible to see the complete picture. Recognise that the results are only as good as the tests so far devised, particularly for function tests like thyroid and liver, which are only partially indicative. There are around 500 functions of the liver, tests only deal with around ten of these. My point is, there is often no guarantee that what is found has any relationship to the symptoms you are suffering.

Remember also, that only those tests requested by your doctor are done in the laboratory. They are unlikely to do more than confirm or deny his ideas, and further tests must often be done, time and again, until a correlation is found.

Also, you have to know that test results vary according to which type of equipment is in use at your pathology lab. Even within the one lab, doctors know to allow for inaccuracy in the equipment and for human error.

I have a friend who has seen fit to put his life totally in the hands of the learned pathologists, and refers to their department as the Vampire Pit. He is right on the mark there. Blood banks, blood taking for tests, transfusions are all evidence of the 'blood-sucking' mentality of the drug companies, draining every last ounce out of the communal coffers. Blood is a commodity like beer and petrol, no longer sacred.

People conform to this idea as a way of life because they have lost (through indoctrination) the understanding that they are worth better than this, there are other ways of getting help, other alternatives to transfusions, toxic drugs and frequent skin stabbing. They suppress their own innate self-preservation instincts and conform to the fear-mongering, bullied into accepting that it is all OK and the best thing to do, and 'you'll be in big trouble if you don't'. Inappropriate loyalty dominates.

The Vampire Pit is another fad that will fade out of fashion as time goes on, once you all begin to take a stand against stabbing, which you will, after you read about Hypericum, Ledum and Staphisagria, and against taking drugs that are so poisonous that their levels in the blood have to be monitored every week, lest you succumb. What happened to 'Safety First,' and 'First, do no harm?'

THE CHOLESTEROL BOGEY

The popular misconception is that high cholesterol in blood tests is a sign of high cholesterol buildup in and on the blood vessel walls, and that this is the result of eating a high fat diet. Wrong on both counts. It is not possible to make an accurate assessment of the state of one's arteries unless you are a kinesiologist, iridologist, clairvoyant or have an angiogram or surgery. If you have a blood test that shows a high cholesterol reading, how do you know that your bloodvessel walls are not in the process of reducing excess cholesterol buildup, thus the blood is containing more cholesterol than usual and carrying it out of the body?

Your body is not static, a test done on one tiny amount of blood at any one time does not always reflect what is constant. The same applies to sugar levels, blood pressure, hormone levels, mineral content, lipids, vitamins and many other components. They vary constantly, to one degree or another. Added to that, there is the recognised 15% inaccuracy in the diagnostic equipment. Don't stress out over test results, stress is the most powerful disturber of all these levels. Blood tests themselves cause shock, and shock can kill. Instead, recognise that while reducing your intake of fats from meat sources will lower your cholesterol levels, it was not the eating of these fats that gave you the build-up in the first place. Fats are not cholesterol and no foods contain cholesterol or can be called high or low cholesterol foods. They simply contain saturated, unsaturated or neutral lipids.

Eskimos living a relatively stress-free existence live on whale blubber and whale meat, very high in saturated fats, yet they are well known to be free of cholesterol build-up in their blood vessels. Stresses like racing against the clock, whatever the job, or emotional stresses of fear of reprimand, guilt and over-responsibility are the reason why the liver fails to break down excess cholesterol in the bloodstream. When you fail to adjust to the stress situation, the Kuppfer cells in the liver, the wonderful little macrophages that break down and cleanse the excesses out of the blood, are prevented, through continuing overload stress, from working as efficiently as they ought for the levels to be balanced out again. The blood then tries to offload the excess on to the larger blood vessel walls in order to protect your brain, lungs and heart from blockages in the finer blood vessels in these organs.

Cholesterol is an essential part of all cell membranes and half the dry weight of your brain is cholesterol. Now think about whether you need to reduce it or not! New research[26] reveals that your brain makes cholesterol. Specialised brain cells called glial cells make it. Cholesterol appears to have a role in regulating where and when brain cells connect or synapse. If the brain makes it, and needs it, considering the millions of nerve synapses that occur each day, we cannot think of it as an enemy that must be fought. Instead, de-stress!

Low cholesterol has been linked to suicide, increased deaths from all causes (including cancer) and physical and mental problems. In fact, studies indicate that certain age groups (such as the elderly) benefit from high cholesterol.

The two forms of cholesterol, HDL (high density lipoprotein) and LDL (low density lipoprotein), are the goodies and baddies. HDL has now been found to reduce LDL in the bloodstream after a heart attack. Furthermore, Professor John Kastelein, chairman of Genetics of Cardiovascular Disease at the University of Amsterdam, has done research that demonstrates that raising cholesterol can help the heart, providing that the cholesterol in question is HDL, and that the protective effects of HDL are as significant a part of the heart disease story as the adverse effects of LDL. It's all a matter of balance.

We might mention statins here, too. These are the range of 'wonder drugs' developed to reduce cholesterol. In Australia the most popular one is Lipitor. I had a man come to me once who had been confounding the medicos with his recurring, transient dizzy spells and blackouts, severe enough that he had lost his driving license. MRIs had found that his brain was full of small mystery spots that looked like tumours. There was no possibility of operating, and no drug for this problem. I conducted the interview as usual, getting all possible information about his history, his food likes and dislikes, climate preferences, standard stuff. Then I asked about medications. 'I've been on Lipitor for 25 years.' I opened my computer and Googled Lipitor, and began to read him all the many adverse effects people had experienced from taking Lipitor. He went pale, then aghast, and after five minutes, begged 'Don't read me any more!' I asked him for a Lipitor tablet and made it up to a 10M potency, the best strength, I find, for antidoting any toxic substance with itself (for what it causes, it can cure, if used in micro-dose). Over the next few months, the fainting turns reduced greatly; and after another year he was on the road, driving his camper-converted truck around Australia with his wife.

UV SUNTAN LOTIONS PROTECT AGAINST SKIN CANCER?

Another great hoax perpetrated against the populations of the world by drug companies is the myth that ultra-violet light from the sun is the cause of skin cancers. Susceptibility is the only reason that some get these cancers and others don't, and the reason for susceptibility is the breakdown of the immune system, which is the greatest scourge of our times and which is a direct result of medical drugs and chemical toxicity in the environment. To imagine that the sun, without which we die, is also an enemy from which we must hide, is the greatest delusion of all time. But there is big money in 'health' pharmaceuticals. Really, this era we live in is going to be laughed at mercilessly in times to come.

Here is some recent research into suntan lotions: A chemical used in 90% of suntan lotions worldwide might be toxic, according to new research by a team of Norwegian scientists. And exposure to the sun could make the UV filter octyl methoxycinnamate (OMC) even more deadly, according to a report published in New Scientist magazine.[27] Tests conducted by the Norwegian Radiation Protection Authority found that half of mouse cells died when they came into contact with a weak dose of OMC, at a much lower concentration than is found in most of the world's sunscreens. Shining a lamp on the OMC-impregnated cells to simulate sunshine made the chemical twice as deadly. NRPA biophysicist Terji Christensen warned sunbathers to use sunscreens with caution.

Quantum mechanics has an answer that may explain why UV light is becoming more of a problem. It relates to the perception that time is speeding up, flying faster than it used to. Time is relative to gravity - the stronger the gravity, the slower the time, and vice versa. Light also changes relative to gravity. A glowing object changes in colour (as perceived by an observer) according to the gravitational power of its environment, becoming red as the gravity increases, or blue as gravity is reduced. Indeed, anything that vibrates changes in the frequency of that vibration when placed in a different gravitational field.

The conclusion to be drawn from these known facts of physics is that time is speeding up because our gravitational field is lessening. A minute, an hour, a day no longer have the same length as they used to. Time is flying faster and faster - only yesterday it was Christmas, now it is mid-year. Our clocks are still measuring as they used to, it seems, the only thing that can have changed is gravity, for when gravity changes, the measuring of time-clocks also changes. Is the planet moving faster around the sun? And is our shift to greater UV light a result of this lowering of gravity, perhaps, as well as a breaking down of the ozone layer? For skin cancer is occurring in many places not close to the holes in the ozone layer.

THE BODY CAN HANDLE ANYTHING I PUT INTO IT?

No way. Life is all about processing - our brains process information, our bodies process nutrients. All life-forms depend on the minerals of the earth, but only plants have the ability to transform those minerals into forms suitable for animal and human nutrition. They do this via photosynthesis, the use of sunlight and water to process minerals into what, nowadays, we call 'organic' form, containing amino acids, carbohydrates, also vitamins, enzymes, hormones and other phytochemicals. These mineral-rich plants are then used by all other forms of life; first-hand by vegetarians, second-hand by those who eat the vegetarians, third-hand by those who eat the carnivores.

The further you get away from plant nutrition, the less the quality of food you consume. Plants contain everything the human body needs from the soil, including clean water. Only clean air and sunlight need be added and you have the four primary, essential elements of life, Earth, Water, Air and Fire.

You will notice that the world's strongest animals - elephants, rhinos, horses, camels, oxen - are all vegetarians. They are not only strong, but have great stamina and lasting power. The carnivorous animals such as the cat and dog families may appear strong to us but depend on their patience and their sprinting speed for their kills. Their stamina is not sufficient to be able to outrun vegetarians that manage to keep in front for a couple of hundred yards. This is the only reason they manage to catch the old, the infirm and the young. They are also useless as pack animals, having no carrying strength.

We have, by design and programming since the dawn of human life, used plants for all our nutrition, be it for food or medicine. When we eat meat it is second-hand plant food, but still containing most of the important plant nutrients (but no fibre). But - when we create medicines and foods out of chemicals that have not been through the plant-processing conversions, we are putting into our bodies substances for which we have no satisfactory methods for processing and elimination. The more you introduce non-plant chemicals, the more confused and congested the body becomes.

Man's natural intelligence has enabled him, through the ages, to choose what is needed from the bounteous table of nature, for both food and medicine. Of course, not all plants can be used for food or for medicine. Some are highly toxic, some are indigestible, some, like soya bean, need fermenting - predigesting - before they can be acceptable, as they are difficult for the liver to handle. (You do not see the Chinese, who have used soya beans for thousands of years, eating them unfermented. They are smart enough to process the beans into bean curd and soy sauce.)

Thanks to greed and loss of sight of the truths of nature, we face an epidemic of man-made disease that is getting out of hand. Modern medicine is manufactured chemicals, processed largely from petrochemical sources that have not seen the light of day, that have lain buried in the bowels of the earth, way beyond the reach of plant roots, for millions of years.

Where is the life-force in that? Only one of the four essential elements of life is present - Earth. The plants that eventually became the crude oil lost their lives long, long ago.

Death begets death, life begets life. You don't need an Oxford degree to understand that.

MAN-MADE DIABETES

Diabetes Type 2 is now one of the greatest killers in the western world, and is often associated with heart disease, capillary and arteriole shrinkage, kidney degeneration, nerve damage, ulcers and gangrene and a host of drug toxicity effects.

But why have diabetes Type 2? There is no need for it. It is not a genetically determined disease (as Type 1 sometimes is), but is, purely and simply, a condition of nutritional imbalance - a self-created kind of malnutrition. Yet, 90% of these people are obese. In the midst of plenty, you may still be starving.

The problem arises out of poor blood glucose control. Glucose is the form of sugar preferred by the body. It is created from the metabolic breakdown of lipids, proteins and complex carbohydrates and natural sugars such as the fructose and levulose in honey and fruits. Glucose is acted upon rapidly by insulin to enable it to enter the cells of almost all tissues of the body as energy;

it is converted into storage forms such as glycogen and fat and brought back into the bloodstream as glucose at frequent intervals, as the brain and body demand energy. Poor blood glucose control is the inevitable result when excessive sucrose from super-refined white sugar floods the metabolism. There is simply not enough insulin available in the pancreas to deal with the oversupply of sucrose that is maintained and perpetuated over years.

This is something that every individual can do something to cure, it is not a medical industry problem but a personal responsibility problem. But billions of dollars are being extorted out of governments and individuals, without giving any hope of cure, and despite the knowledge that you could help yourself if told how, if told about the destructive nature of sugar as sucrose. All you need do is take charge of what is going into your mouth.

The sugar industry grew out of Britain's and Europe's competition for dominance of trade in the seventeenth century. While sugar had been known in older times, the refining processes were comparatively primitive and sucrose remained in combination with many of the great nutrients found in the sugar cane, or in the sugar beet, and was a relatively expensive item. But even in 1670 Thomas Willis, physician to King Charles II of England, commented on the direct correlation between the increase of diabetes among his wealthy patrons and his employer's growing wealth from the sugar trade.

Since those days, refinement has become virtually absolute, the white crystals we think of as sugar are now a non-nutrient that the human body must metabolise into glucose and convert into fat; a toxic, foreign chemical which, like all non-nutrient substances, places a strain on the body's homeostasis processes. You only need look into the rich mineral content of molasses to see what has been removed from the refined, white, crystallised pure sucrose offered to you today. Farmers know the great nutritional value of molasses to their stock. They feed their animals better than most people do their families. In the body, the mineral-free sucrose retains an affinity with those minerals it used to be associated with in the cane, and draws them to itself. Calcium is leached from your teeth, bones and muscles and excreted from the body because of this. Similarly, other minerals are lost, leaving you suffering malnutrition, a deficiency problem, which creates a craving for more food to (hopefully) supply the missing ingredients.

Greed for wealth having initiated the sugar trade, greed in the form of gluttony resulting from sugar addiction finally created a giant opportunity for drug companies. Dr Frederick Banting, joint Nobel Prize Winner in 1923 for discovering and researching insulin, said in 1929, 'In the heating and re-crystallisation of the natural sugar cane, something is altered which leaves the refined product a dangerous foodstuff.' However, greed takes precedence over common sense, and instead of promoting harmless alternatives to sugar refining in order to protect the world's population from this diabetes-causing toxicity, the great philanthropy of the already wealthy drug companies turned to meeting the world's demands for more and more insulin, and food manufacturers found more and more ways of getting you addicted to sugar. So many people make money from the sugar industry that it seems much better logic, to them, to create drug treatments to antidote, if possible, the effects.

According to Patrick Quillan Ph.D., RD, CNS[28], in his self-help booklet *The Diabetes Improvement Program*, a researcher named Dr O'Dea, in Australia, wondered if the modern, refined diet of many aborigines living in Sydney could be causing diabetes. She recruited ten full-blood male aborigines with Type 2 diabetes and asked them to return to the hunter-gatherer diet of their (recent) ancestors. All ten were middle-aged and overweight.

Seven weeks after beginning their ancestral diet, all ten men had lost an average of sixteen pounds in spite of making no conscious effort to lose weight, all had experienced a 50% drop in blood lipids (lowering their heart disease risk) and all had such splendid improvement in fasting blood glucose levels that they were considered cured of Type 2 diabetes.

When people with sugar toxicity problems, even when the only evidence is obesity, put themselves on to low glycemic index foods (foods high in soluble fibres such as fresh vegetables and fruits), low animal fats and unrefined carbohydrates, they achieve benefits far beyond their expectations. Blood sugar levels even out, blood pressure normalises, blood fat levels are lowered, weight normalises, sleep normalises, mood swings and depression lift and energy and wellbeing soar.

Alternatively, the drugs used in Type 2 diabetes can, according to a huge study done by a University Group Diabetes Program[29], elevate the risk of death from heart attack or stroke by 250%. If you buy into this, if you seek drug resolution for your Type 2 diabetes, you are being played once again for the great sucker they think you are. Wake up before they kill you.

OPIUM FOR TEA

The trade in opium, heroin and morphine was begun by the British in India as a way of balancing trade - Indian opium was sold to China as payment for tea, in the 1840s, thus setting off the growth of Chinese opium addiction. British trade was dominated since the time of Napoleon by Rothschild and his Bank of England, which was then, as now, financing and profiting from the production of arms, drugs and the bomb. (Rothschild financed both sides, the English and French during the Napoleonic wars, as well as the slave trade to sugar plantations in the Caribbean.)

Until the 1950s, heroin, a synthetic derivative of morphine, the principal alkaloid in opium, was the gynaecologists' painkiller of choice in major maternity wards in Australia. In 1953, the use of heroin was banned in medicine and morphine, a less rapid painkiller but less toxic to respiration, took over. Both are destructive, and many cancer patients die with the discomforts of morphine poisoning. They are led to believe their suffering is caused by the cancer alone.

Morphine affects the central nervous system in both excitatory and depressive ways. It depresses respiration, causing death by respiratory failure; it is analgesic, which endears it to those who are not averse to risking killing to be 'kind' (some anaesthetists give it routinely so you do not come back to consciousness feeling pain - too bad if it makes you hallucinate for days); it stimulates the spinal cord to convulsions; it stimulates the vomiting centre causing acute nausea and gastric discomfort; intravenous doses produce a fall in blood pressure that lasts for several hours, owing to its causing a release of histamine from the skin and muscles, making it contraindicated in asthmatics; it frequently causes constipation by inducing spasticity of the intestinal walls; and it produces a euphoric state that becomes an addiction that is very difficult to treat - the euphoria, by temporarily overriding awareness of the physical effects, is sought again once this override wears off.

Morphine produces both sneezing and itching of the nose. Coma, pin-point pupils and slow, snoring breathing with long pauses between breaths or death-rattle breathing suggest morphine poisoning. It is mainly stored in the skeletal muscles, although some is excreted by the bowel if that is working. Our homeopathic materia medica detail the toxic effects quite clearly.

What doctors do not tell you is that there are a number of homeopathic remedies that minimise the pain of end-stage cancer, harmlessly, enabling these sufferers to get their affairs in order and reach their end calmly and philosophically. Ignorance is only a partial excuse. Thinking people in the healthcare professions need to know that harmless, unaggressive methods are preferable and are available to be learned.

Is it just coincidence that America's and Australia's military presence in Afghanistan has been so protracted, given that this country is the world's largest grower of opium poppy? And why is it that over the first decade of the 21st century, the use of morphine in Australian hospitals has risen to the point of being the first pain-killer to be offered, to everyone, regardless of the condition suffered, and that everyone over 90 who goes to hospital is put on morphine until death do us part?

IT CAN'T BE ALL BAD?

I have detailed only a few of the many ways that medicine and industry have gone off the track. But if you are still under the impression that pharmaceutical medicine has your best interests at heart (heart?), read on.

The Sydney Morning Herald on February 13, 2001 ran a front page article called The Drug Body Snatchers, in which it claimed that 'Thousands of

Australian patients are being used as guineapigs in drug trials for global pharmaceutical companies without explicit laws to adequately protect their rights. Intellectually disabled men and women, incapable of giving consent on their own behalf, are being used in the trials, which are aimed at getting new drugs to the United States and European markets.

'Pharmaceutical companies are paying private doctors up to $6,000 for every patient they recruit but the patients do not have to be told of the financial arrangements. Some trials are abandoned after reports of side effects and deaths, either here or overseas, or because the drug simply does not work.'

A Herald investigation found that patients are being bought and sold like commodities by doctors and pharmaceutical companies, but are not being told that money changes hands when they volunteer for new treatments.

This information was commented upon with regret by three Australian medical professors. Associate Professor Paul Komesaroff, chairman of the ethics committee of the Royal Australian College of Physicians, said: 'In many cases the industry sponsored trial doesn't have a valid scientific intention. It is eroding research that is truly innovative in favour of research that satisfies commercial purposes.'

Many clinics that treat diseases of epidemic proportions such as STD/HIV claim they could not survive without drug company money. But does this justify using such clinics for trialling possibly dangerous, unknown treatments? (They could survive if they employed homeopathic treatments.)

On the same lines, in the SMH of July 15, 2002, we read the article by Malcolm Brown called 'Doctors ready to test drugs on aged'. 'The medical profession feels that the elderly should have more opportunity to take part in clinical trials', says an expert in legal issues for the aged, ... 'if they are capable of informed consent,' according to Professor Carolyn Sappideen, Director of the Centre for Elder Law at the University of Western Sydney. Professor Sappideen agreed that a powerful argument remained that the elderly were still vulnerable as a group and could be perceived as bearing the burden of drug testing for the benefit of younger people.

The key word here is vulnerable, meaning woundable, able to be damaged or hurt. And the truth still remains, that the trialling of any chemicals on the general public, with or without consent, is fraught with vulnerability no matter what your age, and will, one day, be seen to be what it is, a criminal offense against mankind. It is quite unnecessary when you use homeopathy and test new remedies on healthy volunteers, according to homeopathic principles.

PESTICIDES

We know how the world is writhing from the onslaughts of chemical pest control, against whose toxicity modern, wonderful medicine knows no answers. The WHO claims 3 million people are poisoned by pesticides every year, of which 200,000 cases are fatal. Guy Murchie[30] gives this simple story to demonstrate the chain of events they can produce.

'Even the World Health Organisation botched its well-intentioned effort to control malaria in Borneo by spraying native villages with poisonous DDT before its effects were fully understood. Although the malarial mosquitoes were eliminated on schedule, roaches and caterpillars in the houses absorbed the poison, passing it on to small lizards feeding on them, whose nerves were impaired, reducing their agility so much that not one of them escaped being caught and eaten by cats. But cats are very susceptible to DDT and they all soon died, permitting forest rats to move into the houses, carrying with them fleas infected by bubonic plague. As if that were not enough, the roofs of the houses started falling in because the thatch was being devoured by the caterpillars that were no longer being kept in check by lizards.

'So it should not surprise anyone that no native Bornean could think of any convincing objection when a gathering of local witch doctors was seen making incantations to summon back: good old malaria!'

Pesticides and herbicides are causing increasing numbers of deaths from toxic overload destruction diseases like systemic lupus erythematosis. I agree - give me malaria, any day - much easier to fix.

RECYCLING?

Our local community was once encouraged via radio and newspaper to take their left-over drugs back to the chemists for 'disposal', as they would poison the waterways if thrown down the sink or toilet.

I rest my case.

CHAPTER 4

There is nothing too little for so little a creature as man. It is by studying little things that
we attain the great art of having as little misery and as much happiness as possible.

- Samuel Johnson

THE ART AND SCIENCE OF HOMEOPATHY

Medicine is an art. Physicians and other artists are born, not made. The greatest healers of all times from Hippocrates and Celsus to Hahnemann, Mesmer, Priessnitz, Kneipp, Kellgren, Coué and Sir Herbert Barker were self-taught, and many of them were laymen, keenly interested in the art of healing. In all the arts and sciences, outsiders have been pioneers. The schools produce chiefly mediocrities; Cromwell, England's greatest soldier, was a farmer, and Ulysses Grant, America's greatest soldier, was a shopman. Leeuwenhoek, who discovered the micro-organisms of disease, was a draper; and Pasteur, who created modern medicine, was a chemist. England's greatest medical men, Harvey, Sydenham and John Hunter, were treated as quacks by their orthodox contemporaries.[31]

Samuel Christian Hahnemann, founder of Homeopathy, was one of these radicals. A child prodigy, he graduated from Salzburg University at the age of sixteen, having mastered six languages, chemistry, physics, theology and medicine. His early experience as a medical practitioner was disillusioning - he watched helplessly as the favoured medicines of the day were unable to relieve or cure, and in some cases actually killed his patients. Unable to practice with this amount of ignorance, he gave up medicine and began to provide for his family by translating medical books from other languages into German. While doing this, he stumbled upon an assertion he felt was inherently incorrect, by Professor Cullen, of London. He decided to test the accuracy of the assertion by trialling the medicine in question, cinchona bark, on himself, and thus discovered the law of nature he came to call the Law of Similars.

Hahnemann's discovery, first published in 1810, caught the interest of numerous physicians of the day, but it also incurred the wrath of many others, and also the apothecaries, who felt threatened by Hahnemann's discoveries that drugs worked much better in micro-doses. Fearing that their very profession was at stake, they guiltily forced Hahnemann to leave his homeland and he spent the next fifty years or more in Paris, where his body lies buried. Notwithstanding this opposition, Hahnemann's findings inspired many great minds and his teachings were carried around the globe.

Research scientist Dr Viera Scheibner PhD[32] says 'Modern medicine considers itself scientific. Nothing could be further from the truth. The only scientific medical systems are those which are based on detailed and meticulous observation and knowledge of the human body and which cater to individuality. One does not need expensive and complex diagnostic tools to be able to diagnose the patient's condition and choose the right remedy.

'Without the knowledge of dose-related effects of remedies and without testing these on themselves, the orthodox medical doctors will continue causing more harm than good.

'Hippocrates is all but forgotten. Homeopathy, based on the intimate knowledge of the human body and the dynamics of health and illness, is the medicine of the twenty-first century. Although developed by Dr Hahnemann some two hundred years ago, it is based on the most modern understanding of the dose effects of remedies and the most modern physics of solutions. It is also based on a most intimate knowledge of health and illness.'

Medicine today stands on the threshold of a deep and radical change that has already begun to be felt by most thinking doctors. Some have taken steps to train in one or another complementary or alternative therapy, while still using drugs. Some have gone further and given up chemical drug prescriptions in favour of lifestyle counselling, dietary healing, acupuncture or hypnotherapy. All too few, in Australia, have ventured into Homeopathy. May their numbers increase!

BASIC PRINCIPLES OF HOMEOPATHY

Before we go any further it is necessary to know exactly what homeopathy is. Have a look at the following definitions and compare them.

HOMEOPATHY From the Greek, *homoios*, similar, like, and *patheia*, disease or suffering.

George Vithoulkas[33], arguably the world's leading contemporary homeopath, defines homeopathy as a system of therapeutics based on the Law of Similars (*Similia Similibus Curentur*, 'Let likes be cured by likes'), i.e. the principle that the cure of disease is effected by a substance known to be capable of producing in a healthy subject, symptoms similar to those of the person to be treated. The dosage is usually minutely small.

Historically, homeopathy belongs to the Empirical school of thought, in that empiricists base their attitudes on the hypothesis that pure observation of the patient is the root of knowledge in medicine. Symptomatology is therefore all-important. Observing the patient fully and also the effects of medicines on people allows knowledge that caters for individuality.

Homeopathy offers a reliable technique for distinguishing disease conditions on a symptomatic basis, since the symptoms which point to the remedy also indicate to the physician the disease suffered, by virtue of the whole dynamic pattern presented by those symptoms. No single symptom has significance by itself but only in the context of its companions, which, collectively, as a pattern, tell the practitioner all he needs to know to be able to stimulate the vital force of the patient towards healing. He has no need to treat symptoms individually.

The Law of Similars has been so reliable and successful that remedies discovered two hundred years ago are still in daily use by homeopaths worldwide for the same conditions or symptom pictures for which they were first used. It makes homeopathy the only truly specific system of medicine in the world.

ALLOPATHY From the Greek, *allos,* other, different, and *patheia,* suffering

Treatment by inducing in the body a reaction opposite or contrary to that which is produced by the disease. This is the way of orthodox medicine today and since the days of Galen, who formulated the concept of the doctrine of contraries. While it may seem logical to say, counter a hot condition with cold, this is not a scientific concept.

Allopathic medicine comes under the category of Rationalist medicine, which denies therapeutic clinical experience and relies fully on information derived only from subsidiary fields in the selection of its prescriptions. Patients are not considered as individuals, because individuals are too variable in the manifestation of their conditions. Logical thinking demands a fixed set of signs for each named disease and indeed, a name for a symptom picture before it can even suggest a prescription.

This idea has led to an absolute plethora of named conditions and an even vaster number of drugs supposed to counteract these conditions.

Nowadays, medicines are divided up into categories that define their aggressive intent: anti-biotics, anti-microbials, anti-histamines, anti-inflammatories, inhibitors and blockers - all intended to force the sufferer's body into a state of quiescence rather than stimulate its self-healing mechanisms. Rationalist, but not really rational.

You can see that the reason medically trained people have so much trouble accepting homeopathy is that it is based on a totally opposite concept to their own, with far-reaching, opposing differences in philosophy and application - needing them to throw out a lot of their university indoctrination.

THE LAW OF SIMILARS

The Law of Similars, as a basic rule of nature, had been noticed and mentioned by many medical writers dating back to Hippocrates, but it was not until the late eighteenth century that the noted German physician Samuel Christian Hahnemann rediscovered this truth and scientifically put it to the test. Years of experimentation on many substances enabled Hahnemann to develop a practicable basis for safe, effective medical practice, which has not since been equalled.

In simple terms, whatever mental, emotional or physical symptoms a substance can cause to a healthy individual can be noted and studied, and this symptom picture can be used as a guide to indicate to us that this substance has the power to cure a similar range of symptoms in a suffering person. When we find such a pattern of symptoms in a sufferer, we can be confident that that substance most similar in what it can produce is the one to use, to treat that range of symptoms.

Fortunately, there are a number of plant and mineral remedies in common use, because they have an ability to produce symptom pictures similar to a wide range of common complaints. There are lots of examples of homeopathic similarity in everyday life. For instance, onions have been used for centuries to ward off the common cold - and what do onions cause? Runny nose, watery eyes, sneezing ... symptoms of the common cold and hay fever. Onion (Allium Cepa) is one of our greatest sniffle remedies.

An old man I knew used to swish his arthritic hands through a clump of nettles whenever they pained, and the nettles cleared the arthritis stinging.

Also homeopathic in action is the use of cowpox to provide immunity to smallpox. Even without using microdoses, cowpox vaccination has been successful in eradicating smallpox from the world, thanks to its similarity.

Drinkers of alcohol all know the benefit of the 'hair of the dog that bit you', when they wake next morning with a hangover. Even a few drops of an alcoholic drink will clear the headache and sharpen up the senses.

We are surrounded daily by instances of homeopathy in action.

PROVINGS

Hahnemann and his followers did many 'provings' of substances in common medical practice at the time, many of them highly toxic. Since then, homeopaths all over the world have expanded the knowledge of remedies to create a vast array of valuable tools for healing.

You can see that only healthy volunteers, not mute animals, can give us accurate details of the subjective and objective effects of the remedies being tested. Different types of people volunteer to be provers, thus the widest range of effects of a remedy can be experienced, some by all provers and others by only a few of them. All homeopathic remedies are proven in this way, and even the symptom experienced by perhaps only one person is included in the documentation. It could be of critical importance to someone searching for an elusive remedy.

THE LAW OF THE INFINITESIMAL DOSE

In his early years of experimentation Hahnemann was aware of the aggravation of disease if a material dose was administered. People were usually made worse before the benefit began to set in. Some patients even died, despite the similar remedy being given, from the toxicity of the medicine - a common event even in those days, and still occurring today from drugs.

In order to eliminate these toxic effects Hahnemann began to dilute the medicines, but he reached a point where there was neither benefit nor harm from the dilutions. For a while this gave him much cause to think. Then one day in a flash of inspiration, he came up with a method of diluting which was able to intensify the beneficial action of the remedy, while reducing the adverse effects.

He hit on the idea to dilute (1 part in 100) and to follow the dilution by sharply banging the bottle of diluted remedy several times on a closed book. He then took one part of that bottle and added to 99 parts of diluent in another bottle and repeated the same succussion process. To his surprise and pleasure, the more he diluted in this way, the more quickly and powerfully the remedy healed and the less were the side effects. He had beaten the problem of the side effects of drugs.

Hahnemann did not know exactly why, but he knew that the dynamic energy of the dilution was greatly increased with each dilution and succussion. Nowadays, thanks to nuclear physics, we know that when such a process occurs, electrons of the drug's molecules are knocked off and attach themselves to molecules of the diluent, thus carrying the pattern of the drug on to the diluent at a subtle vibrational level. By the same process, latent energy is made available, more and more with every dilution/succussion repetition. The effect is somewhat similar to splitting the atom to release the power of the atom bomb. We have to call this 'bio-physics'! Furthermore, the amount of energy

71

released from the molecules (or made available for healing) is directly proportional to the number of potentisations made.

Think about the genius of this man, over two hundred years ago, using nuclear physics long before it was ever thought of, and for the purpose of healing, rather than destroying mankind!

POTENTISING - THE CENTESIMAL SCALE

Hahnemann labelled each of his dilutions with its number followed by the letter C, the Roman numeral for 100. So the first dilution became 1C, the second 2C, and so on: a strength or dilution of 1:100 became 1C, then one hundredth of that bottle into the second bottle containing 100 parts of diluent became 1:10,000 parts of the original diluent, known as 2C (1:100x100). 3C then is 1:1,000,000 or 1:100x100x100 parts of diluent, or $1:10^6$.

You can see that by this time the amount of original substance is getting fairly small - and this is only the third dilution. Imagine how microscopic the amount becomes as you continue to dilute. In fact, by the time you get to 12C ($1:10^{24}$), you have reached and passed Avogadro's number and there is not likely to be found a single molecule of the original substance. Yet the medicine is now far more powerful for healing than the original substance was.

This method applies to liquid medicines. Insoluble substances such as metals are ground with 1:100 parts of sugar of milk with a mortar and pestle, taken this way to the third dilution and then dissolved into alcohol, and the process goes on as described above to whatever potency you wish. In common use are 3C, 6C, 12C (low potencies), 30C, 200C (medium potencies), M (1,000C) and 10M (10,000C) - high potencies.

VERY HIGH POTENCIES (MEGAPOTENCIES)

Since Hahnemann's time, many homoeopaths have taken the Centesimal dilutions way beyond the 200th, with ever-deeper, longer lasting benefits from just a single dose, and without aggravation of the existing symptoms. It is at the level of these highest potencies that you see the most amazing miracles in deep-seated problems, in rapid time, often overnight. I like miracles.

Imagine now how the mathematics looks if I tell you that I commonly use potencies of MM, or 1,000,000 dilutions of 1:100. This book is about my use of CM (100,000C), MM and 10MM(10,000,000C) potencies. I also see a lot of permanent physical benefits from 50M (50,000C) and lovely emotional benefits from 20M (20,000C).

I am not alone in this. For well over a hundred years, practitioners have been trying very high potencies with excellent results. It has been the manufacturers who have made it a somewhat restricted practice, the

72

potencies are so time-consuming to make by hand.

Dr Dorothy Shepherd[34] wrote of her conversion, very early in her career, to very high potencies, her first experience being with a CM potency. Her comments were, 'I find that high potencies go deeper and act longer; that is, they act for longer periods and they powerfully stir up the constitution and make a vital difference in the character, temperament and mental make-up of the respective patients. But a word of warning is not out of place here. Let me impress upon lay people that 'high potencies' are not for them to play with. A knowledge of metaphysics, mental philosophy and logic is necessary before one can hope, even humbly, to understand their action from a distance. Let each man stick to his own lasts; the study of medicine and still more, the study of homeopathy is a whole-time and life-long occupation.'

A great deal of ignorance is taught to students about the so-called dangers of high potencies. This is the main reason why homeopathy is still struggling to be acknowledged in Australia. The American homeopath, J. T. Kent's influence in teaching the lovely benefits of very high potencies is the main reason for the success of so many earlier practitioners, both in the US and in the United Kingdom.

Prior to the use of the megapotencies, the original Foreword to CMF von Bonninghausen's Repertory (1846)[34] states, 'Several practical physicians of the highest order have found by a number of the most careful experiments, that not only do the high dynamisations, far from being inefficacious, continue to operate with a force sufficient to cure any kind of disease, but that also the totality of the power of the medicines and the extent of their peculiarities develop themselves by this means in a more perfect manner, and that very often a disease is cured with high dynamisations which had been attacked in vain with the lower dilutions of the same remedy.

'Convinced of the truth of this important discovery, I have used for two years those high dynamisations, the results of which were so satisfactory, that during the last year I have scarcely given any other: since this time my practice, always a successful one, has become still more so, and all those who have taken my advice are enthusiastic in their approbation of this progress.'

He goes on to say, 'It is in the diseases of the skin, of the glands and of the bones that I have observed the most surprising effects from dynamisations of the highest degree and my journals contain a great many perfect cures, particularly of those kinds of diseases, which had, for a long time, resisted the larger and often repeated doses of the same remedy.'

If we are to overcome the deepseated beliefs and attitudes we are describing in this book, it is necessary to use these remedies in very, very high - mega - potencies.

THE DECIMAL RANGE

At some point in history, other practitioners began to use a Decimal scale (1:10) of dilutions, known as the X or D scale, now in common use in Europe. It is not customary to use these potencies beyond 30X, and they are mainly used as potencies below 15X in Australia and England.

THE LM OR 50 MILLESIMAL POTENCIES

Hahnemann only ever diluted/succussed his remedies up to the 200C potency. At this level he found that once again, people were getting to feel worse before they got better. The healing was much more rapid than with the very low potencies, but the aggravations were sometimes very uncomfortable, and sometimes lasted for several days. Nowadays, we recognize that 200C is a potency likely to aggravate some people, with some remedies.

Late in his life, in an effort to prevent these aggravations, instead of potentising to higher levels on the 1:100 scale of dilution, Hahnemann decided to water down the second dilution to 1:50,000 (1 ml in 50 litres). He found that with succussion, this gave a smooth remedy that could be repeated for many months without aggravation, and he developed the 1:50,000 dilution/succussion process up to the 30th potency, which is known as 30LM or O/30. Mathematically, these are very highly attenuated potencies, yet are sometimes thought of as low.

Knowledge of Hahnemann's new process was not made public until 1921, when his final Organon was published, 60 years after it was written, and decades after the very high potencies had been introduced by Kent.

Many modern homeopaths prefer to use LM potencies. I do not, though I did for some time, as I find that most of my patients come to me as a last resort after drugs and surgery have not fixed them. They need powerful help, and they need it quickly, now, without needing to be taking frequent doses of the required remedy over a long time, patiently and hopefully awaiting results to reverse their deterioration. Megapotencies are truly the 'minimum dose', as numerous doctors discovered through the 20th century.

MODERN METHODS OF MANUFACTURE

Of course, manufacturers have developed methods of remedy preparation that mechanise the processing. Yet there are still companies who do the potentising strictly 'by the book', as it were, hand making all their remedies.

And that presents a little problem to traditional homeopaths - because I have found that it is not possible to obtain hand made or commercially made remedies in the potencies needed, for most remedies. No-one makes them, anywhere in the world, my supplier told me, except for a very few remedies.

Australia's largest manufacturer advised me to continue doing what I had always done. I have always made up my remedies using a magneto-geometric remedy simulator, a modern-day instrument that can reproduce an energy with a vibration equivalent to that of the medicinal substance I wish to use, be it plant, mineral or whatever, and applies this energy to a vial of pills or liquid - all within minutes. I can make potencies that would have taken years of diluting and succussing by hand. Because the vibrational pattern is identical, the healing takes place as if the remedy were hand made from the intended substance.

The megapotencies we need can be made on these radionic instruments, which are available for purchase.[36] Many thousands of practitioners throughout the world use them.

Since radionic and radiesthesia research is only eighty years old, and Hahnemann did not invent it, this method of remedy preparation is frowned upon by many purist homeopaths, and they keep proclaiming that such remedies are not homeopathy, don't work or are specious, to say the least. Our own NSW Government is at present trying to have them outlawed as 'not part of medical science.' By contrast, Sir James Barr, a past president of the BMA who duplicated some of the early radiesthesia experiments done by Abrams in the 1930s, described him as one of the greatest medical geniuses of the early 20th century. Many great brains have continued radiesthesia research and developed increasingly streamlined radionic treatment instruments and remedy makers.

I am here to tell you that Hahnemann would have enjoyed greatly the chance to make his remedies so simply. He was forever the experimenter, and would have been appalled to think that no-one ever advanced on his knowledge. He was always interested in energy studies and recognised the life force as a Vital Energy or dynamis. He became interested in the new study of magnetism later in his life. He would have rejoiced at electricity, radio, television and the computer age, would have been fascinated and excited by the study of molecules and atoms, electrons and photons and over the moon about the recent research in psychoneuroimmunology, which is finally demonstrating how his observed body/mind/spirit interconnections occur.

Hahnemann would also have enjoyed the fact that repeat preparations of a radionically prepared remedy are always consistent, they do not vary with the influence of climate on the plant, or the effects of environmental pollution that are ravaging our plant life throughout the world.

ISOPATHY

This is a term used by homeopaths who think there is a major difference between 'similar' and 'the same.' The Greek *homoios* was chosen by Hahnemann to indicate the similarity of a remedy picture to the symptom picture produced by a substance, and it covers a much broader range of substances than the word for identical would have done. But the law of similars still applies in isopathy.

Isopathy is the use of a substance, in potency, to counteract the symptoms that exact substance has caused. We use isopathy, in particular, to clear away the adverse effects of drugs like penicillin or cortisone or the previously mentioned Lipitor, or any for which we cannot find a similar remedy. (We also use drugs in potency for the benefits they can offer, without the risk of building up side-effects or overdose toxicity.)

Common examples of isopathy include the use of Radium Bromatum to counter the destructive effects of X-ray and radium treatment, the use of poisons like Dieldrin in potency to counter their poisoning effects, and in orthodox medicine, the use of anti-venenes after, say snake bite, and the use of small doses of allergens to improve the body's immunity to those allergens.

We do this allergy reduction in homeopathy as well, using much smaller doses of the allergens, which is faster and more effective, cleaner and without residues of serum materials. Some homeopaths get a bit hung up on this as being 'not homeopathy', but it is very effective desensitising. I was taught not to use Apis (potentised bee), for example, to treat bee stings, but it works very well as long as you use a high enough potency to avoid adding more bee toxin to the sufferer. What it causes in crude, material form, it will always cure in potency. I always use 10M potency for isopathic antidoting.

HOMEOPATHIC IMMUNISATION

Homeopathy, since Hahnemann, has been able to give preventive protection against diseases - homeoprophylaxis (HP) - but until recently, the lack of documented scientific research has prevented its good results from being accepted by governments in many countries. A ten-year clinical study by Melbourne homeopath Isaac Golden, PhD (MA), DHom, ND, BEc (Hon), was completed in 1997. The study involved 557 parents returning 1,305 questionnaires over the ten-year period, each questionnaire covering one year of a child's life.[37]

The study found a protection level of 88.8% in cases definitely not suffering diseases after definite exposure and after taking the appropriate remedy. This compares very favourably with claims of the pharmaceutical proponents. Parents reported their children were very healthy, appeared to be

76

in better health than other children, enjoyed taking the pillules, they were very satisfied, the children rarely were sick and if they were, recovered very quickly, and many similar comments. One parent said, 'More parents should be made aware of the alternative to immunisation. I was very pleased with this program. I have a very healthy child.' Another reported, 'D. ate all the remaining pills left over in the kit - suffered no reaction.'

And others: 'We are very aware of the negativity about the program in the press and we have been questioned by health sisters about its effectiveness. We have told them that we find it extremely effective and easy to follow and administer, with no sinister side effects.' 'S. is much healthier than poor J., who was vaccinated by a doctor when young and is now allergic, asthma etc.' 'My husband wanted some type of immunisation. This was a compromise between something and nothing, and one we are both pleased about, and it puts responsibility back on to the parents where it ought to be.' 'Thank you for making this available and following through so thoroughly. I have been totally pleased with it as an alternative to mainstream immunisation programs. Thank you for supporting me and other families in our efforts to nurture healthy, balanced kids.' 'There have been a spate of infectious diseases in our area, and it continues to amaze me that children who have so-called immunity through vaccination contract them, whilst my child remains healthy.' 'Blood tests showed antibodies to the diseases covered by the homeopathic program. Just goes to show you.' 'I hope the work you are doing may be able to change this unjust and unhealthy political situation which says immunisation is a governments' decision, and put it back in the hands of parents.'

Of 345 such parental responses, 79% were similarly favourable. I have used the program for some of my patients, with equally pleasing results. Over the period of the study, Isaac Golden came under legal fire from the Victorian Government who attempted to stymie him, finally disallowing him from sending the prophylactic remedy kits through the mail, anywhere in Victoria. Many parents and practitioners supported his efforts, both morally and financially, through legal proceedings, and as usually happens, time is allowing right to prevail. Most homeopaths in Australia will happily provide your family with the prophylactic treatments you feel you require, as a result of this very difficult, very long and frustrating clinical trial - but by consultation only.

To complete this research, Isaac Golden entered a PhD program at the Graduate School of Integrative Medicine at Swinburne University in Melbourne. This program had four aspects: a review and update of the first ten years, by re-contacting parents who had not responded previously; a national survey to homeopathic practitioners' attitudes to and use of HP; a national health survey of children between five and ten years of age; and a randomised, placebo-controlled clinical trial of HP. This fourth aspect faced difficulties in terms of finding parents who we re willing to go blind into an unknown choice between the HP remedy (Morbillinum) and the placebo, in protecting their child against measles, over a two year period - children from birth to six months of age were sought for this trial. However, orthodox thinking requires this kind of trial if HP is to be considered by public health authorities, so it is thought. Surely, ten years' documentation of clinical usage tells enough? There was never a ten-year trial done of orthodox vaccines.

THE LAW OF THE SINGLE REMEDY

Samuel Hahnemann insisted that remedies were to be used singly as the symptom pictures, the indications, were collected using single remedies in the provings. We have no indications or provings for compound formulae in the Materia Medica. Therefore, technically, we cannot know whether a combination of remedies is going to be helpful or not.

With experience though, and with understanding of what the different potencies are capable of achieving, on which levels of the individual they are working, it becomes possible to use two or several remedies for specific reasons without disturbing the Vital Force or having one remedy over-ride the other. For example, I find it sometimes a matter of urgency to use more than one remedy when a person has had a composite injury requiring bone healing, bruise reduction and joint correction, and even, sometimes, to counteract the effects of fright. There are times when the problem will not be covered by any one of the known remedies and more than one may be needed to give the right resonances to stimulate healing.

It is a big stumbling block for the purists ('classical' homeopaths), who guiltily believe in giving only one dose of one remedy at a time, which, often, must be given months to run its course. Many people could have been fixed much more rapidly and comfortably if a repeated dose or another remedy was brought in sooner. The right remedy works rapidly, and must be repeated as often as symptoms return that still pertain to that remedy. Sometimes, another remedy is indicated very rapidly, and this can then be used without fear of complicating the case.

It is quite often that I find that people have stored guilts pertaining to more than one remedy. Some very complex disease conditions will not give way until all the needed remedies have been given. While it is necessary to select the most urgently needed remedy according to the currently presenting symptom picture, many people benefit from being given their second guilt remedy in the days immediately after the first. Not uncommonly, I also follow these immediately with their constitutionally needed mineral remedy.

I have never found adverse effects from working this way. Occasionally, a patient will say that there appeared to be no change from one or other of the remedies, but time and subsequent changes usually indicate that benefit did set in, subtly. When you understand what the megapotency remedy can do, you can easily see whether it has done so or not, within three weeks if not immediately.

The benefits of working this way are great. Patients, even the most seriously chronically ill, are given confidence that they are fixable after all, and this confidence alone is a powerful contributor to the final cure. Sceptics like to rubbish it as 'placebo effect' - let them think so. If that is the case, I get a wonderful lot of placebo effects as my patients get themselves well. Better that than telling them they have no hope.

All healing comes from within. No-one ever heals anyone else, all anyone can do is stimulate the patient's inner healer to get into gear. Free the guilts, fears and griefs and you free this innate healer to operate. All methods of homeopathy do this to some degree, the megapotencies do it rapidly and joyfully.

COMPOSITE REMEDIES

At this point we must mention the compound formulae that are available on the market today. These remedies usually consist of compatible remedies that would cover most of the symptoms in a disease state (such as influenza) and for acute conditions they are probably quite effective. Purist homoeopaths deplore them, for Hahnemann's reasons.

The system was evolved for the sake of expediency, as busy practitioners were looking for short cuts in prescribing, which often takes quite a long time; and it has value here in acute conditions.

The composite remedies are usually in low or medium potencies, when bought over the counter. They work sometimes by the 'shot gun effect', when only one or two of the remedies included will be helpful to that particular patient, while another purchaser might respond to a different component. The others will have no effect, if not required. Sometimes the remedies grouped together have a synergistic benefit greater than the individual parts. These become great favourites.

I remember an address long ago by a retired Sydney homeopathic doctor, Dr Lindsay Grant, who spoke of his own experience with a problem in his leg. This venerable master of forty years in practice had tried several well indicated remedies to no avail, and eventually, in desperation, was persuaded to try a composite remedy of good repute. To his great joy, the remedy worked like a charm - but imagine his surprise to read the label and discover that the remedy contained several of the remedies he had previously tried singly, without success.

HERING'S DIRECTIONS OF CURE

Constantine Hering was a colleague of Hahnemann whose conversion to homeopathy is worth mentioning. Hering was born in Germany in 1800, studied medicine at Dresden and later at Leipzig. He was a pupil of Dr Robbi, the most eminent surgeon in Germany. Robbi was commissioned by a powerful group of German medical practitioners to write an article critical of Hahnemann, but gave it as an assignment to Hering, to look into Hahnemann and his experiments for the purpose of debunking this new and wacky system once and for all. Unfortunately for them and fortunately for us, Hering studied Hahnemann's writings carefully and repeated many of his experiments. While dissecting, Hering cut himself and developed a gangrenous hand which would not respond to orthodox treatments. Amputation was advised. With the help of a friend who was a student of Hahnemann, he treated himself with a potentised remedy and recovered completely. He was converted, and his subsequent thesis defending the Law of Cure was never published.

Hering was so impressed with the scientific method and attention to detail practised by Hahnemann and the consistently good results from using the homeopathic remedies that he adopted the new medicine and became one of the greatest practitioners of his day. In 1833 he migrated to America where he developed a thriving practice and started homeopathic colleges in six cities in the USA. He was instrumental in forming the American Homoeopathic Association in 1841, the first medical association in the USA.[38]

Hering taught Hahnemann's observation that under the action of the similar remedy, healing takes place and symptoms move in three directions:

- from above, downwards - e.g. head symptoms will go first and action moves downwards causing symptoms to arise further down the body, particularly down the limbs;

- from within, outwards - to the skin, urine, bowels (faeces), mucus linings. From the more inward organs to the more outward, e.g. from liver to bowel, from lungs to skin;

- in the reverse order of arrival - e.g. the most recent symptoms are treated first, these will go and less recent symptoms will re-arise to be dealt with, by the same or another remedy. It often happens that the first remedy will ease the current problems, and old symptoms will re-arise of any condition that could have benefited from that remedy in the past. These will go away and others will pop up, one at a time, dating back into childhood, going away without any need for separate treatment. When this happens, true healing is taking place.

Such a Return of Old Symptoms (ROS) is a wonder to experience and is a sure sign that you are on the right remedy. (Nothing to fear - it is never as bad as the original symptoms were, and clears up quickly.)

Hahnemann had observed that as disease conditions develop, they become more and more deeply entrenched in the vital organs, from the outer tissues towards the internal and generally from below, upward. Cure must reverse this trend, so cure takes place from above, downwards, and from within, outwards. Symptoms disappear in the reverse order of their appearance. This applies whether you practice homeopathy, chiropractic or any other healing system.

To understand the above statements we must realize that disease does not just happen. It is often a culmination of many things. You may have noticed that few doctors take the time to ask you what you had been doing, what had been happening in your life prior to the onset of your present symptoms. The separatist view makes them want to treat all these issues as different issues. The homeopathic way is to look at everything that can be considered:

- inherited constitutional weaknesses;
- mental attitudes and emotions, which can so strongly influence the functions of the body. Many times the illness symptoms can be traced to an upsetting event, a grief or shock, a stress situation, a fright or an on-going fear situation. Also, we are taught from childhood a number of harmful, wrong beliefs that have an unhealthy result in our bodies: such as, that it is bad to express feelings, whether anger, grief, fear, love or whatever; feelings cannot be trusted as much as logic;
- accumulation, or damaging effects, of toxic materials in the body, such as are in food additives, preservatives, sprays, drugs both medical and social, immunisations or vaccinations, injected and ingested medications, environmental pollution in either air, water, or building materials, agricultural chemicals and food animal medications, viral residues from past illnesses and many more;
- poor nutrition - some foods are affected by soil depletion; foods are further diminished in value by manufacturing processes. Foods of low vitality do not add to your own vitality but do in fact lower it, because valuable energy is wasted in trying to process something that is giving nothing in return - even the body likes a good return on its investment;
- previous injuries or illnesses that were treated poorly at the time and the patient has never been well, or as well, since. Such trauma could be of medical origin, such as an infection, a fever, an injection, inoculation, lumbar tap, medication, operation, X-ray or Ultrasound or a mismanaged childbirth; or may relate to child abuse, rape or incest, abandonment or neglect, violence in the home or in the form of motor vehicle accidents and virtually any kind of injury.

81

Sometimes the patient will produce a rash as the result of treatment. This is a good sign as the vital force of the patient is endeavouring to throw off toxic material or viruses through the eliminatory organ of the skin ('from within outwards'). If the patient can understand the process of reversal of symptoms, removing blocks and overcoming constitutional defects, he will understand that this can take a considerable time. Sometimes, symptoms from long ago return, which indicate to us that we are on the right track, healing is in train and the fundamental laws of homeopathy are true.

As an example of this, here is what one patient wrote for my newsletter, under the title of 'Rubbish Removal Within the Ever-improving Subject.'

'You may have read the words 'Health Detective' on Jill's card. Many times I have observed the truth of this with her uncanny abilities as a diagnostician.

'Recently I was troubled by a persistent itch on my left forearm which prevented the wearing of long sleeves during the coldest winter period. At first, I put the symptoms down to insect attack while gardening, but no insect bite lasts for four months!

'Jill decided that the problem could have stemmed from a shot against rabies that I had in the US in 1942, which I had mentioned. Two days following the taking of her rabies remedy, Lyssin 10M, the itch had stopped and I was, thankfully, able to dress appropriately for the August cold weather.'

This is a classic example of 'from within outwards', (a previous remedy having chased the inoculation matter out to the skin), illustrating the emergence of old nasties which surface after a long period of administering healing remedies to a patient. (We treat what comes up, when it shows up. Lyssin suited the symptom picture, and Lyssin did the job.)

It also demonstrates how long inoculated material will lodge in the body - a lifetime - possibly causing or contributing to serious, intractible complaints. I had been treating this patient for ten years, and she had had many gains in health over this time. The Rabies skin itch was yet another of the many levels of illness brought to the surface by homeopathy. As each was resolved, her health improvement took another step forward.

THE CONCEPT OF MIASMS

Hahnemann recognised that some disease entities had the ability to pass down, from one generation to the next, a predisposition to certain kinds of conditions. He was the first to link inherited diseases and familial, constitutional weaknesses to specific virulent diseases, namely syphilis and gonorrhoea.

Long before genes and viruses had been discovered, Hahnemann's theories on chronic disease and its origins and treatment were published and put to use in the successful treatment of a wide range of conditions still regarded today as 'genetic, therefore incurable'. He had discovered that syphilis created destructive factors that could continue to affect succeeding generations for many centuries, these destructive factors being responsible for passing down what we now call genetic diseases, as well as chromosome alterations that pre-disposed people to a wide range of tissue-destructive diseases including tuberculosis, leprosy and cancer, which they would not necessarily develop; but the altered gene patterns are passed down and may cause a large number of complaints if circumstances that undermine strength and vitality trigger them off.

Hahnemann found that this genetic weakness could be mitigated and/or corrected out of the families affected, through the use of homeopathic medicines. Over two centuries now, many excellent homeopathic physicians have proven Hahnemann to have been correct. Why is western medicine still ignoring this knowledge?

About fifteen years ago, it was announced in the Sydney Morning Herald that scientists had (finally) discovered that viruses can get into genes and change chromosome patterns.

A few years later, scientists working on leprosy found it had links to both syphilis and tuberculosis. Surprise, surprise.

Hahnemann actually named three major miasms. These were Syphilis, Sycosis (from gonorrhoea) and Psora, which he saw as being the oldest in history, the 'itch' or skin disease. The first two are of prime concern to us today, as they describe the two main ways in which people manifest their reactions to the world and to life. Both types of people suffer injury shock from drugs and surgical procedures, but in opposite ways. Today, we also describe a Tubercular miasm which is an offshoot of the syphilitic and has similar qualities to it and to the Psoric.

Furthermore, it is the opinion of numbers of experienced practitioners that we are creating a new range of destructive miasms unknown in Hahnemann's time, these being a Cancer miasm (created from some forebear having had chromosomal damage as a result of getting cancer, which then becomes a predisposition, not to cancer necessarily, but to a particular range of destructive characteristics), a Radiation miasm (a genetic mutation leaving the succeeding generations altered in their physical or psychological characteristics), a Petrochemical miasm (similarly, chromosomal damage from very many petrochemical sources in our modern world, none the least of which are pharmaceutical drugs). In addition, medications that were used in standard medical practice years ago - such as mercury, arsenic, lead - have left their imprint on chromosome patterns that produce conditions in today's generations similar to the poisoning symptoms of those chemicals.

There are hundreds of such influences that have disordered our genetic strength over recent centuries. The twentieth century has left much to be repaired as our New Millennium children carry the effects forward. Chemical pesticides, herbicides, household cleansers, paints, building adhesives, pharmaceuticals and beauty products, DDT, 245T, 24D, hydrofluorocarbons - I skim the surface of an ocean of these man-made toxins.

Addictive substances are also creating gene distortions. 'There is a protein, delta fos B, produced by addictive drugs, that accumulates in neurons. Each time the drug is used, more delta fos B accumulates, until it throws a genetic switch, affecting which genes are turned on or off. Flipping this switch causes changes that persist long after the drug is stopped, leading to irreversible damage to the brain's dopamine system and rendering the animal (rat) far more prone to addiction. Non-drug addictions, such as running and sucrose drinking, also lead to the accumulation of delta fos B and the same permanent changes in the brain.'[38b]

All such inherited and acquired changes to gene patterns can be and are being restored to normal by homeopathy, even though, in some cases, it may take three or four generations to see the totality of such healing.

After forty five years in homeopathy, I find it simpler to consider all outside influences on the individual as either constructive-congestive-suppressive or as destructive-fragmenting-expressive - the two major ways in which people diverge away from normal health under the influence of their beliefs and attitudes. So henceforth, since this book is about the psyche rather than the soma, I will mostly be referring to these miasmic influences simply as suppressive or expressive, as described below.

THE SYCOTIC MIASM - SUPPRESSIVE

This is the miasm indicated by certain suppressive characteristics in the individual. The sycotic miasm predisposes the individual to manifest, in all his features, characteristics and symptoms, the qualities of *withholding, retaining, contracting, accumulating*. So we see suppression of eliminative functions, mucus production, accumulation of waste products and thickening of tissue, crowding of the teeth, muscle tensions and joint and disc compression. These are the physical manifestations of suppressed emotions, both the beautiful and the ugly; suppressed anger, guilt, grief, fear, resentment, as well as love, praise, generosity, confidence and joy.

The direction of energy in every aspect of the sycotic person's life is toward the midline, toward the centre, on the midline, keeping to the straight and narrow, holding himself in check, hoarding or withholding for fear of lack. His brain acts mainly from the left hemisphere of logic and rationalising. He has a continual battle going on to overcome this contractive sensation, break out, eliminate from within, express himself, extend himself and stretch to his fullest potential, give out and give away. Somewhat agoraphobic, he fears to lose the security of the close boundaries, preferring limitations, but is imprisoned by their constriction of his bodily functions.

This miasm is under continual expansion throughout our society because of the excessive introduction into the human body of materials for which it has no elimination mechanisms, particularly since the introduction of compulsory smallpox vaccination and mass immunisations in many countries. It is represented on a less biological level by the developed world's excessive desire to accumulate more and more material goods and money.

THE PETROCHEMICAL MIASM

The Petrochemical miasm follows this suppressive pattern also, as well as incorporating the following, the expressive/destructive Syphilitic.

THE SYPHILITIC MIASM - EXPRESSIVE

This miasm exhibits the characteristics of *expansion, flying apart, dispersing, eliminating* more than needs to be eliminated, *destruction* of tissue, decay and necrosis. It manifests in those disease conditions that are associated with mineral deficiency or imbalance, with distortions and imbalances in the musculo/skeletal system, neurological degeneration and malfunctions, faulty cell replication resulting in deformities or genetic, degenerative disorders. The direction is always away from the midline, outward, of loss. Visually, there may be a cleft palate, a gap between the two front teeth, a wide head with open fontanelles and a broad chin, or spina bifida, though not all cases are so obvious.

The expressive person loves sport, has quick responses, loves to move fast and act first, think later. Claustrophobic, he seeks the open air and needs space around him, between himself and others. He has a sense of high electrical energy, of the need to give this energy an outlet, and if this is excessive, increased by shocks, this high nerve energy can make him feel as if he is flying apart, life is disintegrating, all is chaos, he is devastated; the logical, intellectual brain is insufficiently strong for him to pull himself together, to get back under control. Eventually, he swings to the opposite extreme and becomes depleted of nerve power, the batteries run dry.

He is impulsive and thinks from the right, artistic hemisphere of the brain more than from logic or intellect. While he may be clever enough to take on any kind of profession, his nature is always towards the arts, music and creativity. He feels a misfit in the largely suppressive world, which is constantly trying to pull him into its boundaries and make him conform to restrictive rules.

The Tubercular, Cancer and Radiation miasms are of this expressive nature, as is the Psoric, to some degree.

ALTERNATING MIASMS

There are varying degrees of these influences in different people, and also quite a lot of people of mixed miasmic patterns according to their genetic inheritances, and to make matters even more interesting, a person may be corrected of one miasmic influence, only to find himself developing signs that the opposite type has risen to the surface to be dealt with as well.

Many practitioners have observed that over the life of an individual, the various stages of life are represented by specific miasms. So we see that babies and children often begin as expressive, become suppressed by their social pressures and/or medical encumbrances into adulthood, develop blockages and tumours of the suppressive kind and finally, may develop breakdown and degeneration of the 'expressive' kinds in late life.

This follows the common understanding of the progress of disease from acute condition to sub-acute, to chronic, to degenerative, as vitality is diminished and aging sets in. Genetic predispositions create an emphasis in one direction or the another, but the basic pattern seems to apply widely, across the board, unless the vital energy is given restorative support.

FINDING THE SIMILAR REMEDY

In searching for the similar remedy one must look at the totality of the person. No two people react in exactly the same way and rarely do they present the same totality of symptoms, even in an epidemic: their genetic constitution, temperament and environment are different, and even when these are similar, as in family members, differing beliefs and attitudes cause different reactions to the same environmental circumstances.

Provings of remedies have, in many instances, brought out very specific information about the mental, emotional and physical changes being caused by the remedy. We try to find the remedy that not only covers the physical nature of the illness but also the mood, temperament and changes to the thinking processes and emotional outlook. Also noted is reaction to changes of air, temperature, weather, food desires or cravings, aversions, hunger and thirst, sleep patterns and a host of other variables. In short, the full manner in which the sense of wellbeing is changed by the condition.

Often, it is the strange, rare or peculiar symptoms that a substance can cause to appear in numbers of provers that become the favoured features of that substance as a remedy - when we encounter such strange or peculiar symptoms in a patient we know that, more general or specific features matching, we are likely to be on a winning remedy. These are sometimes known as 'signposts' or 'keynote symptoms'.

Surprisingly, we find that when the common injury remedies were proven because of their existing, historical success in herbal medicine for treating injuries, many, in their provings, were found to be able to cause the same sensations and effects as the injuries they had been used to treat for hundreds or even thousands of years. Herbal medicine is often, and ought to be, homeopathic. Homeopathy does not require the micro dose, only the law of similars, to be homeopathy. And the law of similars applies across the board, to all substances.

IN PURSUIT OF PATTERNS

As we have seen, since the discovery of elecromagnetism and the development of quantum mechanics, 'new paradigms of the physical world, new concepts of living matter cause significant shifts in the beliefs about reality and how to incorporate inner experience. The power of these beliefs will shake up every institution in modern society. ... Behaviour on all levels, from tissues to individuals to societies, displays characteristic organisation patterns. And what cells, individuals or communities do is the result of the internal dynamics, not the response to anything external. I strongly believe that the internal dynamics of the most complex biofield, the human energy field, are based on its emotional organisation.[39]

'Emotion provides a force which flows and fluxes; it captains a field organisation to maintain its integrity. Whether the mind-field can continue without becoming disorganised is determined by the strength of the emotion.

'Patterns of the mind dictate complex human behaviours; brain patterns activate simpler ones. Every experience has concomitant emotions, and every emotion temporarily restructures the field. Activated emotions increase the electromagnetic flow of the field. Likewise, emotions arise from an altered electromagnetic environment.'

Similarly, suppressed emotions decrease the electromagnetic flow of the field, often leading to a state of being 'below par' which leads into physical ill-health. Specific beliefs trigger specific changes to our emotional patterns, which can be resolved by matching them up with similar electromagnetic vibrational patterns of remedies.

Provings of remedies provide a pattern on which we can rely, of effects both psychological and physical. When we find, in our patient, a similar pattern of suffering to that of a known remedy, we know that there is a fair chance that remedy will go some distance towards effecting a cure.

Hahnemann believed that the body can only manifest one problem at a time. He meant, by this, that the symptom picture for only one remedy would be showing at any one point in time, which is true as far as it goes. Sometimes only the one remedy is needed, sometimes our first remedy does its part of the cure and leaves us with a new pattern of symptoms, for which we need to find a new remedy to match. This may happen several times before wellness sets in, and it may be very rapid or a very lengthy process.

The interesting thing, I've found, is that some people can manifest a pattern of symptoms that pertain to one remedy, which will present itself in different guises throughout a good part of the person's lifetime.

Even more interesting is that several patterns can be present in each person, overlaying each other. We know that the particular problem that the patient consults us about is often only a part of the picture, and we give a long interview to hear the full story of the person's life events, knowing that these details will provide information vital to our pursuit of the critical remedy.

In my experience, every traumatic event in a person's life, if not treated homeopathically at the time, has had the potential to throw that person off-track, so to speak. The succeeding life and health events are created out of the imbalance or disturbance to vitality and emotions resulting from the trauma.

By adopting a policy of seeking to discover all the emotional or physical traumatic events a person has had in life, and how he has reacted to each of these events, what his attitude was, how he felt at the time of each, I develop a comprehensive picture of the sequence of guilts, griefs and fears that have contributed to today's problems. We are today, the sum total of all the unresolved incidents of our past.

By treating problems at their source with the remedy that had been needed at the time of each trauma, it is possible to get back on track rapidly. Sometimes a pattern emerges for several remedies, each indicated by their own repetition of events over years. Because each aspect of the psyche - fears, guilts, griefs, and the subsidiary guilts of resentment, greed, hate, lack of forgiveness, vengefulness, not to mention the attitudes and beliefs that arise out of social conditioning - can match a particular remedy pattern, my task becomes one of finding the remedy or remedies that are known to have caused such similar psychological patterns to develop in healthy people; and where necessary, to learn new information not previously recorded. Combining this with the extraordinary power of megapotencies, I often see miracles of healing occurring overnight.

HISTORICAL POLITICAL OPPOSITION

Hahnemann's work was well received by thinking men but was savagely opposed by many of the physicians and apothecaries of the day. While homeopathy was being taken to the far corners of the globe in the 19th century, and its successes noted in government statistics in numerous epidemics, the opposition continued.

The rise in homeopathy coincided with a decline in the prestige of the regular profession and a waning of public confidence in its procedures. There was much fear that homeopathy might come to supersede allopathic medicine, which only increased the opposition. The inauguration of the American Homeopathic Association in 1841, followed by the American Institute of Homeopathy in New York in 1844, prompted orthodox physicians to form the American Medical Association in 1846, with the dual intention of increasing the standard of education of doctors and hence squeezing homeopathy out. However, for sixty years nothing was done to improve medical education.

In the early part of the twentieth century, one quarter of American doctors were homeopaths. For purely economic reasons, since the homeopaths were very successful and other doctors feared for their own income and status, this had to be changed. Homeopaths in many states of the US were prohibited from belonging to the Medical Associations they had belonged to, prior to taking up homeopathy. Large amounts of Rockefeller and Carnegie money were invested in the medical colleges, in drug companies and in teaching hospitals. 'Do it our way or you get no funding' was the essence.

In many such ways, homeopaths were crippled and their teaching colleges decimated. By 1930, the last homeopathic college closed in America, and homeopathy remained at such a low ebb for forty years.[38]

In Australia, the picture was similar. We have always trodden the American pathway, and while, at the time of the Gold Rush, homeopathic doctors outnumbered 'regular' ones, by the end of the nineteenth century, thanks to the exclusion of homeopathy from universities, homeopaths were becoming scarce. With the development of drug companies financed by the same financial tyrants, 'regular' drug therapy has become the mighty monster it is today, controlling governments, media and patient choice alike.

In both America and Australia, it has been left to individual enthusiasts to maintain the true and genuine knowledge. Truth will not be suppressed forever, and the time has arrived for us to catch up with other parts of the world and take a stand, vote with our feet by seeking out genuine healing practitioners and refusing to be party to the grand deception.

There is a growing trend, particularly in England, to refer to homeopathy as a 'complementary medicine', as many homeopaths, often conventionally trained medical doctors, want homeopathy to be seen as a valuable addition to the methods used by conventional medicine - rather than a superior alternative. They are trying to have a foot in both camps, to be acceptable.

Homeopathy has been kept alive in Australia by lay practitioners, and is taught almost exclusively by 'alternative medicine' colleges, so the fundamental principles taught by Hahnemann are emphasised without bias or prejudice.

There is no question that Hahnemann believed his methods to be alternative, rather than complementary to the conventional treatments of his day, which he considered suppressive, unscientific, barbaric and detrimental to the health of the patient. (What has changed?) He described the medical practice of the day as 'this non-healing art, which for many centuries has been firmly established in full possession of the power to dispose of the life and death of patients according to its own good will and pleasure, and in that period has shortened the lives of ten times as many human beings as the most destructive wars, and rendered many millions of patients more diseased and wretched than they were originally - this allopathy.'[40]

SCIENTIFIC RESEARCH NOW SUPPORTS HOMEOPATHY

We now find that science can prove the relationship between our physical state and our thinking. It has taken a lot of casting off of false beliefs in the scientific world to get this far, and medical science remains in the dark for this reason, unable to rise free of these Newtonian limitations.

In 1893, the Chairman of Physics at Harvard University boasted that science had established the fact that the universe was a *matter* machine, composed of physical atoms, that fully obeyed the laws of Newtonian mechanics. Within two years of that pronouncement, the discovery of subatomic particles, X-rays and radioactivity toppled the concept of a matter-only universe. Within ten years it was discovered that the universe was actually made of *energy* and its expression could be described by Quantum Mechanics. In 1925, conventional physics was turned on its ear when the laws of Newtonian mechanics were replaced by the laws of quantum mechanics, which recognises that matter is made up only of intangible energy. That little piece of cosmic humour profoundly altered the course of civilization, taking us from steam engines to rocket ships, from telegraphs to computers. Through quantum mechanics it was realized that atoms are not matter, only energy. The body is an energy field, all parts entangled in a mass of energy vortices, which is holism. Every atom gives off and receives energy, vibrating at its own unique frequency and interacting with all other cells within the organism.[41]

Its truth has not yet hit the world of western medicine, except in the field of technological equipment. According to Dr Bruce Lipton, 'To this day, biomedical sciences still use outdated Newtonian physics to describe the 'mechanisms' of life. In failing to accommodate quantum principles, conventional medical science has remained in the materialistic 'dark ages' and is most definitely out of date!'

Dr Lipton describes what he calls 'a cosmic joke': 'A fundamental core belief in conventional biology for over forty years is that the traits and character of organisms are defined by their genes, and that DNA genes 'control' biological expression. Genes are blueprints that encode the structure of proteins, the molecules that comprise the cell. Scientists estimated that at least 100,000 genes would be needed to control and regulate the complexity of the human organism. However, preconceived beliefs in genetic determinancy received a nasty jolt when the Human Genome Project, an enormous project to identify every human gene, finally announced that there were only 34,000 genes needed to make a human - a long way short of the calculations based on the belief of genetic determination, and fewer than some low forms of life.

'In a commentary on the results of the Human Genome Project, David Baltimore, one of the world's most prominent geneticists, said[42]: "... unless the human genome contains a lot of genes that are opaque to our computers, it is clear that we do not gain our undoubted complexity over worms and plants by using more genes. Understanding what does give us our complexity - our enormous behavioural repertoire, ability to produce conscious action, remarkable physical coordination, precisely tuned alterations in response to external variations of the environment, learning, memory ... need I go on? - remains a challenge for the future."

'The 'control' of life is not *in* the genes, it is in the *organisation and activation* of the genes. The brilliant work of many biologists reveal that *environment*, and more specifically, our *perception* of the environment, profoundly influences our structure, behaviour and gene activity.

'An understanding of the newly described cell-control mechanisms will cause as profound a shift in biological belief as the quantum revolution caused in physics. Though mass consciousness is still imbued with the belief that the character of our lives is controlled by genes, a radically new understanding is unfolding at the leading edge of science. By studying how the single cell reads its environment, processes the information, consults with its memory and then expresses a specific behaviour, we are provided with amazing insight into the foundation of (chiropractic's) Innate Intelligence' and Hahnemann's Vital Force.

In 2004, NASA convened a workshop of leading scientists where discussion covered quantum computation and nanotechnology, and the activity of minute particles in life forms. These nanomachines inside living cells such as proteins seem to be there to boost information processing, particularly for self-replication.

Quantum physics is proving to be the interface between the world of matter and that of mind, and it is here we will find the explanations, long sought, of the mystery of Vital Force and how the homeopathic remedy, an information package, is actuallly working.

Chemists are only lately catching up with Hahnemann. In 1988, French biologist Dr Jacques Benveniste published in *Nature*[43] an account of his experiments degranulating basophils using anti-immunoglobulinE (aIgE). What made his experiments controversial was that he continued to observe basophil degranulation even when the aIgE had been diluted out of existence, but only as long as each dilution step, as with the preparation of homeopathic remedies, was accompanied by strong agitation. Benveniste was pilloried by the scientific establishment, who actually brought in a professional *magician* to discredit the experiments, and when he re-submitted similar findings using even more stringent controls, neither *Nature* or *Science* would publish the paper. In an effort to further silence healthy scientific dialogue on this important subject, Benveniste's employer at the French National Institute for Scientific Research in Medicine asked him to stop conducting research into microdose effects, thus losing him his funding, his laboratory and ultimately his international scientific credibility.

We later learned that a pan-European research effort involving Professor Ennis from Belfast and four independent laboratories in France, Italy, Belgium and Holland, led by Professor M. Roberfroid at Belgium's Catholic University of Louvain in Brussels, used a variation of Benveniste's original experiment involving comparing 'ghost' dilutions of histamine against control solutions of pure water. As an added precaution all the experimenters were blinded to the contents of their test solutions, which were prepared in three separate laboratories not connected to the trial, and co-ordinated by an independent researcher not involved in the testing.

The result, which was to be published in *Inflammation Research*, was the same: histamine solutions, both at pharmacological concentrations and diluted out of existence, led to statistically significant inhibition of basophil activation by aIgE. No surprise to me, as in homeopathy we've used hundreds of substances 'diluted out of existence' for 200 years with good clinical results. The article comments, 'The consequences for science if Benveniste and Ennis are right could be earth-shattering, requiring a complete re-evaluation of how we understand the workings of chemistry, biochemistry and pharmacology.'

Perhaps they'll wake up that chemistry cannot be separated from physics and quantum mechanics nor, indeed, from consciousness. What is so frightening about a re-evaluation?

There are experiments that show that photons that set off in opposite directions at the speed of light still appear to have an interaction or an effect upon one another. It is said that there is a non-local connection between them. Photons at the speed of light should not still be interacting according to classical theory. Quantum theory, however, predicts that there will continue to be an interaction, and indeed, that interaction is seen. This is what Buddhism has taught for two and a half thousand years - that separation is an illusion, that there is significantly more connection between consciousness and the physical universe than it seems.

Dr Candace B. Pert has conducted visionary, groundbreaking research into the biochemical links between consciousness, mind and body - the biochemistry of emotion. In *Molecules of Emotion*[44] she describes this research and her journey of understanding, and says 'The neuropeptides and receptors, the biochemicals of emotion, are ... the messengers carrying information to link the major systems of the body into one unit that we can call the body-mind. We can no longer think of the emotions as having less validity than physical, material substance, but instead must see them as cellular signals that are involved in the process of translating information into physical reality, literally transforming mind into matter. Emotions are at the nexus between matter and mind, going back and forth between the two and influencing both.'

Dr Pert goes on to say, 'Aristotle was the first to suggest a connection between mood and health: "Soul and body, I suggest, react sympathetically upon each other." But it is only since the early twentieth century that researchers have had tools powerful enough to discern the links.' She describes how Howard Hall, in 1990, was finally able to show changes at the cellular level, as measured by saliva and blood tests, using cyberphysiologic strategies such as relaxation and guided imagery, self hypnosis, biofeedback training and autogenic training. Hall was the first to show, under strict scientific protocol, that psychological factors, that is, conscious intervention, could directly affect cellular function in the immune system.

So homeopathy's consideration of the patient's mind and emotion symptoms has validation in physics, in biochemistry and in history.

SWISS GOVERNMENT VINDICATES EFFICACY AND COST-EFFECTIVENESS OF HOMEOPATHY

The Swiss Government has undergone investigations into the efficacy and cost-effectiveness of homeopathy, and has confirmed that a significant body of evidence from multiple sources verifies the efficacy of homeopathic medicines, and another body of evidence used to investigate the cost-effectiveness of homeopathic treatment showed that it is significantly more cost-effective than conventional medicine. The significant reduction in health care costs (15.4%) from homeopathic treament represents a potential savings in hundreds of millions of dollars or more in many countries. An independent Dutch study analysing claims from a major health insurer and also found a 15% reduction in health care costs.

In the Swiss report, a study of children with upper respiratory tract infections found that children who received homeopathic treatment had fewer recurrences and lower antibiotic consumption than children using conventional treatment. Further, an economic assessment of 569 patients with rheumatic disorders found that 29% could stop taking their conventional medications, 33% could reduce their dependence on drugs, and only 6% chose to increase their medication once homeopathic treatment began.

Patients of homeopathic physicians were significantly more often "completely satisfied" (53% vs. 43%) with their treatment than patients of conventional doctors.

The Swiss Government's Health Technology Assessment report, finalised in 2006 and published in book form in 2011, asserts that there is substantial appropriateness for homeopathy for the Swiss public.

RESEARCH OR WHAT?

The world is being bombarded with junk science and junk research and it is not always easy to tell what is good. For instance, we have known for a long time that the brain uses glucose as fuel for its neurological functions. In the news one day, we heard that experimenters gave students a glass of a glucose drink, then asked them to memorize a list of items. They were able to remember better than prior to having the drink. This was given as a great news item, as if it were a breakthrough.

When are people going to stop doing 'research' to prove what is already known? Research must take us further into new discoveries, otherwise it is not research.

I have noticed that students are taught at school to do 'research' by seeking out and documenting existing knowledge. That is a good learning experience. But there is no attempt to take this further, to use the information in support of an original concept not previously written about. We need to stop confusing this finding of known information with true, scientific research based on the combined processes of original hypotheses and impeccable methods of clinical observation, thought, experimentation and assessment, if we are to advance knowledge.

Unfortunately, within the homeopathic and other holistic modalities, this research to prove the known has been going on for some thirty years, purely to gain the approval of bigoted, medical pseudoscientists and impress ignorant politicians. Doctors are two hundred years behind homeopathy. As Dr Bruce Lipton, himself a general practitioner who learned more, tells the chiropractors, 'What's with you guys? You are the ones with the truth, doctors are seventy five years behind scientific knowledge and a hundred years behind chiropractic, and you want their approval, want to be like them? Wake up to yourselves!'

CHAPTER 5

The exciting or contributing causes may be legion, but whether mental, physical, mechanical or chemical, if they do not or cannot produce SHOCK, there will be no "Disease".
- Pulford

THE PARAMOUNT IMPORTANCE OF RESOLVING SHOCK

It is essential to understand the concept of shock as being much wider than that of the established medical model. Your paramedic will tell you that shock is always manifested by a certain particular range of symptoms:

- pallor
- cool, clammy skin
- thirst
- rapid, shallow breathing
- rapid, weak pulse
- nausea and/or vomiting
- evidence of loss of body fluids, or high temperature if sepsis is present
- faintness, collapse or unconsciousness
- progressive shut down of the body's vital functions

When any or all of these symptoms are present as a result of injury, heart attack, severe blood poisoning of any kind or spinal injuries, this degree of shock can kill, and must be treated seriously. Without treatment such shock does not resolve itself. Shock is usually the reason accident victims die on the way to the hospital. There would be far fewer fatalities if paramedics knew and used the appropriate remedies as rapidly as possible after the injuries. Homeopathic remedies for shock work instantly to restore order in rapid time, reducing haemorrhage and bruising, normalising pulse, respiration and temperature, settling digestive upset, restoring consciousness and inducing a state of calm. They also begin immediately to restore breaks in bones, nerve pathways, blood vessels, organs and flesh.

SUBCLINICAL SHOCK

Shock can occur to a lesser, sub-clinical degree. In fact, every trauma to the body carries an element of shock, even the tiniest little scratch or pinprick. People vary in the degree to which shock is noticeable at this level. Some people become faint and look pale at the sight of blood, and may even vomit - even though their own physical body is not harmed. Emotional shock manifests quickly in the body for such people, and it can be just as deadly as an injury if the shock comes on top of previous, unresolved shocks.

In fact, it is highly probable that some injury sufferers may go into shock from fright even before the body has had time to lose fluids or experience blows, jarring and lacerations. Shock bears little relationship to the severity of the injury, but relates to the way the endocrine and nervous systems respond to sudden change of circumstance. People vary in their ability to make rapid adjustments.

What is shock? Shock is registered impulse or impact, actual, perceived or anticipated. As Pulford[45] said, 'The exciting or contributing causes may be legion, but whether mental, emotional, physical, mechanical or chemical, if they cannot, or do not produce shock there will be no disease.

'And just what does that shock do? It simply breaks the lines of communication between the central control organisation of the body and its parts, depriving the central organisation of its power to direct the normal functions of the part affected, thereby weakening the natural body defenses and upsetting the normal body balance. The predisposition to 'disease' is inborn, in the form of defective lines of communication, which lines are easily broken by even light forms of shock, thereby the inherited predisposition to disease (is activated). Therefore it behooves us, as intelligent physicians, to refrain from introducing foreign elements directly into the body.'

Unresolved shock, from my perspective and in the view of many other homeopaths, is the primary cause of illness. Even acute, insect-borne viral infections do not develop in people whose adaptability was not shocked into inactivity by the sting or by some previous shock. Shock causes shutdown of control mechanisms, to some degree or other, and further shocks add to the degree of shutdown so that some intruders can run rampant and normal body functions are disturbed.

In cases of inherited predispositions, specific lines of communication are already weakened or defective because of genetic alterations from the previous norm (shock in the forebears), and may be the more easily shut down by even light shock from illness, drug or injury.

We can say that every homeopathic remedy is resolving shock while it is healing the problem for which it was prescribed.

Shock never occurs without some degree of trauma to the non-physical self having occurred at the same time. The subtle, invisible body is, in part or in whole, damaged in its energy pathways by sudden trauma, whether physical or emotional. This causes a break in the flow of vitality to a particular area, and it matters little whether the physical trauma was a first or secondary occurrence.

By their ability to operate on the non-physical plane of the individual and heal damaged energy pathways, homeopathic remedies can effect total (holistic) resolution of shock, whatever its cause and however long ago it occurred. By this means the processes of shutdown are reversed and vitality is restored to normal. Depending on the degree of damage, whether to cells of the physical body or only as blockage of energy impairing function, this can happen virtually overnight.

It might surprise you to know that, armed with this knowledge, I have on occasion treated and resolved life-long problems in the elderly, by treating conditions that developed from birth trauma, using the remedy they should have had at the time of birth. Such is the subtle power of sub-clinical shock to influence the direction of life. Such is the power of the minimum dose to resolve shock and its perpetuating effects, no matter how long ago.

So you can see that it becomes critically important to treat injuries and acute illnesses as they occur, with remedies that resolve the underlying shock derangements, and thereby prevent long-term conditions from developing.

It has been a real surprise as we have gone through our research years, to observe the various ways in which the body develops chronic disease after unresolved trauma. As we go through this book I will be referring frequently to this inevitable relationship.

In homeopathy, we have always known that some difficult-to-treat cases can be resolved once we get the patient to remember what had happened in his life around the time he was last well. Cases of measles, diphtheria, influenza and other such acute complaints, poorly treated at the time, are found to be at the point of origin of the sense of 'never well since', and the remedy for the initial condition must be detected in order to solve the current problem. We also have acknowledged the influence of medicinal drugs and other forms of poisoning in causing long term disturbances in wellbeing.

However, it is not so commonly recognised that this happens also after accidents and medical procedures, and because of social attitudes to medical practice it remains unobserved, or discounted as just tough luck, that many procedures are abusive and an assault on the physical body and the person as a whole. The idea that such procedures result in chronic conditions, of a psychological as well as a physical nature, is never given any thought.

Every medical procedure should be regarded as an injury shock which needs to be treated with the appropriate remedy in order to prevent future problems, which can be very destructive, even fatal.

BIRTH SHOCK

The most common cause of subclinical shock in Australians today is the medical profession and its assaults on the population from even before the day of birth. Later on, you will read about the shock trauma of a needle injected into a baby. How horrifying that this is being done routinely, without even discussing it with the parents, whenever a child is born. For some inexplicable reason, doctors seem to think that all babies have a Vitamin K deficiency at birth, so this is injected into them immediately. No inquiry as to whether it is needed or not. Mothers are often oblivious that they are signing permission for this as they enter the hospital for the birth. From this day, babies are likely to develop any of the complications that follow needle-shock, and these can be horrifically damaging and include bronchiolitis, encephalitis with brain damage, meningitis, tetanus and cot-death. From this day, a steady stream of needle-shocks follows at regular intervals, to the extent that recently, changes to the Australian Standard Vaccination Schedule have seen the number of injections that a child receives before turning two, increase from nine to sixteen.

As if the child is not already traumatised enough by birth! Dr Desmond Morris, renowned English behavioural scientist and author of *The Naked Ape* and over fifty scientific papers and other books, says in *Manwatching*[46], 'during the later stages of pregnancy the baby is sensitive to both touch and sound. There is still nothing to see, taste or smell, but it can feel the snug embrace of the uterine walls, the heat of the mother's body, and can hear the pounding rhythm of her heartbeat, thumping away at 72 beats per minute. These are the primary impressions of human life on earth, and they make a lasting impact. Even if, after birth, the mother is quite unloving towards her baby, she will have given it at least these three signals of parental care. For every child, warmth, embraces, and the heartbeat sound-signal will always suggest comfort and security.

'When the baby is born it experiences a sudden loss of these vital signals. In a typical delivery it is jettisoned into a bright light, assailed with the metallic clanking of medical instruments, feels sudden cold and loss of surface contact, and may even be held upside down and smacked to make it take its first breath. Small wonder that the first signal it gives in response to this treatment is a panic-stricken outburst of crying. For some inexplicable reason, these signs of distress bring a proud smile to the faces of the listening adults. Masquerading as 'normal delivery procedure' the behaviour in some ways could be compared to a primitive initiation ritual.'

Trauma is increased if the unfortunate baby develops respiratory distress or other problems and is rushed away from its mother and placed in isolation in a humidicrib. Suddenly, it is totally on its own against the assaults of a savage world, perhaps jabbed, perhaps having tubes inserted into its tiny body, or even anaesthetic and surgery. These are the only methods available to 'heroic' modern medicine to preserve life. There is no love, no harmless treatment is offered, the belief is that harmless methods are ineffectual. To add insult to injury, the equally primitive initiation ritual for boys, circumcision, may be then performed, even nowadays often without anaesthetic, as though babies are not really sentient humans yet.

Birth trauma is something that is common, to one degree or another, in all of us, but that is no reason to dismiss it. Ashley Montagu, in *Touching*[47], stresses the importance of defusing the tensions of birth shock by immediate fondling and handling (= massage), and nursing. 'When afforded such reassurance through the skin, the effects of the shock of birth are gradually mitigated. But if the infant is not afforded such an alleviation of his shock, the effects of that shock will continue, and will more or less affect his subsequent growth and development.' All too often, in hospitals, babies are denied such shock resolution, and to make matters worse, are receiving further shocks from needles and other procedures, from immediately after birth. Where is humanity?

The long term effects of birth traumae, including the damaging effects to the brain resulting from fear for your survival and oxygen depletion after having been half strangled by the umbilical cord during the birthing, are numerous and can carry through the whole of life if left unresolved.

SURGICAL SHOCK

Surgery and anaesthetics create their own deep levels of sub-clinical shock. Take one greatly overdone operation, the hysterectomy. Dr Lita Lee[48] says 'When menopause is created surgically within a short time, as is the case with hysterectomy, many problems arise. The sudden shock of the surgery causes the remaining organs to try frantically to take over some of the functions of the ones that were removed.' Dr Lee has observed adrenal and pancreatic problems (including diabetes) along with symptoms of menopause such as vaginal dryness and sudden hot flashes, for which oestrogen is commonly prescribed. 'This is ironic, since relative oestrogen excess is one of the primary causes of problems (fibroids, excessive bleeding, endometriosis and cancer) that lead to hysterectomy in the first place,' Dr Lee says.

Not only does surgery traumatise the body but it does nothing to deal with the hormone imbalance that began the problems in the first place. When the immediate shock is not resolved, the endocrine system cannot get itself back on track of its own accord, and chronic hormone imbalances remain and continue to develop into further problems.

Fashions come and go in surgery as in everything else. Hysterectomies are popular with male gynaecologists, and some believe this to be a demonstration of male hatred of women, of fear that women are somehow superior people and must be made less female, cut down to reduce their competitive edge. It is certainly a view that is supported by the competitively aggressive, masculine nature of modern medical practice.

Many of the fashionable operations of today are needless. Almost all problems of the female reproductive system can be resolved safely and reasonably quickly by homeopathy, herbal medicine, chiropractic, osteopathy and other naturopathic methods, long before the patient is reduced to needing the knife.

Some surgical procedures are in themselves the cause of future disease conditions. After thirty five years of coronary bypass surgery, some bright researchers decided to investigate the prevalence (already observed as a phenomenon) of adverse effects to the brain after bypass surgery. Using pre-operative and post-operative neuropsychological testing, they 'convincingly demonstrated' that measurable cognitive dysfunction - poor thinking and understanding - is very common, with an incidence of up to 80% to 90% at hospital discharge.[49] Do such patients, in years to come, begin to get the label 'Alzheimer's'? I've known some.

Certainly, the ones I've known have also had trouble with thoracic pain, both muscular, skeletal and lymphatic, often very severe, resulting from the savage treatment needed to perform the operation. Firstly, the breastplate bone is sawn down the centre with an electric saw. Then the ribs are stretched apart and clamped with powerful clamps to make space enough for the heart to be removed from the chest cavity. This almost always has to be done because the blocked arteries are situated at the back of the heart and inaccessible. The major blood vessels into and out of the heart are severed and attached to a nearby heart-lung machine so that the body can still be operative during the procedure, the blood now bypassing the real heart.

Sometimes the body is chilled down to give the brain a better chance of avoiding damage from low oxygen while this process is done. Meanwhile, veins are being removed from areas prolific in long veins, such as legs, and prepared for connection to the heart's exterior wall, and the offending blocked arteries are cut out and replaced by these veins. The heart is then reconnected to the bloodstream, the joins checked for leaks and when all is in order, the chest cavity is closed over again and the breastplate sewn together with wire.

Do you believe that an operation like this, lasting several hours, can take place without residual effects?

It is a truly heartbreaking experience, both physically and emotionally. The ribs are almost never put back into their correct alignment with the spine (from which they have been dislocated by the opening up of the chest), so they are also out of alignment with the connective tissues and muscles attaching to them, causing repeated pain episodes. (Using the homeopathic trauma remedies helps the body to re-align itself by resolving the shock-created energy blocks.) And ICU nursing staff often have to spend their night shifts comforting the big, tough men whose tears simply will not stop flowing, despite their embarrassment and efforts to control. (Using the homeopathic grief resolution remedies, the heart chakra is re-energised and a great sense of emotional hopefulness is installed.)

And such an operation does nothing to deal with the reasons the arteries clogged up in the first place, which, as we know, are stress-related and often suppressed grief is the stress, so unless big changes are made in the attitudes and consciousness of the patient, the problem will redevelop in the replaced blood vessels and continue to worsen in those that were not replaced. I have known people to line up a few years later for a second bite at this ferociously violent cherry, simply because fear for their life is greater than fear of the operation. There is no need for this fear, and no need to feel that only an operation can help.

Every surgical procedure, however seemingly innocuous, has a degree of shock trauma.

ANAESTHETIC SHOCK

What happens when we are given an anaesthetic?

The purpose of anaesthetic is to prevent pain and sensation from shocking the patient too much while the operation is performed. Many forms of anaesthetic have been developed since 1847 when the Scottish surgeon Simpson first discovered that operations could be performed more comfortably if he gave the patient a whiff of chloroform. Some anaesthetics produce total unconsciousness, others act only on a small local area. Nowadays, anaesthetists have such a repertoire that they are able to select a specific drug to suit each type of operation or procedure. In less sophisticated circumstances, drugs like alcohol and opium, or even a good punch on the jaw have been used to create the required degree of numbness or unawareness. The Chinese do it with acupuncture.

When a drug sends you rapidly into a state of unconsciousness, the same thing happens as if you had been knocked out. The sudden jarring of a KO drives you, your non-physical mind-body, out of its physical residence. You are still attached to this physical by means of an energy cord, but you can go anywhere you like from here, without the encumbrance of the physical. Some people report rising to the ceiling and observing the operation, listening to the conversations of the surgical team. More often, we do not remember where we have been once we return to consciousness.

Returning to the body can be a source of future problems if you fail to realign yourself correctly, the etheric you with your physical body. When you wake up you may have a sense of headache, of disorientation, of things being not quite right somehow, quite additional to the sorenesses of the surgery. Homeopathic remedies clear this.

Some anaesthetists like to give a few doses of morphine after an operation, to minimise pain on recovering awareness. These opiate drugs, in common use, create after-effects of hallucinations, disorientation and delusions that are embarrassing and confusing. I use homeopathic remedies to antidote these rapidly, otherwise they may go on for a week or more.

EMOTIONAL SHOCK

With or without physical injury, emotional shocks throw us out of kilter, so that body functions cannot operate as well as they ought. We all know the immediate effects of a fright make our heart race and our breathing shallow, but what about in the long term? If fright shock is not resolved, heart problems may develop, or chronic breathing problems set in. Worse, trying to reason oneself out of being still afraid can cause damage in the brain and bring on mental derangements. Fear can also be for your financial or other material welfare, following loss of a provider, or a business or investment collapse.

Grief shocks also can throw you out of gear, and lead to lung disorders, blood disorders including leukemia, lymphatic disorders, heart conditions, hysteria and uterine disorders.

Guilt following accidents can be a profound cause of chronic conditions.

Indignation, inner rage and indignities perpetrated against you - all situations from stored anger and outrage, including rape, medical and dental procedures (bodily indignation), social injustices and even accidents - lead straight into pituitary imbalance that extends to the whole of the endocrine system, affecting any or all of the major glands and leading to chronic immune deficiency and fatigue, thyroid and parathyroid disorders, adrenal and pancreatic disorders, almost all the common reproductive system malfunctions and hundreds of minor, difficult complaints.

If grief and indignation traumae are not resolved, they can lead to a chronic storing of resentment or grievance that also contributes to ill-health. Lack of forgiveness is one of our world's major problems, and you will love how homeopathy dissolves this away. Grief can also lead into deep inner loneliness, the major forms of this are: the feeling of being abandoned, separate from others, unvalued; fearsome parenting that created an intense grief over lack of love; and a lack of unity in a team or partnership, the grief of lack of support.

INJURY SHOCK

Injury shock usually results from sudden impact, for which homeopathy can be used to bring body and soul back together again in perfect realignment. This can occur even where there is no unconsciousness, the damaged areas are jarred into a state of relative misalignment of etheric and physical that slows the healing processes.

Some injuries have a significant effect on only one system of the body, which, if you treat that, will find the rest of the systems healing as well. This happens particularly with the central nervous system, the brain and the spine and all the peripheral nerves originating from the spine. Often, when you treat the injured nerves, healing of flesh wounds, bones and other damaged tissues follows. Some remedies are very broad-spectrum in this way.

You will be reading a lot later on about the nerve shock effects of puncture wounds such as injections, and about the effects of spinal jarring in violent accidents. The same remedy is used if you are having surgery or other procedures that only require small holes to be made in the flesh - canulas and such things.

Other injuries require shock remedies - fractures and bone jarring, bone ulcers and tumours after injury, and failure of the bones to heal or knit; puncture wounds (bites and stings); flesh wounds; ligament weakness or damage, cartilage and spinal disc injury; the tumours that arise from blows; spinal (coccyx) damage. All of these injuries, if not treated well at the time, can lead you into chronic disease, which you will read about in depth as I describe many cases with the remedies described in this book.

ACTIVATING HEALING

In the process of freeing up chronic conditions, we find the appropriate remedy can shift the body into a state of acute activation. The chronic condition must be activated into an acute one before it can be resolved. A chronic condition exists because the body's usual energy for dealing with injury, or foreign life-forms and contaminants, whether bacterial, viral or of chemical toxicity, has been undermined by shock and is insufficient to keep up the work required.

All the guilt release remedies provide the energy needed to reactivate normalisation, which is the natural, self-healing way of things. Evidence of this often comes as a fever or inflammatory state which may last from a matter of moments to as long as two weeks. During this time, the patient re-experiences many symptoms of old events from the past for which that remedy had been appropriate but never received. After such a fever, it is unlikely that the remedy that brought it on could ever cause such a reaction again, the normalisation process will have been (or be nearly) completed, and the chronic disease will have been immeasurably altered for the better, permanently. If symptoms persist, the practitioner then assesses whether the same remedy still is applicable, or whether the remaining symptom picture requires a change of remedy.

As a result of the release of stored emotions, attitudes change, perspective changes, muscle tensions release and allow full nerve and blood flow to return to affected organs and healing begins to repair tissue damage.

This is all the result of adding powerful light energy via the megapotencies, and enlightenment on a spiritual level is its natural accompaniment.

Even brain cells can be regenerated. It has long been taught that when brain cells are damaged, they cannot restore themselves to normal. This is the natural expectation, when you know that no drugs or orthodox treatments had been successful in achieving this; but it is not a truth, as in clinical practice, when hospitals have been able to get extra oxygen to the brain as soon as possible after cerebrovascular 'accidents' (CVAs) the risk of permanent nerve damage is minimised and in many cases, full recovery has occurred quite rapidly, from total hemiplegia.

In the Sydney Morning Herald of September 10, 2002, on page 4 is a report by Ruth Pollard that people with a brain injury may be able to use their own neural stem cells to repair the damage, reversing the long-standing belief that the brain has no capacity to regenerate. Researchers, led by the neuroscientist Simon Koblar of the University of Adelaide and the Special Centre for the Molecular Genetics of Development, say they have discovered a neural 'guidance mechanism' that directs the migration of stem cells in the brain. In areas of the brain damaged by, for example, a stroke, Parkinson's disease or accident-related trauma, it may be possible to use the guidance mechanism to redistribute stem cells to the damaged area and repair it, Dr Koblar said.

'The beauty of this is that the cells would be derived from your own body, rather than from embryonic stem cells or pig cells, for example,' he said. 'That means there would be no need for immuno-suppressants (to prevent rejection of cells) - it would be a far superior method.'

Pointing to evidence of stroke victims being able to regain some functionality, such as hand movement, he said the mechanisms for neural stem cells to repair limited areas of brain damage may already exist. 'If this is the case, we need to explore ways of stimulating and guiding them to help the brain repair itself.' Dr Koblar presented the research at the annual scientific meeting of the Haematology Society of Australia and New Zealand in Adelaide, the previous day.

As you will read as you go further through this book, homeopathy has just the ways to stimulate the brain to repair itself, without needing to do it via stem cell technology, which, Dr Koblar says, could take another ten years yet to develop.

See what I mean about science being light years ahead of drug medicine?

Research in neurology, immunology and endocrinology is providing more and more evidence that the living body has its own self-healing mechanisms. All the researchers need is to keep quantum mechanics in mind, examine the impact of vibrational energies (including thought) on the activity and function of cells and great insights will come to them, as it has to others in the healing fields, as to how energy can be provided to stimulate this self-healing mechanism. It will not come through the decadent, bullying methods of chemical drug therapy or surgery.

THE PSYCHOLOGY OF INJURIES

The psychology of injuries is very interesting, and relates directly to the psychology of chronic disease patterns resulting from injuries years before, that had a common psychosomatic origin. Yes, injuries are psychosomatic too. I don't mean we are all hypochondriacs. The word psychosomatic simply reflects the interconnection between *psyche*, mind, and *soma*, body. In respect to injuries, I was fascinated to discover that particular kinds of guilts or fears attract specific types of accidents.

We all know, for instance, that rugby footballers tend to get muscle injuries (strains, bruises and corks), joint (ligament and cartilage) sprains and tears and the occasional broken bone. Some will get the full range of these injuries, others will only tend towards one or another. The injury, and the remedy needed to fix it, must both be related to the same way of thinking, or attitude. In the case of footballers, the attitude is frequently, 'I'm OK, I'll be right'. Such people have a belief that it does you good to get a good belting now and then, so they keep lining up each week for their thrashing. They have to prove how tough they are, how much they can take.

What we discovered was that when we gave the muscle damage remedy, Arnica, in very high potency to the people who had frequent recurrences of muscle injuries from blows or falls, the guilt release stopped the person from getting muscle injuries again. This remedy changed the belief and allowed the person to stop having to prove how tough he was, or how much punishment he could take. In some cases, this release of guilt allowed him to hang up his boots for the last time, no longer needing to get beaten up. This proved to be the case for every type of injury - the appropriate remedy cleared the mindset or attitude and the injuries stopped happening.

I have also noticed that in a car accident involving several people, one whose constitution is in need of the remedy Silica will attract the fragments of glass, one whose attitude is always of guilt if he is not working will get the broken leg and be kept off work for weeks or months needing Symphytum, and the fun-loving, reckless, daredevil speedster will get the spinal damage and need Hypericum. The one who staggers out of the car declaring he is OK and then falls over, needs the blows remedy, Arnica - he still thinks it is OK to get a good bashing and believes he can take it, although he is undoubtedly concussed!

Once you realize the mental attributes of the remedies it becomes much easier to read the signs that enable you to choose the right one quickly.

I have spent a lot more time treating the adverse effects of old injuries than I have the injuries themselves - acute injuries do not come to me as often as chronic disease; but I have learned a lot through being associated with Bryan in his osteopathy practice, where they often turn up. Through this association, also, I have been able to observe and document the specific spinal and muscular changes that are taking place when a particular remedy is needed. Through repeated observations of the same phenomena, we have come to some very clear realizations about the injury remedies themselves, far and away beyond what was previously known about these remedies.

As a result of this work, I have come to treat many acute injuries with the megapotencies, simply because they were injuries that were recurrences of similar injuries. It was from this repeated observation that I came to realize that an unresolved attitude or belief was causing the repetition of similar injuries, and that this attitude was probably stemming from a guilt or fear based teaching, a misunderstanding or ill-treatment in childhood. In most instances, the patients were able to discuss freely the type of child and teenager they had been, their parents' attitudes, and the nature of events in their past that stuck in their memory with a particular emotion attached.

Less obvious was the evidence that chronic illnesses were resulting from these same injuries. We found that the muscle injury remedy was a primary one for heart muscle disease; that hyperactivity often began with the sting of the hyperdermic, and that this and many, many problems arose from bodily indignation, the shock effect of the trauma being one where the body 'takes offense' at things done to it by going into a kind of go-slow or shut-down of some functions, allowing others to run haywire. We found also that the opposite was happening, that the injuries were occurring after an illness that needed the same remedy had been suffered some time before.

There is an inextricable link of vibrational resonance between the psyche, the real self or mind, and the physical body, that attracts accidents, injuries and illnesses to match the thought patterns. Healthy, optimistic thoughts create healthy reactions in the body and resonate with safe living practices.

CHAPTER 6

It is estimated that as few as ten remedies could free the world of its major guilts.

- Gonjesil

THE TEN MAJOR REMEDIES FOR GETTING BACK ON TRACK

Most of my ten research remedies are in common use in every homeopathic first aid kit for treating injuries and grief. Only Hydrastis had not been appreciated as an injury remedy before I discovered its broad usefulness. Conium is not used much in first aid, although it could be, once we become clear on how its symptom picture can be interpreted in acute conditions. It is usually only brought in after tumours have developed from blows, though it is very useful for children's coughs and other problems.

Here follows a summary of the main features of each of the ten, in terms of our new discoveries. This list and the personality pictures in the following chapters are meant to be used in association with the information found in any comprehensive homeopathic materia medica. While I am encouraging you to look for yourself within such texts, I also must stress the importance of finding a competent homeopath to help you get the benefits of what you are learning here.

Homeopathy is a life-time study and this work only gives a minute fraction of the available knowledge. We all started somewhere, and in Australia, for many of us it was without the benefit of a teacher - yet from the first application of homeopathy in my life, I was able to help myself, and later my family, with every problem that arose. I have no hesitation in giving credit to the many home users doing the same, and to the many practitioners in other fields of alternative and complementary healing and medicine who, even from a limited range of remedies, are able to solve many problems using homeopathy to great advantage.

Everyone interested in any kind of healing, personal or collective, needs to know how these remedies can re-green the planet by re-greening the people.

ACONITE

CAUSATIVE GUILT: that fear indicates a mental weakness or inferiority, the intellectual mind must be strong enough to protect against experiencing the emotion of fear, so fear must be over-ridden by logic

- Physical and mental effects of sudden, life-threatening fright, any cause
- Fear for life, your own or someone else's, whether a single, frightening incident or prolonged fear - of abuse, of getting beaten up, of men, of torture, of death
- Fear for your survival (as mother or baby) during a prolonged, difficult birth, cord around the neck strangling you, or breathing difficulty after a premature birth, fear of not being strong enough to survive the hardship of the labour. History of such life-threatening birth trauma (cord around neck, heart defect, prematurity) - wherever the child had cause to wonder if he would survive, even if the parents were confident
- Fear of life-threatening illness or other harm to self or loved ones; fear of epilepsy, or of going mad
- Fear of the dark, the unseen, the supernatural, religion, evil entities, dangerous men waiting in the dark to get you. May be superstitious.
- Fear of reprimand and punishment for not being good enough or perfect in the eyes of parent or God. Fear of Hellfire and damnation.
- Atheist. Suppressed fear of God causes denial of God; intellectual logic takes over and denies any higher Intelligence; intellectual arrogance, snobbery, while the God Within, the heart and soul of the person goes unacknowledged
- Intense, suppressed grief that much-craved love is never perceived to be forthcoming, particularly from parents, who are perceived as always critical
- Fear of intuitive knowledge, of trusting the right side of the brain, distrust and ridicule of others' or one's own intuitive or psychic abilities or spirituality
- Trust only for logic and intellectual thought, emotions can get out of control; all fear feelings suppressed by over-riding logic - 'nothing to fear, silly' - or from expectation of further punishment or harm if fear is shown
- Dreams of violence, of harm or death about to strike oneself or a loved one

- Mental/brain illnesses - schizophrenia, bi-polar disorder, paranoias, depression, epilepsy; from fear, from fright, from radiation, from marijuana, all of which cause disconnections of neurones between the hippocampus and the cerebral cortex
- Severe, chronic hypertension, extremely constricted blood vessels
- Paralytic weaknesses, numbness in body parts, from stored, repressed trauma
- Severe heat flushes often mistaken for menopausal
- Inability to conceive or carry to term. History of miscarriages from faulty cell multiplication in the foetus, resulting from fear paralysis of cell division
- History of life-threatening accidents or illnesses
- Chronic asthma, dyspnoea
- Childhood eczema
- Anorexia
- Crohn's disease
- Chronic kidney disease
- Addiction to alcohol; it gives Dutch courage and banishes the fears of life
- Sleep often broken in the night, especially around 4am, or many times, often at two-hourly intervals, 12am, 2am, 4am. Dreams of harm to self or loved ones, actual or threatened
- Many Aconite patients had changed their name, in a vain attempt to give it better energies to improve their life

Facial feature: a prominent bridge to the nose, sometimes almost squared sides to it, rising straight into the profile of the forehead without concavity.

Followed well by: Arnica; Conium; Ledum; Ruta; Staphisagria; et alia.

ARNICA

CAUSATIVE GUILT: a soft heart is a sign of weakness. Life's tough, you have to be tough to survive. Guilty if not able to take life's blows strongly - must be tough

- 'I'm OK, I'll be right, I'm tough'
- Feels mentally all right but the body is letting him down
- Soft-hearted but will not admit publicly to any softness or gentleness, which shows embarrassing weakness and could be construed as effeminacy; fears this
- Touches others only in sport or aggression, will not be touched affectionately in public; can be rough, unable to handle gently
- Can be tough in disciplining the young, to toughen them up to take life's knocks and blows
- Chronic heart conditions, muscle disorders, circulatory disorders of thickened muscle and blood vessel walls, hypertension; ischemic heart and cerebrovascular attacks, aneurism.
- Haemorrhagic tendencies, ready bruising - cortisone toxicity
- Chronic effects of birth trauma, blows, falls, fights, rugby football and hockey injuries, most childhood injuries, motor vehicle accidents
- Concussion, unconsciousness, coma, anaesthetics, shock - chronic effects

Body indicator: Thoracic vertebrae 2-4 are anterior to the rest of the thoracic curve (dipping towards the breastplate). The Arnica flesh is muscular, thickened up by the need to be tough. The heart muscle becomes tough and can lead to breaks at the blood vessel connection points.

Followed well by: Aconite; Conium; Hydrastis; Hypericum; Ledum; Ruta; Staphisagria; Symphytum; Natrum Muriaticum; et alia.

CONIUM

CAUSATIVE GUILT: of not being able to provide for oneself independently. Dependency on financial support, fear of having to provide for one's livelihood. Dependency on others to provide, support, assist in any and every way. Fear of loss of independence.

- Strives for independence, believes he/she is independent, often works for himself but worries about where tomorrow's money or help is coming from, and whether it will come or not
- Dependent on government financial support, or community welfare support
- Dependent on medical and nursing support, drugs, crutches or wheelchair; addiction; fear of lack of supply
- Mental enfeebling: memory lapses, slow thought processes; or fears, with hysteria
- Reversion to childhood physically and mentally, eventually to babylike inability to feed or dress oneself
- Paralytic weakness beginning in the lower spine and legs and rising up the body as years go by, finally paralysing the ribcage and diaphragm
- Traumatic sacro-iliac weakness. Toxic brain and spinal poisoning (lead)
- Mouth, throat and cough disorders; sleep apnoea. Tumours, cancer, stone-hard glands

Facial feature: the eyes slant upwards at the outer corners - a cat's-eye look; the sphenoid bone at the temples is pulled in towards the midline, causing a high, vaulting palate and narrowed maxilla. Often one eye is higher and more slanted than the other. While the eyes are initially rounded, they may become more slanted and half-closed in later life.

Followed well by: Arnica; Hydrastis; Hypericum; Staphisagria; Symphytum; et alia.

HYDRASTIS

CAUSATIVE GUILT: of responsibility or over-responsibility; lack of self-forgiveness. Guilt over causing or allowing harm to oneself or others, or over harm caused to one's race or community or to other nations, races or communities; or suppression of these guilts.

- Guilt of not having been able to prevent a harmful occurrence - personally, or guilt carried on behalf of race or community.
- Over-responsibility towards other people, carrying their loads. Big Brother attitudes of governments and support organisations, multinationals - 'Let us look after you'
- Injuries of any kind to any part of the body - when 'my own fault'
- Spondylolisthesis - the lumbar spine shifts forward through carrying the loads and responsibilities of others, physically or psychologically, or through prolonged guilt, causing injury
- Domestic violence, physical and verbal aggression; morose, bad-tempered
- Aggressive behaviour while intoxicated; guilt of this; denial through guilt
- Diabetes following injury shock, when 'my own fault'
- Liver disease, effects of alcoholism; chronic constipation
- Drug damage to the liver - antibiotics, many others
- Chronic post-nasal catarrh that can be drawn into the mouth by sucking; after vaccination, antibiotics, other drugs
- Cancer of bowel or liver or skin
- Depression. Guilt suicide - family or business guilts - 'my fault'

Body indicator: lumbar vertebrae 4-5 are anterior to the sacrum and to their normal alignment in the lumbar curve, usually without rotation of the vertebrae or pelvis. Pain is equally left and right-sided across the lumbar spine - lumbago.

Followed well by: Arnica; Conium; Hypericum; Ledum; Staphisagria; Natrum Muriaticum; et alia.

112

HYPERICUM

CAUSATIVE GUILT: low self value is the message this one gets from life's experiences; believes others consider him worthless; may have been abandoned.

- Devastated by loss; yet will abandon others
- Lack of respect for others, or for their property
- Never responsible, always someone else to blame
- Disparaging of all except those below him on the social or business ladder
- Sympathetic only to underdogs, children, the disadvantaged, loses interest if they reach his level. Must cut down the tall poppies
- Must prove himself best in order to feel he is good enough
- Competitive, loves to win at any price - second place is still worthless, in sport or business
- Must create the biggest and the best, and kill out opposition - multinational companies, monopolies, banking kartels, the western medicine machine
- Only fun and games matter in life - work is separate from fun but competition makes it more like fun when you win over others
- Loves speed, takes risks, fears aging and loss of beauty - 'Live fast, die young and have a good-looking corpse'
- Unconscious of risk to others; accepts no blame for their hurt; often no sympathy
- Panics, runs away from trouble without looking back
- Enemy/victim consciousness; wages war on all forms of life - him against the world - divide and conquer.
- Suicide bombers; terrorists, whether anti- or within the administration
- Extremist - has to go overboard, to excess; out of balance
- Bored; boring as he labours a point; often misses the point
- Effects of puncture wounds from sharp, pointed instruments - bites, stings, injections, bullets, knife stabbings, keyhole surgery, cannulae, etc.
- Fever and restlessness, tetanus, encephalitis after puncture wound shock
- Sudden infant death, meningitis after medical puncture wound shock
- Hyperactive nervous system, out of balance, over-reacts, cannot slow his mind down to reason clearly

- Cannot wait to get into the next moment in time - always racing into the future, ignores the past and fails to reflect and learn from mistakes, his own or others'
- Insomnia - the brain stays in logical thinking mode (beta waves) most of the night even though the body is asleep, giving an illusion of wakefulness
- Hypertension, hyperglycemia, hyperthyroidism, hypersensitivity, over-reactions
- Spinal injury shock from speed and recklessness, explosions, bombings - paraplegia, quadriplegia, hyperaesthesia
- Viruses, particularly from puncture wounds, including from mosquito bites, ticks

Facial sign: a single, vertical crease centrally above the bridge of the nose; in the young, this is a faint depression of the forehead above the bridge of the nose; sometimes a gap between the front teeth; a rounded hairline and oval face and head, doming at the vertex; often the upper and lower teeth meet only on one side of the mouth, the jaw or maxilla diagonally displaced.

Body indicators: Thoracic scoliosis, distortions of the trunk from unequal tensions in the diagonal muscles latissimus dorsi, trapezius, psoas, teres; winged scapula; tension in the balancing muscles of the limbs - gastrocnemius, sartorius.

Followed well by: Arnica; Conium; Hydrastis; Natrum Muriaticum; Rhus Tox, Calc Carb, Calc Fluor et alia.

Complementary to: Pulsatilla, the primary endocrine partner for the Hypericum Central Nervous System.

Antidoted by: Staphisagria 200, which takes the 'bodily indignation' out of any remedies wrongly used. Refer to Chapter 11 for notes on accurate prescribing of Hypericum.

IGNATIA

CAUSATIVE GUILT: The plans have been changed by unforeseen circumstances beyond your control and you can't see where to go next, the previous plan is no longer an option; feeling stymied, thwarted, unable to get ahead.

- Deep sense of inner sadness and disappointment on this account; always suppressed and held tightly within
- Inner tension, even while seeming relaxed to others - can reach breaking point and become hysterical
- Often someone's death or illness caused the loss of opportunity; or redundancy, business closure, divorce, accident, war, any major trauma beyond your control
- Sadness and disappointment from any cause; may be on behalf of someone else
- Thoughts tend to be of the past, the present is hampered by past events
- A sense of being at the end of the road - nowhere to go, can't see any future track to take - failure to see opportunities because of this, that could get you back on track
- Fluid imbalances - dryness, wetness; urination problems, sinus congestion from suppressed grief tears; fluid retention, anywhere in body; hayfever; lymphoma
- Blood and heart disorders from being disheartened, disappointed or griefstricken

Facial features: Two vertical lines rising from the sides of the bridge of the nose at the eyebrows; a sad turn-down of the corners of the mouth; there is a definite and visible sensation of pulling downward of the cheek muscles towards the jaw, even when there is no conscious awareness of a grief issue. This is not as long or pronounced as the strong grudge or grievance lines seen on some who need Ledum, despite being the same muscles in action. May need both remedies.

Followed well by: Ledum; Hydrastis; Hypericum; Staphisagria; Symphytum; Natrum Muriaticum; et alia.

LEDUM

CAUSATIVE GUILT: Inability to let go and move on. Carries grievances or resentment, harbours grudges. Lack of forgiveness. Misplaced loyalty.

- Unforgiving resentment that perpetuates disharmony and war; holding of grudges and grievances
- Cannot forgive someone who acted against his interests or his wishes, beyond his control. Lives from the past, cannot put things behind him and move ahead. Suppressed, internalised grievances
- Intimidation by threats, fear; prolonged cruelty, torture, mental or physical
- Grief - cannot let go of a deceased loved one (even despite trying)
- Extreme loyalty, whether to a person, a cause or ideal, a nation, even blindly unto death. Inappropriate relationships are held onto too long.
- Fears loss of emotional control: grief, anger, love, joy
- Some become begrudging of praise, gratitude and appreciation
- Must be in control - life or wellbeing depend on staying in control, of having the circumstances all on your own terms
- Cannot let go, must hold on at any cost, fears someone or something stronger than he might overcome him
- Tenosinovitis, repetitive strain injury, tendon tears - from chronic tension in the 'holding on' parts of the muscles
- Tendon injury from puncture wounds - nails, stings, needles - tetanus
- Gout and gout-like complaints in the extremities as the body holds on to uric acid
- Often people whose work tools - power tools, heavy vehicles or animals - must be kept under control, kept on a tight rein

Facial features: a set mouth, sometimes just a horizontal slit; often with Staphisagria forehead and Ignatia lines; or a very disgruntled, resentful downturn of the corners of the lips. A long, narrow face more often than any other shape, with teeth close or crowded. May have a strong Nat Mur chin.

Followed well by: Arnica; Hydrastis; Ignatia; Ruta; Staphisagria; Symphytum; Natrum Muriaticum; et alia.

116

RUTA

CAUSATIVE GUILT: a sense of need for power and strength from numbers; lacking this strength of unity.

- 'We must all pull together - united we stand, divided we fall'
- Grief/guilt over lack of unity - family, work, community and nation; team spirit is important
- All must do their bit, pull their weight; we want no free-loaders
- Insensitive to personal hardship, of self or others
- Desires the perceived strength of unity, as of NATO, the Commonwealth of Nations, United Nations, conglomerates, unionism
- If he tackles big jobs alone and no-one wants or is available to help, no co-operation, the body fails by weakening at the joints, particularly load-bearing joints
- Ligament weakness, spinal subluxations, disc compressions and herniations, and ligament and cartilage damage, all joints; lift-and-twist injuries; sciatica; hernias to integumentary tissues of the pelvis; from workplace and sporting injuries, road accidents or similar causes
- Chronic bowel problems, constipation, haemorrhoids, cancer
- Pelvic ligament prolapses, whether uterine, bladder, intestines or other
- Bowel and rectum prolapses

Body indicator: Lumbar vertebrae 4-5 rotated, sometimes with lateral shift, sacral deviation, traumatic lumbar scoliosis and oblique or horizontal iliac crest levels. MRIs may show disc bulging. Muscle strength over-rides ligament strength.

Followed well by: Arnica; Ignatia; Ledum; Staphisagria; Symphytum; Natrum Muriaticum; Sepia; et alia.

STAPHISAGRIA

CAUSATIVE GUILTS: a belief in Right and Wrong; a belief in Justice and the Law; helplessness in the face of authority; anger is unacceptable, fear of upsetting others, of not receiving approval; peace at any price

- Lives by the rules, obeys the law, always does the 'right thing' according to the socially accepted highest standards of right and wrong, judgemental if others do not also live this way; takes charge of others 'for their own good', without their permission - 'do-gooders'
- Life is full of reasons for indignation or anger, but it is unacceptable to show anger, so he/she keeps it down to a level of silence or of whinging
- Acceptance of situations out of a sense of helplessness to alter them
- 'How dare they? How can this be happening? Where is the justice in this? But I'm only one voice, what can I do about it? It's not fair.' Frustration
- Inoffensive, harmless, sweet-natured, nice, proper, peace-loving
- Suppressed indignation and outrage at offenses done to one, whether physical or mental. 'There should be a law against it.' Believes he knows what right is, how things *should* be, in all circumstances, for himself and everyone else - self-righteous; the word 'should' is used often
- Conformity to standardisation, whether in the 'free' world or in communist countries, manifest in nationalisation of health services and similar public services as well as de-nationalisation into the hands of conglomerates, to 'make it easier for us to look after you, knowing what is best for you'
- Hypocritical; the highest standards demanded of the children and others, but a different rule for himself, secretly. Seeks to protect others' feelings by keeping truth from them, even if it means lying, he/she cannot see that the lie, the secret, is more offensive than any truth would have been. White lies are a normal part of life for Staphisagria
- Intolerant of misdemeanours, seeks the power of the Law in getting justice or righting false accusations. Impatient and intolerant of imperfection; cannot live and let live, no allowing - love is suppressed
- Fears to speak out in case the words offend and lead to dissention which makes him feel helpless to fight back, he always loses the argument and hates anger, suppresses his own anger and seeks peace at any price
- Offenses to the body in the form of antibiotics, steroids and other drugs, surgery, anaesthetics, injections including immunisations, dental and orthodontic work; physical force

- Often the perpetrators of these offenses need Staphisagria, too, as they are blinded by their belief that they are doing the right thing or upholding the law
- Accumulation in the body of viruses and toxic pollutants from inoculation serums, auto-intoxication from retentive bowels and bladders, distorted and inefficient foreign cell recognition and destruction, leading to allergies as severe as 'Total Allergy Syndrome,' a man-made condition
- Suppression of anger and outrage causes pituitary malfunction leading to irregularities, even tumours, in any endocrine glands: thyroid deficiency, parathyroids (osteoporosis), thymus (allergies, coeliac disease, chronic fatigue, all immune deficiency diseases), pancreas (hypoglycemia), reproductive system (all conditions arising from male or female hormone irregularities including high or lost sex drive and homosexuality), adrenal hormone irregularities even if congenital
- Pain and abnormalities remaining after operations, other procedures. Hormonal imbalances remaining after taking The Pill or HRT, or steroids
- Hysterectomy after years of medical abuse - antibiotics -> glandular fever and/or Candida albicans proliferation, -> chronic fatigue, painful, excessive periods, -> endometriosis, -> uterine collapse
- Rapists and sexual harassers. Many Staphisagrians are obsessed by thoughts of sex, which many suppress guiltily (not nice, you know), others cannot, the guilt coffers are too full and the energy cannot be contained
- Rape, incest, physical abuse of any kind. The body takes offense at things done to it. The Staphisagria person is too embarrassed and guilty to speak of the outrage, and stores the emotional energy in the facial muscles and in the offended organs, causing pituitary malfunction. Sexually transmissible disease - Gonorrhoea, Human Papilloma Virus; cervix erosion, cell abnormalities in PAP smears; 'honeymoon cystitis'
- Skin conditions - rash like chicken pox; psoriasis; vaginal and penile rashes
- Sacral area - fluid, puffiness; sacro-iliac joint subluxation causing sciatica, worse right side. Any joint subluxations from injuries where a sense of injustice is felt - shoulder, neck, cranial joints. Or back may be strained by coition

Facial signs: horizontal creases across the forehead; raised eyebrows; jaw tense and laterally out of alignment, retracted jaw, teeth cramped and misaligned. A surprised or mystified look. A sweet, bright smile.

Followed well by: Aconite; Arnica; Conium; Hydrastis; Ignatia; Ledum; Ruta; Symphytum; Natrum Muriaticum; et alia.

119

SYMPHYTUM

CAUSATIVE GUILT: that a living has to be worked for, only work earns the right to life. 'I feel guilty if I am not working'

- The language is full of the word 'work' - everything is seen in relation to whether it works well, badly or not at all
- The body is not working well enough, or a single part is not working - muscles have to be worked hard, especially after injury that put the person off work
- The workaholic must break a bone in order to give himself a break from work. Unemployment, redundancy and retirement are feared and create great guilt
- A medicine, remedy, tools, electrical or mechanical gear or a solution to a problem must 'work'
- Brain and spinal nerve reception problems causing organs or parts not to be able to heal - the brain is not receiving the message that there is a problem to be fixed, so no messengers are sent out to initiate the healing. Calcium ions are switched off, not working, in the afferent nerves.
- Throughout life, tendency to bone breaks and disc damage from injuries; soreness still in old bone injuries; connective tissue brittleness; arthritis
- Children with genetic abnormalities. Elderly people whose bodies are beginning to break down
- Abnormal, or lack of, cell proliferation and replacement. Faulty function of cells, not from congestion of toxins but from damaged DNA/RNA. Toxic chemical destruction, mutation of cells. Radiation damage to DNA.
- Liver necrosis, chronic hepatitis, cirrhosis, alcoholism. Kidney cell distortions. Cancer
- Leucocyte abnormalities. Rheumatoid arthritis. Genetic diseases of bone and nerve - Paget's, Huntington's, Parkinson's; organ malformation and degenerative diseases
- Ulceration, deep-seated abscesses, chronic bacterial infections, recurrent outbreaks of tissue disintegration or haemorrhages. Failure to heal, chronic lesions - skin, eye, ear, breast lumps, bone pain, jaw and gum affections

Facial sign: horizontal crease or creases across the indented bridge of the nose.

Followed well by: Arnica; Conium; Hydrastis; Natrum Muriaticum; et alia.

NOTES

- Hypericum and Symphytum are the only remedies of the ten that are truly Expressive in nature; yet they are opposites in some ways-Hypericum hates work, seeks fun, Symphytum finds enjoyment in his work. Hypericum types can become Symphytum when age catches up with them.

- Aconite, Ignatia, Ledum, Ruta and Staphisagria are Suppressive remedies that release volumes of congestive energies and matter. These can be the hardest to recognize, because the person himself does not register that emotional reactions to life have been suppressed.

- Some people have mixed inheritances and may need remedies from both groups, including such opposite remedies as Staphisagria and Hypericum. The face will show the indicators for both. In such cases, I use Hypericum first and use Staphisagria immediately after.

- Arnica, Conium, Hydrastis and Natrum Muriaticum are remedies that can be applied to any miasm. While some remedies have an affinity for certain inheritance patterns or constitutional types, there are many that are useful to all.

CHAPTER 7

The only thing we have to fear is fear itself
- Franklin Delano Roosevelt

ACONITE - 'I WAS FRIGHTENED, NOW I'M DEPRESSED'

Homeopathy has plenty of remedies for fears of different types, including our wonderful Conium, Hypericum and Staphisagria, but none compares with the mighty Aconite for the acute, paralysing effects of terror and its aftermath, depression.

Aconite (aconitum napellus, *Monkshood,* N.O. Ranunculaciae) is not a remedy that is used in herbal medicine, owing to its deadly toxicity in its raw form. According to Mrs Grieve, Gerard says, 'There hath been little heretofore set down concerning the virtues of the Aconite, but much might be said of the hurts that have come thereby. Its power is so forcible that the herb only thrown before the scorpion or any other venomous beast, causeth them to be without force or strength to hurt, insomuch that they cannot moove or stirre untill the herb be taken away.' Even then its paralysing nature was observed.

Mrs Grieve also noted that 'the tincture of Aconite in the British Pharmacopaeia of 1914 is nearly double the strength of that in the old pharmacopaeia of 1898'. Even more toxic by then.

In the early 20th century, in the days before antibiotics, western medicine practitioners used to use Aconite in tincture form, drop doses, as they did many other toxic herbs such as Belladonna (deadly nightshade) and Conium (hemlock). They had learned about these medicines from the homeopaths, but failed to appreciate that the micro-doses worked much more effectively without risk. As with modern medical attitude, the more toxic the better, if it can kill it must be good for you. Finley Ellingwood[51] found it to be efficacious in fevers, but warned to minimize the dose. 'One drop of the specific medicine in a four ounce mixture, a teaspoonful every half hour or hour, will sometimes produce the best results in children under twelve years.'

It is the half-remembered guilt of using such toxic herbs that causes medicos to tell you, nowadays, that herbal medicines are dangerous and poisonous. None of the herbs used in modern botanical medicine are poisonous in the generally accepted understanding.

But the really poisonous plants that are not used in herbal medicine make very powerful healing medicine when converted to the micro doses of homeopathy - for what they can cause in the crude forms, they can cure in potency! Ellingwood admits that 'Homeopathic physicians class it as one of the most important agents and their dosage is always minute. In such dosage, with small, feeble, frequent or corded pulse, in adynamic or asthenic fevers, it may be given with excellent advantage.'

ACONITE IN HOMEOPATHY

Aconite has always been known to homeopaths as the great remedy for calming people after a severe fright. Wherever there is a perceived threat to life, whether yours or someone else's, Aconite removes the fear and expectation of death or harm and restores order to the nervous system. For this reason, homeopathic hospitals give Aconite as routine emergency treatment for heart attack sufferers and their families, and for those involved in or witnessing terrifying events such as floods and earthquakes, war, rioting and violence, severe accidents and any situation where life is threatened. It calms the injured, the ill and the on-lookers. Aconite has also been used successfully for the treatment of conditions that arise, sometimes months later, following such a fright - conditions such as pneumonia, asthma, heart irregularities or recurrent fevers. In these cases the patient usually tells the physician that he has not been well since the fright, and it is immediately clear which remedy to use.

There are other common uses for Aconite. It is included in first-aid kits for its excellence in treating rapid-onset, acute fevers and inflammatory conditions, such as colds and chills from icy cold, dry, winter winds, pleurisy, asthma, pneumonia, croup, membranous laryngitis, pyelitis, local inflammations anywhere, heart attack, injuries threatening life and generating fear.

History records a typically Aconite situation in the death of Francis Bacon, whose love of science was his downfall. From the diary of John Evelyn, a contemporary, we read: 'He was taking the air in a coach with Dr Witherborne (A Scotsman, Physician to the king) towards Highgate, snow lay on the ground, and it came into my lord's thoughts, why flesh might not be preserved in snow, as in salt. They were resolved they would try the experiment presently. They alighted out of the coach, and went into a poor woman's house at the bottom of Highgate Hill, and bought a hen, and made the woman exenterate it, and then stuffed the body with snow, and my lord did help do it himself. The snow so chilled him, that he immediately fell so extremely ill, that he could not then return to his lodgings in Gray's Inn, but went to the Earl of Arundell's house in Highgate, where they put him into a good bed warmed with a pan, but it was a damp bed that had not been laid in about a year before, which gave him such a cold that in two or three days he died of suffocation.'[52] Such is the rapid onset and extreme severity of the Aconite chill.

The acute Aconite problems, and the acute episodes of chronic disease where Aconite is needed, all have characteristics from the following range:

Fear (of death, of darkness, of bed, night, ghosts, the unreal, the intangible) even to predicting the hour of death. Frights. Anxiety, worry, restless anguish, acute distress, fear or terror; from real life or nightmares; something awful is about to overcome him. Temperature variations - chills and heat flushes.

Clarke[53] gives the following list of Aconite's discovered uses:

Clinical.- *Amaurosis. Anger. Apoplexy. Asthma.* Blindness, sudden. *Bronchitis.* Catalepsy. Catheter fever. *Chest, infections of.* Chicken pox. Cholera. *Cholera infantum. Cold. Coldness. Consumption.* Convulsions. *Cough. Croup.* Cystitis. *Dengue fever. Dentition.* Diarrhoea. *Dropsy.* Dysentery. Dysmenorrhoea. *Ear, affections of.* Enteritis. *Erythema nodosum. Excitement. Eye, affections of.* Face, flushing of. *Fear, effects of. Fever. Fright, effects of.* Glands swollen. Glossitis. Gonorrhoea. Haemorrhages. *Haemorrhoids; strangulated. Headache. Heart, affections of. Hip-joint, diseased. Hodgkins' disease. Hyperpyrexia. Influenza.* Jaundice. *Joints, affections of. Labour. Lactation. Laryngitis.* Liver, inflammation of. *Lumbago. Lungs, affections of. Mania. Measles. Meningitis. Menstruation, disorders of. Miliaria. Miscarriage. Mumps. Myalgia. Myelitis.* Nephritis. *Neuralgia.* Numbness. Oesophagus, inflammation of. *Paralysis. Peritonitis. Phlegmasia alba dolens (acute lymphatic oedema in the legs). Pleurisy. Pleurodynia. Pneumonia. Pregnancy. Puerperal fever. Purpura. Quinsy. Remittent fever. Roseola. Scarlatina. Shivering. Sleeplessness. Smell, disorders of. Stiff-neck. Testicles, affections of. Tetanus.* Tetany. *Thirst. Throat, affections of. Tongue, affections of.* Toothache. *Traumatic fever. Urethra, spasmodic stricture of.* Urethral fever. *Urine, suppression of.* Uterus, prolapsus of. *Vaccination, effects of. Vertigo. Whooping cough. Yawning. Yellow Fever.*

To this I can add: Anorexia. Confidence, loss of. Depression. Eczema. Ego-centricity. Enuresis, by day or night. Heat flushes. History of burns or scalds. Essential hypertension. Mental illnesses.

Hahnemann[54] tells us that all chronic diseases are conditions, first acute, but never recovered from, and that they are only to be cured by the remedies that show symptoms analogous to the original, basic, never annihilated malady. Yet in common homeopathic practice, Aconite is one of the most frequently used acute remedies and definitely the least used, though frequently needed, chronic disease remedy. Confusion has arisen from the observation that Aconite works rapidly and fully effectively, and we are taught that if Aconite has not completed its cure of the acute condition in 24 hours, we must continue treatment with another remedy, that its action is only on the violent acute stage. Fair enough, but in cases where Aconite was needed but never given, life-threatening acute conditions may become suppressed into chronic disorders that bear no apparent resemblance to the original, highly active acute disorder, and in high and especially very high potencies, Aconite is still the remedy of cure for these diseases.

ACONITE IN MEGAPOTENCIES

Let us look at what happens when you face a sudden, life-threatening situation. Your sympathetic nervous system prepares you for fight or flight to enable you to get out of danger or fight off aggression. Less urgent body functions like digestion and urination are slowed down, while blood flow to the muscles is increased and your heart beats faster. Coronary arteries expand, to replace the blood volume in the heart muscle, lost when blood is being sent to the more peripheral musculature to power the escape from danger or conquer the adversary. Increasing the heart's blood supply in this way enables it to stabilize its tachycardia (another result of fright) sufficiently and energise it to pump more blood to the limbs. You start breathing faster, you may feel sweat trickling on your back or forehead, your mouth goes dry, your pupils dilate and your responses and energy are swift and strong to enable you to get out of the way as fast as possible.

All this happens under the influence of the perceived threat, which activates the hypothalamus to set the SNS neurons into gear, releasing epinephrine and norepinephrine (commonly called 'adrenalin') from the adrenal medulla for quick action. Once the threat is perceived as gone, ceased, the parasympathetic nervous system cuts in and tells the neurons to stop the whole process and relax. The neuro-transmitters are gradually destroyed by enzymes.

An acute, severe fever requiring Aconite carries many similar symptoms, with the belief that death is imminent.

The long-term effects of prolonged fear, suppressed fear, are another kettle of fish. What if the fear is a frequently felt part of an on-going life situation? What happens when there never comes a time when you can feel out of danger, no longer at risk? What if you are a child with nowhere safer to go, no-one else to look after you than the person or people you fear? What if you are a woman with a violent, alcoholic husband, or if you live in a war-torn area where danger is always present? Maybe you just live in fear of making someone angry, or of going to Hell if you are 'naughty'. In order to survive, you must somehow convince yourself that it is OK to stay in the vicinity of the fear-source, that it is not going to harm you as much as you fear it may. The fear gets suppressed by the logic brain, the cerebral cortex, which, in the modern world, is very strong.

Let us now examine the chronic heart disease that is so well benefited by Aconite. It stems from very ancient times, when our ancestors had constant need for vigilance and their bodies had powerful survival mechanisms for escaping danger, which we still have today. Fear and fright were translated rapidly into powerful physical action, muscular action like running or fighting.

Fear kills. When fear responses are activated faster than the body can clear away the residues of the previous fright, a situation of over-dose sets in. Technically, the increased output of epinephrine, the body's natural adrenalin, causes a range of changes including a constriction of the peripheral arteries in order to push more blood into the heart arteries. Over the last few hundred years of modern civilization, we have become so intellect-dominated that our logical cerebral cortex has taught us to cancel out the physical activity directed by the fear centre, the amygdala, that activates the adrenals. Our stresses are not always physical threats in the corporate world, in the workplace, school or community. To the Aconite person, to fight or to flee is now to give in to unacceptable emotion.

The inevitable physical result is that, while fear situations still arise, we over-ride them, and the adrenalin (that was released to activate muscle action) which is normally used and gone from the blood as soon as action is taken, remains in the body and its volume is increased with every suppressed fight or flight situation.

Because the Law of Similars applies universally, the unused adrenalin remaining in circulation begins to have an opposite effect on the blood vessels and the heart. Instead of expanding the coronary arteries and constricting the peripherals, it begins to cause constriction of coronary arteries and expansion of the volume of the peripheral vessels.

Continuing to suppress fear equates to continuing to constrict the coronary arteries, with the result that they become chronically unable to supply enough blood to the heart for normal functioning, blood pressure rises and cardiovascular ischemic attacks begin to occur. The very neuro-transmitters that had been generated as a life-saving device become your greatest threat, turning into fear toxins that disturb the normal function of your viscera and brain and cause degeneration of tissue to set in.

It was only after ten years of researching these remedies that I reached the understanding of Aconite as a guilt/fear releasing remedy, and when enlightenment finally dawned, wow! what a magnificent change it made to those to whom I gave it. The reason it took so long was because people who suppress fear, who have strong intellectual minds that can apply logic to override fear and get on with life, usually have nothing to offer when I ask them what kinds of fears they have. They are so successful in rising above fear that they cannot think of much at all, and I found I have to ask them what they used to fear in earlier life.

The answer to this is always the clincher. Such Aconite people always have had some terror in their childhood and youth. Here are the most frequent responses:

'My father. He was always drunk and often in a rage.'

'My father. He didn't hit us but he was very critical and would shout at me if he didn't like the way I did things. Even if I did them his way it was never good enough. I grew up thinking that everything I did had to be perfect and even then it would not be good enough. I live in constant fear of not doing things well enough, so I don't do anything.'

'My father. He must have hated me. He never praised me in any way and all he ever gave was fault-finding and criticism, never affection. I could never find anything to do that would please him. All I wanted was to love him. My parents shouted at each other all the time. It was terrible.'

'My parents were Catholics and kept telling us the Devil would get us if we didn't behave.'

'My father was very demanding of perfection, always critical. My mother had a nervous breakdown and he took us and left her. When he remarried, my step-mother was cruel. She used to keep me out of the house until he came home from work. I used to think my brother and I were part of some kind of experiment to see how much we could take, that one day they'd have the results they wanted and it would all end, but it never did.'

'Hellfire and damnation were big threats. I used to burn myself sometimes, I'm sure it was because of that fear. I am really frightened of bushfires.' (Aconite is a plant remedy closely related to the mineral remedy Sulphur, the brimstone of volcanoes, the burning fires of Hell.)

'I was always frightened to go out in the dark in case the bogey man got me.'

Children whose parents treat them harshly are forced to suppress fear. 'Stop that crying or I'll give you something to cry about' are words a lot of parents say. When a parent can never be pleased no matter how hard the child tries, many such children will give up trying and change to anger and rebellion in the belief they are not loved. Fear chases love out. When parents behave only from love the child never knows fear from that source and will never rebel. The deep sense of lack of love in childhood is often a part of Aconite patients, and it transposes into an inability to love unconditionally, following the pattern set by the parent.

Many people who began life as highly intuitive, psychically sensitive or clairvoyant children have shut down these abilities because they have been told they are making things up, imagining or just plain daft. Guilt allows the left brain to take control and convince them they must be intellectually based in their life. Freeing up this guilt allows them to give these faculties greater expression again.

Guilt over loss of the ability to feel love as a powerful, energising emotion becomes a heavy burden. The out-pouring of love towards others is shut down, replaced by fearfulness and a belief in being unloved. At its extreme this can develop into a recluse attitude, there is a great lack of self-confidence and the sufferer withdraws from society into a lonely situation of his creation, unable to move ahead as a useful part of a community.

127

Life has not shown them that the best loved people are the greatest lovers of people - not that the best-loved people are loved and then love back, but the opposite - they love, then are loved greatly in return. Early life has shown them that even when they love greatly, it is not reciprocated, and their love is suppressed in the presence of too much fear.

Shutting off emotions altogether is a result of trying to protect oneself from this deep sense of grief that there is no love for them. The suppressive person tries to understand life from an intellectual viewpoint, because he has been led to believe this is the way to be, society has said so for three hundred years. But this focus eventually fails because of the extreme imbalance of its head and heart weighting. The result becomes emotional illness. Life becomes dispersonalised to the extreme, for some, of schizophrenic dissociation - detachment from feelings, total devotion to intellectualising in an impersonal manner, dissociation from emotions altogether as life is too painful to be felt and can only be analysed coldly. This is the remedy par excellence for all of the major mental illness suffered nowadays - conditions like schizophrenia, paranoia, bi-polar disorder (manic-depression), obsessions, obsessive-compulsive disorder, many phobias (especially agoraphobia), suicide and voluntary euthenasia.

Paralytic inaction of many forms, indicates Aconite. Four of the first five women to whom I gave it had reached the age of forty without having any children. When I began to see a pattern in this, I asked the fourth why this was so. 'My parents were very religious', she said. 'They put the fear of God into me as to what would happen to me if I ever came home pregnant, so after I was married I found I just never could conceive.' Fear had paralysed the egg release.

When normal fertilisation occurs, cell division and replication is rapid, but when fear is dominant, the processes are distorted causing malformation and spontaneous abortion. Many women living in fear-filled situations have miscarriages for no apparent reason.

Paralytic inaction also occurs in respect to undertaking new business ideas, starting a new job, taking on or being able to complete educational courses, following through on resolutions that could change their lives (such as giving up smoking or alcohol) and many other ways. Physically, inaction occurs, particularly, in the skin, the kidneys, the heart and the bowel.

The fears include fear of the unknown in disease, in giving birth, in going to new places, open or isolated areas; fear of heights and of flying, fear of sudden death by heart attack or of cancer or other deadly ailments, of abuse of any kind, fear of either parent, of reprimand or punishment, fear of men, fear of the dark and of the unseen, fear of entities, spirits, the supernatural and anything that logic cannot explain. Paranoia is common, and phobia for spiders, sharp knives, snakes, deadly animals, sharks and reptiles, as well as burglars and muggers. Doctors and some scientists need Aconite for their fear of anything that might prove their existing beliefs faulty. When all else fails, ignore the facts. Data that does not fit is categorically rejected. Professional sceptics are dead-scared.

With Aconite, there is always fear of reprimand, punishment (on Earth or in Hell) through not being good enough, of physical harm, torture or death, but these are put to the back of the mind.

We need to contrast these Aconite fears with those of Gelsemium, which is another remedy that has paralytic inaction. With Gelsemium, the main emotion is apprehension over anything in the future, which may or may not prove to be a harrowing trial - exam nerves, court appearances, meeting the prospective in-laws, but also over such fear-inspiring ideas as Armageddon, the end of the known way of life, hardship and disasters through powerful climatic changes, earthquakes and tsunamis - which leads to indecision, paralytic weakness in the legs, trembling weakness of muscles generally, double vision, blank thinking processes, brain fevers and occipital headache.

Fears of offending and the repercussions and retaliations of offending, of war, anger and dissention, of the law and authorities, can also cause inaction and indicate Staphisagria.

Fears of being close to others, of crowds, of small enclosed areas, of being trapped, of marriage, of commitments to others, of responsibility all indicate Hypericum.

Grief-fright over losing loved ones, fear for one's own sanity if loved ones were lost, can create hysteria, and then Ignatia is needed.

Fear, panic and hysteria over lack of money is always Conium.

Fears of losing control - of your life, of tools, of animals, of vehicles, of situations, particularly of enemies, of forces and other large bodies of people, of emotions, all suggest Ledum.

Only Aconite people suppress the fear of death.

Suppressed fear paralyses the ribcage causing asthma; the digestive tract causing Crohn's disease; the pancreas causing diabetes; the kidneys causing functional failure followed by damage to tissue; the heart and circulation causing excessive hypertension and risk of clots. The brain suffers disconnections between the cerebral cortex and the fear-reception centres that result in mental illness. The right messages are not being sent, or not received.

Lack of unconditional love when love is craved is the big issue. When parents think it is OK to offer a child judgement, demand perfection, create fear rather than confidence, criticism rather than encouragement, they are doing more harm than they know. The child grows up with a sense of being quite alone, with no emotional support. Receiving no help or understanding creates a huge, black hole of inexpressible isolation that can end up in schizophrenia or bi-polar disorder.

Aconite problems occur in families and societies who worship the intellect above all other faculties. The community or family are sometimes atheist and great respecters of logic, and can be insufferable intellectual snobs. Showing emotions, even love, cannot be allowed, emotions are inferior to mental strength. Such people, when faced with life-threatening challenges, are often the ones who would rather die than seek love-based healing therapies. In such an environment, the Aconite sufferer feels like a misfit, craving love but not perceiving any.

It is our perceptions that count, not the reality. Often, the parents of this kind think they are acting from loving concern, and if you ask them, they reply 'Of course, we love our children. Don't we always try to do our best for them, to instruct them how to be, teach them how to conform to rules and regulations so they can become good citizens?' But there is little communication of love to the child. Remember, fear cannot exist in the same space as love, it simply manifests, screamingly, the absence of a predominant sense of love.

This happens in many subtle ways in today's society. Most people have to suppress fear every time they need to go to the doctor or dentist, or to hospital. In western society, these events have become so frequent, for some people, that they accept them with a sense of pride, and fear is given contempt. It is still there, buried in the body, however well it may have been suppressed - for fear of harm to one's person in such circumstances is a natural part of our survival mechanism. Most of us override the fear with logical arguments like 'It's for the best' or 'What must be done must be endured, I must just get on with it.' But the intuition believes that no amount of harm, however small, is for the best, and it knows that 'the best' cannot result from harmful procedures and practices.

Aconite people are terrified of death and dying, terrified of cancer, terrified of mental illness, too terrified to believe that anything can overcome these all-powerful evils. Therapies that heal are too terrifying to be considered. Life is terrifying. But all this fear is suppressed, over-ridden by the cerebral cortex, the logic brain, which says 'Stop being silly and emotional, you are not acceptable like this.'

Using Aconite helps them reclaim confidence and lose their distrust of things that could heal. It gives them the ability to get on and apply their newfound confidence to the creation of a grand new life. For some it is a long process, but the improvement is evident from the first dose.

When you live in fear for your life, or for a member of your family, over a prolonged period of time, the fear becomes suppressed because you just have to get on with things. The cerebral cortex, the intellectual, logic part of the brain, over-rides the fear. But prolonged fear perception can cause damage to the link between the hippocampus, the fear recognition part of the brain, and the cerebral cortex which keeps saying 'it's OK now, the danger is gone'. While the cerebral cortex is saying 'nothing to fear,' the hippocampus is still creating fear molecules. The production has not been switched off, and the person develops a chronic state of paralytic fear perception. This disconnection causes mental and physical chronic illness.

According to Dr Candace Pert, 'the body *is* the unconscious mind. Repressed trauma caused by overwhelming emotion can be stored in a body part, thereafter affecting our ability to feel that part or even move it.'

Aconite in megapotencies deals with the following chronic effects of fear:

- A paralytic freeze of the emotional processes
- Focus on technical perfection - computers, mathematics, science, accountancy, banking - in order to keep the fear below consciousness by avoiding human emotional interaction. Often they live alone for the same reason.
- Idealism, grandiose schemes, the mind is highly imaginative while the emotions remain untrained. Without the ability to add creative emotional energy, the schemes never amount to anything, the ideas never materialise.
- As a result, we see depression, bi-polar disorder, schizophrenia, psychoses, obsessions, paranoia, or paralytic shutdown of kidneys, lungs, heart, even nerve supply from the brain.
- In the schizophrenic, we find the faculties of the right brain, previously suppressed by the more powerful intellect now disconnected, beginning to rise to consciousness - hearing voices, instructions from God, fearsome messages from the Devil, seeing and being frightened by entities of the lower astral plane. After Aconite, clairvoyance is purified.
- This kind of brain damage can also result from smoking marijuana which can, in the Aconite/Sulphur intellectual, cause the same fear repression and cortex disconnection.

Aconite reconnects the intellectual mind and frees its block on the right brain allowing it to develop creative talents, intuition and eventually, genuine extra-sensory perceptions - clairvoyance, clairaudience, telepathy. Some Aconite patients have these faculties, but they are always distorted and confused by their wildly exalted imagination.

By removing the stored fear, Aconite begins instantly to integrate the left and right hemispheres. All the supression-release remedies do this. I noticed the change more with Aconite than any of the previously studied remedies, probably because Aconite released fears of the unknown, of the spiritual realms, thus making it possible for people to approach and enter into discovering their spiritual selves and their unity with the Universal Intelligence. It has been a great and exciting adventure for them, opening up new healing and self-healing skills and opportunities.

Aconite people, people needing Aconite, are characteristically self-absorbed, self-obsessed. The ego, from perceptions of lack of love from others, seems to feel it has to love itself greatly to make up for the lack. This makes it hard to demonstrate love for others. Psychologists would say this is because of parental patterning of how to be an adult. It is purely from love-deprivation, but it makes it hard for others to love them, they don't allow much room for others to get close enough. 'I know I love him,' not 'I feel great love for him.'

For the Aconite/Sulphur person stuck in the yellow chakra of fear, the intellect dominates life. Intellectual thought is logical, technical, mathematical, rigid, narrow-minded and ego-oriented. The intellect-dominated person, to one degree or another, prides himself on having a 'good brain' that can think things out. Whether his field is literature, law, science, engineering, medicine, technology, business, or just living, ego is big. And with ego comes fear.

Fear is present in such people because our society has given them to understand that intellect is greater than emotion. Our education systems for three hundred years have been focusing on the development of the intellect and rational, logical skills in conjunction with the material and practical skills for living. The trinity of life (Mental, Physical, Spiritual) has only been a duality of mind and matter. Any intuitive skills, emotions, psychic skills have remained undeveloped and untrained and therefore, very erratic and uncontrolled, leading to fear that has resulted in their over-control.

Now that we are into the freeing energies of the 21st century, it is time to get out of society's intellect-dominated base and develop our third great faculty, the emotional/spiritual segment or our totality. Once we lift ourselves as a society, up and out of fearfulness, image consciousness (ego), suppressed love and self-centredness, life will achieve the perfect balance. True intelligence creates the perfect material world from an equally strong heart and head.

My guide, Gonjesil, who, for decades, has been the one prodding me with clues (often missed or misunderstood) to the wider knowledge of these remedies, said 'Fill historically self-absorbed people always with Aconite. Free lots of fears, we think, with repeated doses of Aconite 10MM, interspersed with Sulphur 10MM. Feelings are, this will mightily give them freedom to love unconditionally. Love is suppressed along with the suppressed fear.'

Fear, as I have said, is simply the absence of love. As dark is to light, it cannot exist once love is switched on. Aconite lights up the heart to lift the fearful out of the yellow-bellied solar plexus fear centre into the energies of the heart chakra. Love and intuition are then opened up, and real progress can be made.

Frequently also, Staphisagria is needed to override the conditioning of their Staphisagrian parents and our Staphisagrian cultural impositions. Many will also need Ledum, to help them let go of the past, and forgive.

As a patient, the Aconite person loves to analyse her life as it is impacted upon by others. She needs to tell you all the detail of the day, all her thoughts, and talks without expecting much reply. She is full of fears, and talks a lot

132

about the things she fears, without ever mentioning that she has fear. Her way of dealing with it is to try to find logical reasons for all that is going on, to get the left brain to override the feelings. Consequently, some of these patients have been people who have rung me frequently - even daily - with full reports on what is going on, according to their perceptions.

After years of this, I finally realized that fear was a factor, so I started using Aconite, with such brilliant results that now, when this happens, I am able to suggest they take another dose of Aconite 10MM, which gets them another step closer to true understanding of the way their fear is shaping their reactions. We are finding that the doses are holding well for anything from three weeks to six months, and that total cure of even the worst is possible within a few years.

Notice how most of us are reactive to our circumstances and to others and create our lives in accordance with what we think others expect of us, or what we have been led to believe, reacting to life as our own weaknesses and failings of understanding dictate, rather than with our inner knowledge of who we are and what is best for us. The Aconite ego is very good at denial of Self.

It was only as late as December 2000 that I first began prescribing Aconite 10MM for several patients. One was a woman in her forties, L.M., who had been suffering bi-polar episodes for ten years. I had, in fact, been treating her on and off for over fifteen years, and once we began the megapotency guilt-freeing research, I had had measures of success using Staphisagria and Conium, Hypericum and Ignatia. The bi-polar disorder and the other life-paralysing effects of fear suppression were still a problem, but as she never had talked about fear before, never said the words 'fear' or 'frightened', I had not realized that was a factor to consider.

Finally, on this day in January 2001, she rang and launched into one of her lengthy discourses. This time, it was approaching the start of the school year. She had begun a course the previous year in designing web-sites, and because of her fear-paralysis, had not completed the assignments required. She had been allowed extra time in concession to her illness, but knew that the two assignments had to be in within the next two weeks or she would not be allowed to move on into the second year of the course. She felt guilty over vegetating, feared not knowing enough for success in the website design course, feared getting less than perfect marks, and I suddenly asked 'What's your history of fear?'

L.M. literally leaped at the opportunity to talk about fear. 'Oh, yes, haven't I told you? Massive fear in my childhood, of my father. Nothing I ever did was good enough, I could never please him, even when I did things his way. I became terrified of doing anything in case it got him shouting again.'

I sent her Aconite CM. It saved the day. The next day she woke with a number of acute Aconite symptoms - feeling chilly, even to goose-pimples and this was mid-summer; cold feet, particularly. She had pain in the solar plexus which affected her diaphragm, causing very tight breathing. She stayed in bed all the morning and practised a breathing technique she remembered from the past. She was able to do this until a breakthrough to a moment of supreme peace, after which she could breathe easily. With the dyspnoea went the fear, the 'cold feet.'

She rang me excitedly. 'Guess what? I've just realized, I don't have to do these assignments, I don't want to spend my life sitting in front of a computer, I want to work with people. What can I do, to get into working with people?'

What a revolution! This woman had had her nose glued to the computer screen ever since the first Macs came on the market, she knew the ins and outs of every model and often had helped me sort out my problems. It was all an escape from having to deal with people face to face.

On the second day, she experienced a lot of yawning, sighing and burping and felt sleepy and lazy, still not knowing how to go about getting training in the new lifepath, although she was very keen to begin. On the fifth day, she reported that all dread had totally gone. She began to get lots of dreams of death or harm to others, which went on for a few months. Also, fright symptoms developed in the solar plexus - nausea, griping pains, faintness, which went on also for some time until another dose of Aconite stopped them - a wonderful Return of Old Symptoms.

She was able to describe, now, that every time fear had taken hold of her, she would get a sense of extreme tension in the muscles of the chest, neck, arms and legs, and all these would relax with a dose of Aconite CM. She told me how the bi-polar depression had given her the feeling that she would never get better, that she would lose her mind, and that the fear that she was deranged inside led to her being deranged. When depressed, all her childhood issues would come to the fore and she could not get past them (I had given her Magnesium Lacticum for this, with some benefits). After Aconite, these issues were no longer present in the mind, 'they don't exist now'. She was striding out confidently, where she had been tentative for so long, paralysed into inertia.

Fear of mental illness or brain disorders is paramount among intellectually strong people. L.M. was back in hospital within a few weeks, and I sent some Aconite 10MM immediately I was told. This time the hospitalisation was much more successful, she recovered in record time and spent a lot of her time there helping other patients. That was the last manic episode for two years. Previously, she had spent ten years with very little work, unable to create anything her mind was imaging, living in retreat from life. Now, her confidence was back.

In addition, a ten-year sense of alcohol addiction disappeared. Two months prior to giving L.M. the Aconite, I had prescribed SRQ 10M (spiritus rectus querci, or alcohol from acorns), a few drops several times a day for up to ten days, to clear the effects of alcohol and hopefully, remove her interest. The effect was excellent. 'Amazing benefit,' she had told me on the fifth day, 'I had alcohol cravings all one day, plus *extreme* fear of failure. Then depression, followed by increasing confidence and a sense of being able to do anything required without baulking.'

Interestingly, clearing alcohol effects from her body had brought back the old symptom pattern of fear of not being good enough, that had caused her to use alcohol for Dutch courage. The fear was still there and the cure was not lasting until Aconite was given. Seven weeks after getting her first Aconite, L.M. told me her interest in alcohol had completely gone. 'Furthest thing from my mind,' she said. 'I had a red wine at two different people's homes lately, and felt no inclination to have more, then or at any other time. I'm so relieved.'

Is Aconite a major remedy for alcoholism? One of them, but you must consider Hypericum, for those happy drunks who just do not know when to stop when they are 'having fun', Staphisagria for the nice, innocuous drunks who simply get more affectionate, and for those whose sexual urges go as far as rape once alcohol frees their inhibitions; Conium for inherently dependent people, and Hydrastis, the major guilt remedy for angry violence and the liver damage caused by harming others and themselves while intoxicated. (While there are other homeopathic remedies for alcoholism, these remedies free the guilt and allow the others, if needed, to work faster and more permanently.) The Aconite ones are those who have used alcohol to override their fears and gain the confidence needed to face life.

Image is often a problem with Aconite people. Image consciousness is ego/fear-based. L.M. had been obsessed with image, and all through her illness made preparations for the time when she would be able to run her business as an image consultant, advising companies in getting the best impact from their stationery, logo, all aspects of presentation.

Once she was healing, this began to be supplanted with ideas that were closer to her heart rather than her intellect. Image is a big issue with all ego-based people, and most of the guilt release remedies have some contribution to make towards freeing this up so they can focus on the genuineness rather than the glamour. They may not lose their love of good presentation, but it ceases to dominate their existence.

Immediately the benefits of Aconite began to show forth I found myself prescribing it for numbers of people. In the fifth week of the study, I awoke at 4am with an image of an extraordinary machine in my mind. It was the third time this image had come to mind. It was a rectangular, boxlike apparatus with lots of tubes hanging from it. It changed into a taller, thinner cylinder shape, which I noticed had two red tubes and two blue tubes attached, as would depict arterial and venous blood. I knew that these images were representing a kidney dialysis machine and a heart-lung bypass apparatus.

Aconite relates to heart, lungs and kidneys. Could it be that Aconite is the major fear-release remedy for coronary artery disease and for kidney degeneration? Already stunned by the amazing benefits to the mentally ill, I began to look into the potential for Aconite in these severe, chronic diseases.

Dr Parimal Banerji of Calcutta, who teaches Advanced Homeopathy based on his sixty+ years in the field, uses Aconite 200 routinely for heart attack victims brought into his hospital, and claims it to be more than 80% successful in resolving the attack, without residual damage to the heart.

At the time of my revealing image, five patients had already complained of sharp pain in the lower sternum or heart area. Four had also had pain in one or both kidneys. All five had lived in fear in earlier life: L.M., already described, had developed a paranoia over perfection, and fear of punishment if not perfect in everything she did; the second had been terrorised, according to her perception, by both her mother and her father; the third had been brought up in fear of her father and of the wrath of God; the fourth suffered fear of the dark, of being alone and of men, all her life, and she remembered through a meditation, having been terrorised in a concentration camp in 1940 and finally shot, returning to life in the material world very soon after; the fifth was so fearful of getting pregnant before marriage, because of threats from her religious, self-righteous parents, that when she did marry she was unable to conceive. Only one of these five women had had any children at all, and all were at least forty years of age.

You could argue that fear of punishment is common to all. For the Aconite person, fear of punishment causes inaction, paralytic inability to get anything done, to take the first step needed to achieve anything. It is the paralysing helplessness of absolute lack of self-confidence.

Fear of entities, of the dark forces, and even fear of good spirits was found as commonly as fear of God's punishment. One little boy had been scared out of his wits on waking up in the early morning to see his deceased grandmother sitting on the end of the bed. His lung problems have been greatly benefited by Aconite.

In another case, a farmer who had had benefit from Staphisagria and Sulphur, came in for another pick-me-up just prior to the start of avocado harvesting, a laborious process. He talked of how, in childhood, he, his sister and brother all believed there was a ghost in the home, and they were all frightened about it. His sister says she saw it. As he is a man who bases his life on logic rather than intuition, he now says he doesn't believe in ghosts, but admits there were poltergeist-like effects going on in the house. He had been brought up a strict Methodist, and admitted to no fear of the church or his father, only the ghost. Aconite 10MM and its companion mineral remedy, Sulphur, benefited.

In a third instance, a girl of 13 was brought by her mother for help for her eczema, which she had had since the age of four months, the age at which she had been weaned. She had had many antibiotics all her childhood, for ear infections and tonsillitis, and had had asthma since about six months old. This had mostly left her at age 2 and the eczema had set in more severely since then. It was worse in hot weather, and she would hit her face with both hands as an alternative to tearing at the itchiness. She felt hyperactive, could not sit still. Her fears were of spiders, the unknown, the dark, potential enemies, of worrying her mother by doing anything risky. Her fear ('a real phobia,' she said) also was that someone she loved might die, and this influenced her dreams, in which dangers threatened her family. This lass had been frightened by seeing her deceased grandfather one night in her bedroom.

All this indicated Aconite, but the real clincher came when I asked about her birth. She was born overdue, but was very scrawny. She had suffered malnutrition for a couple of weeks before birth, from a blockage of supply from the placenta. The poor kid was starving and dehydrated. Surely, this was a case of fear for her survival? She has had Aconite in megapotencies every once in a while, with immense clearance of all her problems.

In homeopathy, it has been known since Hahnemann's time that the suppression of skin rashes with topical applications, or with suppressive drugs, would lead to kidney stress and sometimes total breakdown. There is good reason for this. Skin rashes are, in most cases, an expression of toxic material on its way out of the body. The skin is a subsidiary elimination organ (via sweat glands) which is called into extra work if the major elimination organs, the bowel, liver, kidneys or lungs, or all of these, are too overloaded or inactive to handle the amount of toxins needing to be eliminated.

Skin is very clever at this. Relying on no chemical actions, it simply lifts toxic material from its inner base layer out to the surface of the body in the normal progress of skin cell growth and sloughing, a process that usually takes about a month for the lowest of the seven skin cell layers to make its way to the outside. By trapping waste materials between these layers, the body takes the pressure off the already sluggish kidneys or lungs, to give them a chance to catch up. However, while this process may be healthy, it is also itchy and unsightly, and people carry a massive amount of guilt if their ego-image is offended like this.

A skin specialist once told me he 'went into skin' because it was one aspect of medicine where he would be guaranteed patients for their lifetime. He knew he had nothing to offer them that would ever cure their problems. All he could do was try to drive the offending toxic material back into the body so that the skin would look beautiful, but it would be bound to break out again, and he would get another consultation.

Our literature abounds in cases where this has caused death. Infantile eczema, when suppressed, is frequently followed by bout after bout of bronchitis and asthma, pneumonia or kidney disease. Few mothers connect this development to the clearing of the eczema. In one instance on record,[55] the mother had had pyelitis in the later months of pregnancy, and 'was well dosed and injected with various drugs during her stay in hospital, and when the baby came, its scalp was one mass of corruption, but *such* a nice, happy, smiling baby. Soon the skin trouble spread behind the ears, down the forehead, and crept further and further over the face, deep, raw cuts with many crusts appeared and scales formed. The baby was getting on well, gaining weight steadily.

'The mother wept, father scolded, the neighbours jeered, the district nurse, full of the latest medical knowledge, was indignant that the skin should be left in the state it was - and combined public opinion - how few are strong enough to stand up to the opinion, often so wrong, of the herd! The combined pressure took the mother to the skin hospital. Coal tar ointment was applied, the cracks were healed with silver nitrate, and the child's head no longer showed any blemishes. Three weeks later a severe attack of bronchitis followed; two months after, at the age of seven months, the child was taken very ill with albumen in her urine, and was kept in hospital for weeks and weeks.

She never gained an ounce for months after the skin trouble was dealt with so drastically, and what was obvious, too, instead of being a happy, smiling baby she was always fretful and grizzling. At the age of eighteen months she had been in hospital three times with pyelitis, and at age two and a half years she died of inflammation of the kidneys. The mother had been warned in the early days; but she preferred a clean outside and a diseased inside. 'What the eye does not see, the heart does not grieve over'.' (Until too late.)

I had such a case come to me, a woman in her forties, who was being driven mad with an aggravation of her chronic psoriasis. I had given her Hypericum 10MM and a vial of Hypericum 10M, on the grounds that seven brothers and sisters were not speaking to her since mother had died 12 months prior. They had always been close, until then. She felt totally abandoned by them. The Hypericum 10M 'seems to help immensely with the torture I am going through, nearly every part of my body' and she sent for a second vial. However, the skin situation was bad and she was persuaded to go to hospital. Two years later, I was talking to the patient who had referred her, and asked if she knew how the woman was. 'Oh, she died', I was told. Odd, people don't usually die of psoriasis. 'No, it was not from the skin. That cleared up well after the cortisone. No, she developed kidney disease and died after eighteen months of suffering.'

In my own family, my nephew, who had had lots of antibiotics in childhood and also a bad fright at the age of two, developed mild teenage acne. For this he was prescribed Bactrim, a sulfa drug, which he took for six months at the age of sixteen. The drug was finally stopped because it was making him ill, and no longer benefiting the skin. By age eighteen his kidneys were so bad, one totally shrivelled and the other very low in function, that he was soon on dialysis, and the dead kidney surgically removed. Nowadays, I find, the small print that comes with Bactrim warns against taking it for longer than two weeks. At the time, twenty years ago, no responsibility was accepted and genetic inheritance was incorrectly blamed for his kidney problems, they even tried to claim he had probably been born with a shrivelled kidney. Who knows whether this destruction had been initiated even prior to Bactrim, perhaps by the fright, or by the other antibiotics? (But Bactrim has been blamed for kidney failure before.)

Fear for your survival is a common problem among soldiers, who have to over-ride their fear and get on with the job. Aconite has proven to be a mighty resolver of frights suffered by Vietnam War veterans, whose fear was heightened by never knowing who the enemy was (all Vietnamese looked alike, they could not distinguish who was on their own side and who was the enemy), or where he was, the jungle allowed too much proximity for comfort. And I have followed it up with Sulphur, to cleanse the accumulated effects of defoliant poisons sprayed prolifically in that war.

Another aspect of veterans of jungle warfare has been the recurrent sweats created by prolonged dosing of anti-malarial drugs. Elderly men who had been in tropical areas in World War II were still suffering fever recurrences even when they had never had malaria. One Vietnam veteran I remember seeing in 1991 had had lots of anti-malarial tablets which had not stopped him getting a very severe bout of fever in Vietnam, and he was still getting returns of fever with malaise, hot and cold sweats, aches and pains in his fingers and toes, a constant headache behind the right eye and extreme sensitivity of the right side of his head, to the slightest touch.

The homeopathic remedy we always use to clear this effect, whether it is caused by the malaria or by the anti-malarial drugs, is CHINA OFFICINALIS, and I've used it for many tourists with the same drug-induced symptoms. So much for 'preventive' medicine. China (cinchona bark, the quinine tree) cures the problem and completely stops the recurrences, as well as being a safe prophylactic.

Many Viet Vets came back psychologically and chemically traumatised to such an extent that they were unable to sustain any physical effort for long, and could not keep a job. They complain of feeling trapped in a shell, fearful of ambush in busy streets or in crowds, are scared by cars backfiring, by the smell of diesel which takes them back instantly to Vietnam. In an ABC-TV series, *The Brain*, in 2002, we were told that some Viet Vets studied in America were found to have a visibly smaller hippocampus. Constant terror had changed the structure of the brain. The cerebral cortex was not active in the area that usually shuts down the fright responses initiated by the amygdala in response to messages from the hippocampus. They were trapped in the emotions of the past, with a hair-trigger to fear. This is classic Aconite fear.

Many of them found that marijuana eased their trauma - it can cause exactly this same pattern, by damaging the etheric body in the same way as shock trauma does, causing the same brain disconnections as Aconite fixes.

Homeopathy in action, what it can cause, it can also relieve. Over the years, I had found that every Viet Vet I treated had needed Sulphur, which was always a remedy needed for the marijuana users' complaints as well. This was before I realized you could use Sulphur's acute remedy, Aconite, as a mighty important chronic disease remedy.

I have had to treat several children with attention deficit and concentration disorders whose fathers were long-term users of marijuana, and one remedy I have used has been Cannabis Indica, with some reasonable results. Are these children getting the effects of passive pot smoking, possibly via their mothers while they are still in utero? It would seem to me that some children suffer embryonic brain damage in the first few weeks after conception. Does marijuana get through the placenta and also through the blood/brain barrier, which is not such an impermeable barrier as first believed? Does marijuana alter genes, as well? Are these embryonic effects to the central nervous system going to prove genetic?

You will notice that the people who keep using marijuana with the insistence that it is doing them no harm are, frequently, intellectually oriented people who like to reason away any fear of risk. Bravado. They like to ridicule the poor fools who see the damage happening. And, of course, this varies from person to person.

One of my patients, not a regular user, had been given a joint at a party once, which caused all her suppressed fears to surface. She became anxious, jittery and jumpy, ill and sweating, with a sense of only having three days to live. Three weeks later, these fears arose again and led to her having a nervous breakdown. She never used marijuana again but never lost the suppressed fears until they rose to the surface four years later, when she consulted me and received her Aconite. She was on the verge of another breakdown, not coping, not sleeping, had burning urination and a hot, burning sensation in the sides of her ankles and feet. Fear was causing inactivity of both her kidneys and her mind.

Although she had a lot of Staphisagrian features (raised eyebrows, forehead furrowed, contraceptives problems, guilt over an abortion some time earlier and she had unjustly been taken to court) her current symptoms were all Aconite: 'I feel as though I'm about to die. My heart races, I feel nauseous, I'm sweating. The sweats come about four times a day and last for half an hour at a time. Often I only get two hours sleep at night. For two weeks I've been afraid to go to sleep. I'm not normally fearful, would happily hit an intruder to knock him out, but not lately.' This girl's mother had been cruel, belted her a lot, and she had fears still of being punished. Mother had finally left, she felt relieved then. 'I still can't please her,' she said.

When pregnant with her only child, a daughter of three, she had suffered hypertension and toxemia, and said she still gets high blood pressure. I gave her Aconite CM daily for three days, then Staphisagria MM daily for three days, as I knew it would soon be needed. After the three days on Aconite, she rang to tell me of her symptoms - sleeping very well now, but very nervous, trembling in the body, feeling overwhelmed, not by fear this time but thoughts of the abortion were playing on her mind. These were all Staphisagria, and after taking that she settled beautifully.

Many people I have seen in the past need Aconite and I never realized it at the time. If you are one of them, if you recognize yourself in this chapter, get stuck into Aconite now, in 10MM! Your life will charge ahead, believe me, with great confidence and success.

Aconite has also a lot to offer people who have been in violent accidents. While Hypericum types get nerve shock from injuries of violence, Aconite people suffer pain and inflammation which, if not treated homeopathically, can store in the damaged area, latent, for many years. One of my patients, when given Aconite 10MM for more obvious reasons, developed an unexpected return of an old symptom: her ankle, which had been injured coming off a motor bike years ago, became very painful to touch, with limping, and she could hardly walk for a few days. Aconite was clearing out the stored fright of the accident. It made me realize that the commonly used injury shock remedies are not always enough, we need to use the fright remedy as well, after accidents and also after operations.

Bryan and I do a fair number of long distance drives, and to make the journey pass more quickly, we play story CDs. Early in my realizations about Aconite and mental illness, I bought a 'talking' book, *The Surgeon of Crowthorne*[56], read by the author, Simon Winchester. The story describes the life of an American doctor, William Chester Minor, who, early in his medical career, went to the front on the first day of the Battle of Gettysburg, during the American Civil War. The horrors of battle witnessed, combined with the requirement thrust upon him that he be the one to use the branding iron on men deemed traitors - Irishmen who had signed up purely to get a pay-packet and found the slaughter too much to take, who had deserted in fear of their lives, been caught and brought back to camp - threw the surgeon's brain into turmoil.

Minor became paranoid that the Irish were always on his tail to get retribution for their countrymen. His persecution complex stayed with him, manifesting only at night, when the dark held many terrors - the Irish were always around him, hiding under the floorboards, in the ceiling spaces or lurking around the house waiting to get him. He departed America and went to London, and was still besieged by the terrors. One night, he woke to the sense that someone was in the room, about to kill him. He seized his gun and rushed out into the street, saw a man nearby on his way to work, shot and killed the innocent man. Henceforth, he was consigned 'at Her Majesty's pleasure', i.e. for life, to a mental asylum, Crowthorne.

Being a clever, educated, refined and basically gentle man, Minor was assigned two rooms, one of which he furnished as a library, having his books sent over from America. He befriended the wife of the dead man and gave her financial assistance, and in return she would bring him more books from London.

At that time, work had begun on the creation of the Oxford English Dictionary, and an advertisement was put into The Times asking for people to read for the dictionary, to search old and significant works for all the meanings ever used for each word in a specific tiny segment of the alphabetical order, that would be allocated to them, starting from A, Aa, Ab and so on. Minor applied to be included in this collation, and became one of the most prolific providers of words and their meanings in context, contributing to the mighty work over a period of thirty or more years. His schizophrenic paranoia never dissipated, but also, it never prevented him from carrying out his intellectual pursuit to a high degree of excellence. This is typical of the educated Aconite fright sufferer.

I have told you about my first Aconite case, L.M., who suffered from bi-polar disorder until Aconite began to help her step out of it. The second case was a woman of forty who had major difficulties with her partner, always fearing that he was going behind her back, that he was, as a marijuana smoker, always carrying evil entities with him that were undermining her energies. She suffered from fibromyalgia, was addicted to cigarettes and coffee, and suffered great collapse of energy after spending time with her partner, who, she felt, was using deliberate psychic tricks to undermine her life-force. She was convinced for a long time that he was dying, having been told he had motor neurone disease, and sometimes she predicted when this would happen, another Aconite indicator. In addition, there had been major (perception of) lack of love in her childhood. She had been diagnosed schizophrenic after attempting suicide.

It took me five years to realize that her fear was something I could eliminate using Aconite. It seemed that all her problems were within her own intellectualising mind, and I came to believe it was fear of her lover and of his death that had thrown the balance of her mind, so I gave her Aconite 10MM.

The benefit was amazing. After three weeks she rang me again. 'I have had the most amazing three weeks of my life,' she said. 'Every fear I've ever had has come up in my mind to be looked at. I can't believe I've been so *stupid!*' (A typically intellectual judgement of herself - to be 'stupid' is unacceptable to the thought-oriented person.) An opportunity came to attend seminars in a form of life-healing by visualisation, which she did and followed it through by doing the teacher-training as well, which she would not have had the confidence to attend previously.

This woman had been so frightened of life (a victim of her parents' critical, judgemental, Staphisagrian religious hypocrisy and her own fearful, out-of-control thoughts) that she suffered massive guilty terror that healing treatments would kill her, so every time she was given healing, even by Reiki, she would develop violent reactions, swear off the healing and instead, smoke more heavily. She decided that in a past life, she had given healing to people who had promptly died. She believed that she was programmed not to receive benefit from the remedies, and furthermore, could not bring herself to eat healthful foods. As a result, she suffered from anorexia, her fear preventing her even from buying foods that would support life, let alone eating them. Her vitality was ebbing away to zilch. Fortunately, the true genius of Aconite over-rode this destructive belief.

In both the cases described so far, I found that anger was a common outlet for the suppressed emotion. Fear, suppressed, converts to anger outbursts. Anger is not as unacceptable to the Aconite person as fear is, they can allow themselves this kind of energy release when the going gets too tough. L.M.'s manic episodes were all of volcanic build-up of rage, which she would discipline, being a Staphisagria Libran, to the point where her brain would snap, behaviour would get quite out of control and she was usually taken by the police to the nearest psychiatric hospital. Such is the nature of mania.

In the second case, the anger was always directed towards the one she loved, who took it all meekly, lied to say what pleased her and tried to change the subject, which would only make her more angry. Several times she broke off the relationship, found she could not cope with being without him and would be back again in a short time. On one of these separation occasions she tried to end it all with drugs, fortunately rang me before much harm had set in and we were able to get her stomach pumped out. Fear of death had saved her life after fear of life had nearly killed her.

We used Aconite for eighteen months, and her whole life was turned around. Thanks to Aconite, then Staphisagria, the 'helpless victim of circumstances' remedy, which could not do enough for her until the fear of death and wellness was removed, this lovely woman began to take a positive stand for what she really wants out of life. She has now lost the fear of her partner, and through Ledum, has been able to leave him behind and shift into a new freedom. She is totally healed and charging ahead, helping others to help themselves.

The Sydney Morning Herald of November 20th, 2000, printed a report from the New York Times that German researchers had found that mice exposed to radiation during pregnancy (the equivalent of ten medical X-rays) produced pups that, at one month old, showed some evidence of single-strand breaks in the DNA, and at six months, the equivalent of twenty years in human life, there was a significant loss of cells in the hippocampus (which is the fear-reception centre of the brain). The researchers suggest the problem stems from damage to mitochondria, which generate energy for cells. They think the mitochondria are increasingly unable to provide energy to repair the DNA damage. Christoph Schmitz and his colleagues at the University of Aachen think their findings may provide important clues to the development of mental illnesses such as schizophrenia that appear in adulthood.

Mr Schmitz's team wanted to know if events in the womb could account for unexplained mental illness in adults. They told a medical conference in New Orleans of recent reports that children who were born within nine months of the Chernobyl disaster had abnormal hippocampuses They were also more likely to have behavioural problems and were considered to be at high risk of schizophrenia. They warn against subjecting unborn babies to radiation during medical X-rays or intercontinental flights.

I had thought that this Chernobyl effect would have been a result of fright in the mothers, but we do not know whether the mice were frightened by the radiation or not. So we have another potential cause of Aconite problems to add to our list.

The best way to find out what a substance can cause is to do a homeopathic proving on it, and this was done for Radium as long ago as 1904, only six years after the discovery of radium, using the 30th potency, by John Henry Clarke, M.D., whose *Dictionary of Practical Materia Medica*[57] is the one I rely on mostly for the fullest range of provings symptoms. Clarke mentions another proving done by Dr William H Dieffenbach et al and published in 1911 after ten years of investigation. The results of both were similar.

Dieffenbach records that one of the provers, who had developed eczematous eruptions, cracks, scaly excrescences and wart-like outcroppings as a result of previous experiments using X-ray and radium, found these gradually disappeared after the proving using 6X. In the provings of both studies, it was also noticed that naevi disappeared - one of the complaints that the rays are used to destroy, and for which we ought more often to be using homeopathic Radium to eliminate. It is now well known that radium, like X-rays, can cause as well as cure cancer - lupus, epithelioma, carcinoma of the cervix and urethral caruncle. Why use it in toxic amounts when the micro doses cure without harm?

The provings for Radium Bromatum, described by Clarke, contain skin symptoms similar to those of Aconite and even 'sharp pain in the left chest, comes and goes' and constriction of the chest in the heart region, pains, lameness and numbness in the extremities and a general feeling of being 'hardly able to move about, unable to work properly'.

Boericke[58] documents the effects of repeated exposure to Roentgen rays (X-rays) thus: skin lesions often followed by cancer; distressing pain; atrophy of ovaries and testicles; sterility; changes to blood, lymphatics and bone marrow leading to anaemia and leukemia; psoriasis; burns refuse to heal. There are also stiffness, cricks and pain in the neck, fullness and ringing in the ears, general malaise and tiredness. How much of suffering today, of skin cancers and blood disorders, can be attributed to repeated X-rays?

Yes, I would suggest that Aconite is so similar in action to Radium that it can be regarded as an antidote to some of the adverse effects of radiation and X-rays. Generally, homeopaths have simply used Radium Bromatum or X-ray isopathically, with good results, but I believe that when we can find a similar remedy of plant origin we often get wider benefits. The similarities may also account for the fact that some people seem to lose their fear of death from cancer after ray treatment.

Many of the Aconite sufferers I treated were people, particularly women, who had lived a long time alone, either at the time of the consultation or in previous years. Even those in relationships felt quite alone. Somehow, their deep perception of lack of love in youth had predisposed them to this loneliness.

Fear of being left alone is another aspect of this. My first little grandson, at the age of three, spent his days in a kindergarten while mum was at work. It was a good situation as the kindy was opposite the place of work and his mother was able to go and have lunch with him. He became hysterically distraught one day, though, when mum had to go out by car during the afternoon. He saw the car drive off and thought she was going home without him. In no time, his screams and tears had led to runny nose, coughing, nausea, and a temperature. Mother was called in and had to take the rest of the afternoon off to take him home, where he continued to be clingy and miserable until he received Aconite. It quickly restored order after this fright.

An older boy, about ten, had long had a problem of inability to sleep, for thinking about fearsome entities in the dark since he had seen one, years ago, in the bedroom; he also developed boils on his left leg and enuresis, and Aconite was given with benefit.

Aconite proved to be very helpful for another bedwetter, a girl of fourteen who had always had the problem. I have found that in the Aconite cases, some great fright has caused disconnection of nerve cells in the brain, so that the message to the bladder sphincter to keep closed during sleep is not being sent out. In this girl's case, her gestation period had been good but her birth was rapid, and the umbilical cord was wrapped several times around her neck, so that she was going blue by the time she was born. She had been well all her life, only one short-lived ear infection around age three and no adverse effects from immunisations. As a toddler, she had no control over her urine but had learned to hold on consciously - not very helpful once she was asleep.

I first began to treat this girl in August 2000, before I had learned about Aconite and brain damage, so I had given her Staphisagria to stimulate bladder control by increasing the anti-diuretic hormone from the pituitary. It worked well, it seemed, but only for a couple of weeks, then a relapse set in. I looked back on the birth trauma and gave her Arnica, which was of no benefit. Next we tried Calc Carb, a good remedy for self-consciousness and embarrassment, as she had been unable to go and stay overnight with friends or go on camps. This helped for a month or two, but failed, also, eventually.

By this time I had learned of the brain-damage effects of Aconite frights, and thought she may well have been frightened for her survival at the time of birth. I asked more about fears, and found that she was scared of heights, violence, reprimand (though never reprimanded for wetting the bed), and she feared for her siblings, that some harm might come to them. She was not afraid of the dark, she said, but had already told me the previous year that she did not like dark nights. To boot, she had been very frightened recently climbing Ayers Rock, a kilometre high, had only managed to get one third of the way up and her father had to bring her down.

I gave her Aconite CM, which gave some gains, and when it lapsed I gave her MM plus some more Staphisagria, as her eyebrows were looking raised again. She did very well - three weeks totally clear, then two months with only the odd wet night. Aconite 10MM gave a further six weeks clear. We were getting somewhere!

The benefit resumed after Aconite 50M, and she remained free of wet beds until her first period came on five months later. We had a bit of trouble getting her back on track then, until I eventually gave her Aconite 10M followed by Sulphur MM. After two months, another relapse, and despite our repetition of these and then resorting to other remedies, no further gain was made until we went back to first base and gave Staphisagria 10MM and Aconite 10MM. When you are dealing with whole-of-life problems, you must be prepared to be patient.

A mature-age student, one of the childless-over-forty, had consulted me a couple of years ago for anxiety and depression. She had done well on Staphisagria and Ignatia, but continued to have problems getting on with her final thesis. She still had some hot flushes and kidney pains, and various lesser issues. Staphisagria had enabled her to tell a friend she'd been annoyed with her ('pissed off', her words), without causing offense, and this was progress, but she was still prone to anger.

After getting Aconite 10MM, here is what she said: 'I feel really grounded and clear, a great sense of well-being. I'm concentrating on my thesis, and progressing really well. People are telling me I look younger - I really feel alive! I've lost the craving for chocolate icecream, my hot flushes have gone after a quick return, my kidney pain is gone - what a relief! My arm is straightening more fully, my ankle is still a bit sore. People's negative vibes no longer affect me, I can move away unchanged. I feel in touch with my essence, my real self. I had been feeling as if my whole body was on shut-down, on hold and not moving on. When Aconite freed the kidney pain, the whole feeling went. I love the way it works on a spiritual level, real and authentic, giving insights.'

Suppressed fear often comes up as frightening dreams, dreams where life is at risk. One of my elderly patients had reported, before my Aconite realizations, suffering a recurrent dream when in very deep sleep, of choking. The dream would terrify her and wake her, and she would find herself really choking, and would have to sit up and cough it out. The cough, she said, 'comes from very deep down, and it is all very frightening.' These dreams would come on at any time of night. She did not have respiratory problems otherwise. It was possibly an Aconite type of reponse to fear, and shows how swiftly our bodies respond to the emotions even of dreams.

Most of the Aconite patients have reported dreams of harm to others, a death in the family, or of some form of terror for their own life.

When I took Aconite myself (I always take the megapotencies of a new guilt remedy to experience what I can first-hand), after some time a memory came up of something I had completely forgotten. At age five I had been taken, one Saturday morning, by my father to have a tooth removed. In those days, the anaesthetic was in the form of gas. I can remember this as horrendously scary, and I was frightened of anything covering my face for years. I screamed my head off all the way home, a distance of at least five miles through the suburbs, a pathetic little kid in the back of a large car, and my father, who had to drive, was of no comfort.

Surely we all must have some suppressed frights like this?

A young lad of eleven was brought to me in December 2000 after spending nine months sick since a 'viral complaint' which had manifested as asthmatic breathlessness, great weakness, and later swollen glands in his neck. Glandular fever had been ruled out but other viruses showed in the blood test. Later, he developed nausea and headaches and continued to be so weak that he often had to have a week off school. He had dark circles under his eyes, and his vision had suddenly gone from perfect to long-sighted with the virus. There were a lot of Hypericum symptoms - he had a hyperactive, thinking brain that prevented sleep, he had had lots of needle stabs as a baby, and would develop a 'very negative attitude' if not winning, his mum said. He loves music, plays the saxophone and the clarinet in the school orchestra, and is very quick mentally. He also plays lots of different sports. The virus came on after he was told his beloved teacher from last year was leaving the school.

I gave the lad Hypericum 10M followed by his constitutional remedy, the wonderful brain and nerve remedy Phosphorus 10M, as he is quite clairvoyant (a feature of Aconite and Phosphorus patients).

On his return visit five weeks later, there had been marked improvement. 'I could feel the energy flowing through my body', he said, 'especially after I started the Phosphorus.' His mum said he was jumping out of his skin while taking this, and the dark circles had gone away for a while, now returning, as was his tiredness. He still had tight muscles in the neck and shoulders and felt a bit squeamish again lately. He craved sweets and had hypermobile, clicky joints in all limbs, even the shoulders. He was sleeping much better but still waking sometimes between midnight and 4am. At this point I gave him Natrum Phosphoricum 10M, which covers all these characteristics.

This remedy did well, he had a lot more energy and felt more positive.

The new school year was underway and he was very happy there, stronger and more positive and socialising a lot more than last year, and his vision was improving. But the benefit lapsed a little and his right shoulder was very easy to dislocate, he could do it deliberately and loved showing off about it.

People always tell me what I need to know at the time, and his mother then told me how he likes approval, hates getting into trouble and is always on the straight and narrow way (unlike Hypericum). I looked back over his notes and was reminded that he had been born a twin, by Caesarian and eight weeks premature, and the brother was stillborn.

He had felt extremely assaulted by his first immunisation injection. 'Never again,' mum said. He grew well enough and was always very bright. The first year at pre-school was traumatic and he did not enjoy playgroup, too much open space. He loved school for the intellectual aspects but hated the bigness of it. 'He won't do something unless he knows he can do it. And he is fearful at night,' Mum said, 'he came and got into bed with me last night. He is sometimes afraid of non-physical things he sees and hears.'

By this time I had discovered Aconite. On the assumption that he had suffered fear for his survival as a newborn, and the information that he was agoraphobic and had fear of being wrong and of the unknown in the dark, I gave him Aconite 10MM, which completed the cure. He spent the full year at school without losing strength, even though his father contracted cancer and died within six months. When next I saw him, eight months after dad's death, it was to prescribe Ignatia and Natrum Muriaticum for grief effects. Aconite was not needed again.

Essential hypertension is the name given to the condition of chronic, very high systolic and diastolic blood pressure readings. It seems to be that this condition is the direct result of living with a situation of fear, either for your own or someone else's life. Another patient who has a very spastic son was found to have extraordinarily high blood pressure readings, so high the systolic was beyond my instrument's ability to register. It came down to normal within a month of getting Aconite 10MM, and stayed down for eight months. She still has a dose once in a while, as the concern for her son is an on-going issue.

After giving Aconite 10MM to my 'Vampire pit' friend who has developed complications of obesity, blood pressure, heart disease and diabetes after a lifetime of suppressing fears, he came down with a good Aconite flu and was sick for a week. After recovery, the doctor decided that one of the many drugs he was on had been overdosing, and this was reduced. Aconite has this Sulphur-like quality of cleansing out toxic residues from drugs, and may do it by means of a good fever.

Intense fright for your life, if not resolved at the time, can end up threatening your life. I gave Aconite last year to a young man suffering from pneumonia, who had been severely traumatised six months earlier by a gang of thugs threatening to kill him.

Suppressed fear internalises sometimes into the bowel, and we have been getting great results in a case of Crohn's disease, a kind of burning and blistering damage to the linings of the upper bowel that causes abdominal pain and nausea, and frequent loose motions. This woman had had the problem for several years, but since Aconite 10MM, had only a very slight return of the diarrhoea after four months, was given Aconite MM and has improved psychologically and physically, to the point of feeling virtually cured. Her whole life is turning about, with a new relationship as well.

I cannot end this chapter without telling you of the exciting benefits we have stumbled on, using Aconite in megapotencies for people who have been suffering heat flushes. Now, I have to say that it has long been my contention that heat flushes are not necessarily signs of menopause. I have not found any menopausal men yet, but men do get heat flushes, and quite a number of men. They don't like to say so. Aconite 10MM (and/or Sulphur 10M) has totally stopped heat flushes in several intractible cases, male and female - to their great joy.

One of these women had suffered severe, frequent flushes of heat for over a year on any exertion, along with increasing fear for the life and wellbeing of her sister who was spinally weak, on crutches and going downhill with kidney deterioration, facing dialysis. Her fear had brought her into a state of depression and she felt she could not cope, although she was the one her sister depended on and she knew she had to stay strong. Staphisagria helped somewhat, but the fear was the real problem. They lost touch with me while the dialysis training was instigated and the machine was installed in their home, and when I finally heard from them again it was to find a situation quite unenviable.

This woman had become quite hooked on Arapax, a serotonin uptake inhibitor given as an antidepressant. She hated taking it but the withdrawals were worse than the hyped up feelings it caused. We tried using Arapax 10M which helped to counter the side effects but did not alter her fearful depression. I had already seen Aconite stop hot flushes so I gave her Aconite 10MM. On enquiring nine days later, I was told 'Hot flushes, what are they? Depression? Gone, gone. I feel wonderful!' We had already started her sister on Aconite and other remedies for her complex problems, and things were looking as though they might start looking up all around. Depression came on again four weeks later, with a repeat of anger, impatience, intolerance and a feeling of going mad, and another dose of 10MM set her back on track overnight. When this lapsed, we used Sulphur MM.

Fear is introspective. It can cripple the fearful one and leave him unable to put love out to others, he can only see his own self. Fear and ego go hand in hand. All who are self-obsessed need Aconite to clear their fears away and free them up - free them to help the world engage in the great planetary cleanup under way this century. Self-healing is the first major step to take. The self-absorbed person is always looking for influences that affect him, whether friendly or harmful, and is in a prime position to start getting the extraordinary benefits of Aconite.

When a parent behaves to a child in a manner that frightens, love is crippled then in the child, as it had been in the parent. Break this cycle with Aconite and fearless love returns. Use Ledum if necessary, for forgiveness, afterwards.

Crippled functions and crippled minds may need Aconite to free them from paralytic inaction. Thinking is greatly improved, and handicaps in speech and communication are loosened up, when problems have arisen from fright - for example, one man I know of lost his fluency of speech and has stammered, ever since, as a child, his twin brother died of an asthma attack. Aconite would fix this.

The people who need Aconite seem to be basically very spiritually conscious people whose expression of spiritual ideals has been restrained by the paralysing effects of fear. As fear is the opposing emotion to love, while fear dominates, love is crippled into inaction. It is an intellectual thought only, with no true feeling. Freedom from fear brings the opportunity for loving intentions to become reality, and for love to be a real, heart-felt sensation.

Suffering gives knowledge. Once the fear is released and love replaces it, the previous suffering directs the new, strong person outwardly to areas where he can lovingly assist others to heal themselves. 'Been there, done that, and there is a way through it!'

The Pakistan People's Party Leader, the beautiful Benazir Bhutto, daughter of Pakistan's first Prime Minister Zulfiqar Ali Bhutto, was a shining example of positive Aconite. She said[59], 'I am often asked the question, 'What's the difference between men leaders and women leaders?' I think men go into politics because they love the power, whereas women do it for the approval of the people. I would rather rule by love. I'm always accused of being too forgiving, but then, I don't feel the need to instil fear.

'Men think you've got to take revenge because then you will be feared. That's what the current Prime Minister is doing, he's taking revenge against me for having once beaten him at the polls. He's taking revenge against bureaucrats and businessmen who helped run this country smoothly, and that's a very male mentality. I can't speak for the world, but I can speak for Pakistan. The theory that operates here is that fear intimidates and fear commands respect. But I've never felt the need to take an action that would intimidate.' (Unfortunately, assassins caught up with her.)

Another historically well-known visionary Aconite figure was Joan of Arc, Jeanne d'Arc. Clairaudient and clairvoyant, Jeanne had received word from Saint Catherine and Saint Margaret, at the age of only 13, that she was destined to lead the French army in ousting the English and thus end the Hundred Years War. The English had held the city of Orleans under seige for six years when Jeanne, at age 17, through the force of her supremely confident personality, persuaded the Dauphin to allow her to accompany his forces and lead them into a successful storming of the city. By this time she had had numerous visions and instructions and was able to impress many with the accuracy of her predictions. Fearlessly, a slip of a girl incited such renewed courage and determination in the demoralised French that they were able to free the city and put the English to flight.

Thanks to her visions and Voices, Jeanne knew how things were going to turn out and was never afraid of the task ahead of her. 'Lying in bed at Orleans on the night of April 29th, 1429, she knew some things for certain. She knew she would relieve the siege; she knew she would be hurt; she knew she would not die. She knew she would lead her Dauphin to Reims for the supreme ceremony of his coronation, a consummation overdue for seven years, since Charles VII had succeeded his father in 1422. She knew all these things, because her Voices had told her about them, and her Voices were not to be discounted or disbelieved. ... These things lay before her.'[60]

Having fulfilled her prophetic instructions from God, Jeanne lost a good opportunity to completely decimate the English by refusing to enter battle on a Sunday. After seeing her king crowned, she lost her fire and sank into months of tame submission and compliance, no longer able to maintain the enthusiasm of her troops or the King, and when the English joined forces with the Burgundians to defend their hold on Paris, the King turned his back on the city. While still fearlessly militant in her ideals, Jeanne's practical confidence was gone and her Voices were silent. Such is the switching nature of bi-polar depression. Finally, she was captured by the enemy. Her Voices returned, but she paid no heed now to their advice and wilfully tried to escape by fearlessly jumping from a castle tower rather than be sold to the English. Unharmed, she was nevertheless knocked out and failed to make her escape.

Political leaders at the time were strongly influenced by members of the Roman church, who were still engaged in the Inquisition and relentlessly seeking to destroy anyone who had knowledge of God or of healing that varied from the dictates of their Papal rulings. Jeanne was captured and brought to an iniquitous trial, not on a charge of high treason against the King of England and (in their sight) France, but on a charge of heresy, blasphemy, idolatry and sorcery. Although the trial lasted over a month, with an extraordinary number of witnesses for and against, Jeanne was convicted of being a witch and a heretic and was burned at the stake, fearless and spiritually attuned to the end, thus rendering her a martyr and a heroine forevermore. In a strange reversal of belief, the same church canonised her as a saint in 1920.

There is no record in what is known of Jeanne's childhood, of any bad fright or prolonged fear that could account for her visionary states as schizophrenia; not to say that there was nothing, given her instruction in the Catholic faith that, particularly in the 15th century, ruled by fear while demanding faith and obedience. No, from her own and others' accounts at her trial, she was a girl of the utmost trust and confidence in the word of God that promised victory, and it was this singlemindedness that had inspired her followers.

Although, initially, she had been through some period of disbelief that such a lowly soul as herself should be expected to save the country and crown the rightful king, she kept silent about her secret mission throughout the years prior to her actualising of the dream. In her personality, the forcefulness of her inner direction was maintained, never diminished for all that time. This may be regarded as obsession today, but unlike mental illness, there were no sinkings into depression and doubt, no lapses of self-confidence, until after the main predictions had been fulfilled.

This, I believe, is where the Aconite sufferer can expect to be, once converted from fear to faith and confidence by this magnificent remedy - able to push through to a glorious fulfillment rather than be paralysed into inaction by the inner fear.

Nowadays, the intellectualism of medicine and psychiatry has given the term 'schizophrenia' to anyone who hears voices, as if clairaudience is necessarily a medical illness of the brain. It certainly can be associated with damage in the brain, as is often seen in those who tell us that, under the effects of (anti)social drugs like marijuana, God told them they must kill or commit some other mischief. We must learn to draw a line between spiritual awareness and drug- or accident-induced psychic hallucinations and brain damage resulting from fear. We know that God, or Good, does not incite people to harmfulness, but certainly can incite them to the dedicated pursuit of an ideal. My observation is that many people through history have been spiritually open to visions and voices or music, giving them enlightened knowledge and instruction from their inner at-one-ment with the universal pool of knowledge. We often call these people geniuses.

Fred Alan Wolf[61] postulates that for schizophrenics, somehow the electrons of the brain's atoms could be spinning so fast that consciousness could be shooting into a black hole and entering a parallel universe, an altered state where the individual experiences a reality different from 'groundedness.' It would seem to me that this is what happens, also, when the bi-polar person switches from depression ('spinning' too slowly) to mania, a 'spin-out.' L.M. always talked of her manic episodes in this way, she could see herself as from outside and tell me what would be happening whenever she felt herself starting to spin out, and how it would speed up beyond her control. After Aconite, she learned to nip it in the bud, and quietly focus on calming the brain by meditation, music and affirmations. When Aconite had run its course, Anhalonium continued the improvements.

Wolf says, 'If we could enter an electron, we might see just the kinds of things that might be seen when entering a black hole as predicted to exist by general relativity. So far, this is just a speculation, of course. If true, then it would be very possible to witness other worlds by somehow tuning in to our own electrons.' In this way we can also communicate with the past and the future. Is this a hint of an explanation for clairvoyance and clairaudience?

Inner peace is the profound benefit of Aconite. Living in a state of fear, whether this is simply an individual, personal condition or fear suffered by a mass of people as a result of political conflict, terrorism or major calamity, it is impossible to experience any sense of peace or true joy. When fear dominates, love for others on a broad scale is overshadowed by love/fear for oneself and one's family. In countries where life is threatened frequently, where terrrorising is a tool for power, there is little love-in-action to be seen. The terrorised person never ceases to crave the love that is missing from his outer life, and the peace that is missing from his mind.

Humanitarian ideals are always in the hearts of the Aconite sufferers. Free the inner terror, free the suppressed fears, heal the effects of fright and watch the miracles of inner peace and joyful confidence shine forth. Watch the fears created by doubting intellectualism fade away in the light of intuitive knowingness, and see a new wave of spiritual understanding flood through the governments of the world, the churches, the schools and the universities, the repositories of knowledge and initiators of research.

Great planetary healing will be effected by this remedy. Fear is everywhere, at all levels of education and development. Millions are waiting to be set free - and once enough are freed from fears, watch out! The world will become a very different place!

CHAPTER 8

For touch, touch, by the holy powers of the Gods! is the sense of the body.
- Lucretius, in 'De Rerum Naturae'

ARNICA - 'I'M OK, I'LL BE RIGHT'

Arnica (arnica montana, *mountain daisy*, Asteraceae, N.O. Compositae) is found on mountain slopes all over the globe - the Andes, the Central European Alps, in Northern Asia and Siberia, and even in Australia's Snowy Mountains. In Germany it is called 'fallkraut', the plant for falls, because of its excellence in reducing swelling and bruising after falls and twisted ankles, and blows from any broad or blunt source. It is seldom used internally, because of its irritating effect on the stomach walls, but was sometimes used as a tea for low-grade fevers (like typhoid) and paralytic affections.

Max Wichtl[62] warns against its oral use and lists the side effects as 'gastro-enteritis, dyspnoea leading to cardiac arrest and death, due to slowing down of calcium transport out of the heart muscle. In prolonged external use, the tincture can cause oedematous dermatitis, with the formation of small vesicles. Hypersensitivity can occur in those sensitive to other members of the daisy family such as chamomile, marigold or yarrow - the allergy symptoms being painful, itching and inflammatory changes in the skin.'

Arnica was first mentioned in literature in the writings of Saint Hildegard of Bingen[63], who was born in 1099 and placed in seclusion with a holy woman in the Rhenish mountains at the age of eight. Here she was taught music, theology, medicine and natural history at a time when the knowledge of the ancients had been all but lost to Europe. Hildegard was a seer, claiming that many of the statements and sayings in her writings were revealed to her by angels. Her reputation spread all over the continent and she became a very powerful woman whose inspired wisdom was sought by the royal houses of numerous countries; she was later canonised by one of the Popes.

St Hildegard, through a life of prayer and meditation, was able to break through the veil which hides the life of the spirit and the secrets of nature from those whose vision is limited to the coarse, everyday happenings of the physical. She has long been vilified by the modern, materialistic scientists, but her truths and the beauty of her inspiration can no longer be denied and are once again becoming available - firstly through her music and now, also, some of her writings are translated into English and in print.

The virtues of Arnica were highly commented upon by this holy woman. Later, in the sixteenth century, a Professor Joel in Goettingen was the first medical man to recognise its importance as a healing herb, but it remained a folk remedy for the most part.

Ellingwood found that 'In sufficient dose, it causes vomiting and catharsis. It is also diuretic, diaphoretic and emmenagogue. In poisonous doses, it causes a burning sensation in the stomach, intense headache, and violent nervous disturbance, with marked abdominal pain. The pulse is reduced and often fails. There may be convulsions of a bilateral character, and ultimate death.' Nevertheless, medicos used it internally as well as externally for bruised, sore, lacerated, contused muscular structures, whether from disease, childbirth, injury, over-work of muscles, surgical fevers and shock. These extended uses were gained from homeopathic provings, but those doctors were too blinkered to potentise the tincture to a more powerful, safer medicine and get greater, faster benefits.

In modern herbal medicine, Arnica is only used externally, as diluted tincture or ointment, and only on unbroken skin, for its benefits on swelling and bruising, sprains and strains. However, its benefits are greatly extended and more powerful when taken internally in the homeopathically potentised forms.

ARNICA IN HOMEOPATHY

Seven hundred years after Hildegard, Hahnemann proved Arnica as a homeopathic medicine and it has become the must-have of all homeopathic first-aid kits throughout the world. It is one of the few remedies in homeopathy that can be given in any case of injury, without the detailed observation of symptoms and signs needed generally, and in the vast majority of cases it will give relief. This is the one remedy above all others that could be used (and is used, in many countries) for every patient undergoing surgical, dental or any other forceful procedures, anaesthesia, and for the relief of shock in emergency wards, ambulances, the home, the workplace and sporting fields everywhere. Yet orthodox Western medicine still has not appreciated it. How blinkered can you be?

No-one who has experienced Arnica would go into these situations without it. Even many who fear causing displeasure to their doctors will sneak the Arnica in and get the benefit of it, and enjoy the surprised looks of the uninitiated when they see the rapid improvement.

I mentioned spurious research in Chapter 4, and another example of this has recently come to light, in which, in a British study[64], Arnica was given to 62 patients undergoing wrist operations and their recovery measured against a group taking dummy pills. The result showed 'no significant differences' in pain levels, bruising or swelling. Of course! Arnica works on the body of the muscle, and the wrist contains only bones, tendons and ligaments, no muscle bulk. Arnica works on the damage to the muscle body from blows by blunt instruments, not on the painful spillage of blood by a sharp scalpel, for which you need Staphisagria, or the cutting of tendons, for which Ledum might be needed. Come on, lads! Try again! After 2 weeks of therapy, those taking Arnica felt 'significant reduction in pain', which, in my opinion, had no relationship to the Arnica, which always works immediately when it is appropriate to the injury.

I often think of Arnica as the homeopathic ice pack. It has the same kind of benefits as an icepack gives when applied to sprains and muscle injuries - strains, bruises and corks. But it works much faster, resolving the shock aspects while resorbing spilled blood from damaged blood vessels (bruises) and fluid leaking from damaged joint capsules into the surrounding tissues. The following list from Clarke gives you an idea of its extensive uses:

Clinical.- *Abscess. Apoplexy. Back, pains in.* Baldness. Bedsores. *Black-eye. Boils. Brain, affections of. Breath, fetid.* Bronchitis. *Bruises.* Carbuncle. *Chest, affections of.* Chorea. Corns. *Cramp. Diabetes.* Diarrhoea. Dysentery. *Ecchymosis (blood-blister).* Excoriations. *Exhaustion. Eyes, affections of. Feet, sore. Haematemesis (vomiting of blood). Haematuria (blood in urine).* Headache. *Heart, affections of. Impotence. Labour. Lumbago. Meningitis.* Mental alienation. *Miscarriage. Nipples, sore. Nose, affections of. Paralysis. Pelvic haematocele (blood-filled cyst or tumour in the pelvis). Pleurodynia (rheumatic pain in the ribcage). Purpura. Pyaemia (fever). Rheumatism.* Splenalgia. *Sprain. Stings. Suppuration. Taste, disorders of. Thirst. Traumatic fever.* Tumours. *Voice, affections of. Whooping cough. Wounds. Yawning.*

To this list I can add: Anaesthetics, effects of. Bladder weakness. Coma. Concussion, semi-consciousness and unconsciousness. Restless, disturbed sleep from soreness. Encephalitis. Gout. Golden Staphylococcus sepsis. Shock, traumatic. Thrombosis. Transient ischemic attack. Traumatic amnesia. Vertigo.

Arnica is one of the first homeopathic remedies anyone ever learns about. Its use in the household and traveller's first-aid kit is widespread, being the first remedy thought of in times of any injury. My own family often had need for it, as most children do.

Back in 1975, my second son, Wade, at age two, fell from an upstairs balcony to the brick paving below, landing on his front. As I ran down to him, he was already picking himself up, yelling loudly. An egg-sized swelling was developing on his forehead. I gave him a dose of Arnica 30 and took him to my bedroom. Ten minutes later, he was still yelling, so I gave a second dose and he relaxed and fell asleep. Three hours later he awoke, bright and cheerful, no sign of the 'egg-head', and no bruising. It was as if nothing at all had happened, and he returned to play with the other children.

My elder son, Rowan, at age 28, was riding his motor bike home one night on a country road when, turning a bend, he was confronted by a few cattle on the road. Swerving to avoid them, he crossed a ditch and ended up in the nearby paddock, somewhat battered and unconscious. A following vehicle saw the accident and called an ambulance, and I received a phone call around midnight - 'Mum, can you come and get me out of here, and bring the Arnica!' Current policy is to keep all head injury patients in hospital overnight for observation in case of slow haemorrhage in the brain. I had to sign a release form, the staff were very reluctant to let him go. However, the Arnica 10M did its usual wonderful work and all risk was averted. (Why don't all hospitals use it? In addition to the obvious benefits, it would prevent Golden Staph from developing if given routinely after surgery.)

I remember, before I learned of homeopathy, I was influenced by the 'wisdom' of a senior ENT specialist to have my tonsils out, at age 24. The effect of the anaesthetic was so prolonged that I remember to this day the delerium I experienced, trying to regain consciousness. I kept tossing about the bed, drifting in and out of awareness, and in typical Arnica form, was able to drag myself back just long enough to comprehend and obey instructions from the nurses and conk out again. It was hell, I really hated being in this no-man's-land and could do nothing except live through it, struggling for three hours to pull myself together. The whole experience was designed, I now see, to show me how it is, to be now in and now out of your body, in that place called limbo, and not be able to wake up fully. If only they had given me Arnica in the Recovery ward! It works so fast in such circumstances.

Arnica, as it repairs shock damage to the etheric body, causes broken blood vessels to stop bleeding and speeds the breakdown of the escaped blood cells - the bruise - into their component parts, which are then taken back to the spleen to be used in making new blood cells. Arnica prevents clotting and stops haemorrhage, thus reducing the after-risks of injuries, as particularly head injuries can be fatal if these factors are not eliminated. Shock from jarring, falls and blows causes the physical body and the non-physical, etheric and astral bodies to part company, causing unconsciousness (if partial) or death (total severing of the silver cord connecting the physical and non-physical bodies). While the silver cord is still intact, the patient is alive and unless there is too much tissue damage, can still be brought back to consciousness, even after months in a coma. Arnica acts as a magnetic bridge to ensure that the subtle bodies realign perfectly with the physical.

I was once asked to help a boy of 18 who was in hospital, three months in a coma, after a car accident. He had been driving, and his passenger, his grandmother, was killed when the car collided with another vehicle. I sent one dose of Arnica M, the pillule to be slipped between his lower lip and the gum. He regained consciousness within 24 hours and was soon sent home, physically well.

When I ran my ten-week first-aid class back in 1985, my eyes were opened to the wider magnificence of this remedy by one of my students. This lady was a simple, uneducated soul with a heart of gold. She worked at the local hospital as a menial, an aide, a tea-lady or some such job, and was therefore in contact with quite a lot of people.

After the course, I often ran into her in the shopping centre, and she would enthuse greatly on the benefit Arnica had given to one person or another to whom she had given a dose or two. The problems ranged from cough to headache to flu to backache to hangover to palpitations to ... you name it, she gave *everyone* Arnica, and they all got better! It was the only remedy she remembered from the whole ten weeks. I used to go home bemused, and check out the textbook for the complaint she had mentioned, and sure enough, Arnica covered it, though the remedy is only thought of, generally, for a limited range of issues. I owe a lot to this great woman, who taught me to cut through the complexities of detail in homeopathy and keep it simple. She was the first to make me realize that homeopathy need not be difficult, confusing or complicated, and as a result I have spent many years seeking to clarify the common remedies. They say in marketing, eighty percent of your sales come from twenty percent of the existing clientele. In homeopathy, more than eighty percent of cases can be handled by far fewer than twenty percent of the remedies.

You can think of using Arnica in low or medium potencies for injuries and illnesses of the kinds mentioned, affecting any part or all of the body: for the headaches and bruised soreness of passive jarring as from travelling in or on a vehicle or on horseback, the swelling of the gum after a dental extraction, the exhaustion and muscle soreness of prolonged gardening, sports training, fitness exercises, being on your feet too long, jogging and marathon running, mountain hiking and climbing; lifting and carrying little children, schoolbag, or the shopping, lifting heavy weights in your job, e.g. in carpentry, farming, labouring; truck driving and heavy implement handling where the arms are kept out in front of you, pulling all day on the steering; jarring to the eardrums from loud noise, and even for the head symptoms of a hangover, where alcohol has separated you somewhat from your physical self, and the room spins when you put your head to the pillow and close your eyes.

Any of the above can give you characteristically Arnica symptoms of, among others, the bed feeling too hard, the head feeling as if a nail was pushing out through the skull, the bladder sphincter is weak and exertion causes leaking, or the injured part is very tender to touch - fear of being touched.

From the list of named complaints previously given, you can see that it is not the name that matters but the cause. In every case needing Arnica, there has been some degree of dislodgement of the non-physical self from its correct alignment with the physical, whether of the whole body or only a small area, usually by jarring from falls, blows or travel, exhaustion of

158

muscles, sometimes from the use of anaesthesia or other drugs, or the shock of surgery. And it matters not, how long ago the trauma occurred.

The wonderful art of osteopathy has at its foundation, the first dictum of its founder, Andrew Taylor Still, 'Structure Governs Function', and his second dictum which is, 'The rule of the Artery is Supreme.' Chiropractors like to argue that Still's third dictum regarding 'the Integrity of Nerve Supply' should be paramount, that the central nervous system is the first and main area of consideration in creating and maintaining health.

In placing the blood supply in the higher position, Still was considering all the qualities and functions of blood. Blood is the carrier of life around the body. You can be brain-dead, have no measurable brain activity, yet while the heart still pumps blood, the body can remain alive, as life-support machines have demonstrated. Some people have returned to consciousness after months in a dead coma, even when brain impulses had not been registered. The heart has its own pace-maker nervous system, separate from the CNS, specifically so that if anything happens to the general nerve supply, the heart can still keep beating. This fact in itself must prove that the body itself, in its very design, values the blood most highly.

By the same token, a remedy whose primary action is on the heart and circulatory system and the construction and reconstruction of blood cells has to be one of the most valuable remedies in the world.

ARNICA IN MEGAPOTENCY

The one feature that has been known about since Hahnemann did the first proving is the strange sensation of being quite all right, even when quite ill or badly injured. 'I'm OK,' they say, 'If it were not for this (whatever the complaint), I would be perfectly all right. Don't worry about me, you see to someone else.' It was this feature that showed me the real guilt behind the prevalence of Arnica problems.

The main benefit of using megapotencies is to get to the guilt behind the chronic disease so that even the most intractible complaints get a chance to be set on to a path towards healing. For, while most people can benefit from Arnica at the time of an injury, not everyone who has an injury develops a chronic problem (one that is not self-healing). This develops when the guilt is great. From the previous paragraph, you can see that the bruised and battered person feels guilty that he or she has not been tough enough not to be hurt by a mere blow or fall, or whatever is affecting him. He does not want to admit that he is soft, sick or wounded. He believes it is a sign of weakness, and if male, a sign of not being masculine enough, if he cannot take all of life's blows without moving a muscle, without a flinch, so he keeps asserting he is OK.

'Life wasn't meant to be easy', former Australian Prime Minister, Malcolm Fraser, said - but it *was*! Life *is* easy, once you know how to play it.

It is wonderful little Arnica that is going to free the world, in time, of great guilt over soft-heartedness. In the Arnica mind, it is unacceptable not to be tough. This idea gives some of them the foolish belief that it is also not acceptable to be kind-hearted, that this is only a weakness. Many an Arnica person thinks you have to knock people into shape, be cruelly hard on children (including corporal punishment) to harden them up for the knocks that life will offer them, as if emotional scar tissue is a strong preparation for life. 'Life is tough, and you might as well know it from the start.'

Touch, especially loving touch, is essential for life. Ashley Montagu (in *Touching*) describes how orphaned babies dumped into uncaring children's homes and left in their cots all day without handling or touching from other humans except to be fed and changed - given no love - simply withered and died. Touch is the most powerful proof of love.

More recently, scientists were removing baby rats from their nest, handling them for a while and then replacing them. Within a week each baby rat showed signs of a sudden increase of intelligence. The scientists put it down to the observation that the mother rat had spent a lot more time grooming them after the separation than she had before.

It presents a warning to parents not to leave their babies lying alone and unhandled if they want intelligent, well adjusted children. Children who receive no loving handling will play up on their parents 'to get attention', as even unkind touch via a smack is better than no touch at all.

The enlightened Arnica (having received his megapotencies) learns to be firm, kind, able to discipline and teach children without bullying, able to keep order in a community without police brutality. There is a mental toughness that Arnica imparts that enables you to stride purposefully through life without fear of being harmed by it. You give up on feeling bruised by life's knocks, all that happens in your life is taken in your stride and you lose the need to feel you must be tough. Life ceases to be a series of knocks and blows and becomes smooth sailing. You have learned to live without having to prove how tough you are, you are it, you know it and you love it. At this point, kindness is freed up and you can fearlessly be as kind as you like, able to 'love your neighbour as yourself.'

Typical Arnica thoughts often expressed are: 'It does you good to get a good belting now and then,' 'I'm OK, there's nothing wrong with me,' 'Life is tough, you just take it and get on with things,' 'If I didn't have this bad heart (or whatever problem) I'd be perfectly well'.

Arnica parents: 'Stop that crying or I'll give you something to really cry about'. 'A good beating never hurt anyone.' 'Only silly girls cry, stop being a sooky baby.' 'You get better respect once you have knocked them into shape.'

Our former NSW Premier, Neville Wran, is well remembered for his quip, 'Balmain boys don't cry,' inferring he was like the tough footballers of his Balmain constituency. Football players, particularly in Australia, love to play rough. Rugby is a game that requires constant tackling, bumping, jostling, jumping high and landing hard. Muscle injuries are an expectation in every game, and many players suffer injuries to other parts, cartilage tears and head blows being commonplace. Every year someone dies from one of these, who would not have died if Arnica had been given on the field.

Physical strength is often socially important to Arnica, especially teenagers. This is the remedy for thinking that it is strong muscles that give you sexy desirability - 'Mr Universe'. It is the main reason for their great love of all the sports where muscle is more important than brain. The majority of Olympic sports are of this type. And a lot of young people, girls and boys, feel that strength is a necessity for manliness, and that a slim or puny body will never attract a good partner.

The male of the species has a lot to learn about women, doesn't he? Because for most women, a big heart and personal integrity count for a lot more than the temporary worth of youthful strength and vigour.

Toughness also predominates over inter-sexual relationships for the Arnica male, and this young man spends his leisure time 'with the boys', drinking or playing men's games, doing men's work, the girls hanging on if they wish but not missed if absent, and not welcomed into the male domain. Often this is made explicitly and rudely clear. In Australia, this means that for most of our history, at social events the men congregated at one end of the room and the women were ignored, forced to chat together at the other end. Talking to women was thought to be lapsing into softness and gentleness, and this was not to be done in front of your mates!

They must continue to prove how tough they are, even if it kills them. For many, their childhood has been devoid of physical touch of an affectionate or approving kind. Hugs and embraces were forbidden, being 'only for women and girls - sissy stuff'. Only on the field, the opportunity is there to combine the demonstration of toughness with physical contact. They rough each other up, then the winners or point-scorers get embraces and pats on the back, hugs and even, I have seen, kisses! from their team-mates. Their soft centres are allowed, only on these occasions, to be seen through their hard shells. It is the only time the excitement, the emotion of the moment bubbles up to over-ride the intellectual guilt of having loving feelings. For once, the left brain gets drowned out by the heart.

A friend told me how, when he was at a country agricultural high school, football was played five days a week. There were tough boys and even tougher teachers. The tough kids paid into a collection every time they got the cane, and at the end of term, the one who had had the most cuts of the cane collected the lot.

Bryan gets a lot of footballers coming in for treatment. By observing and comparing, we learned a great deal about Arnica. One of the most interesting observations was that after we had given them a good dose of Arnica MM,

161

not only did they cease to attract the Arnica types of injuries but in many cases, where age was really starting to tell on them, they were able to give up on the need to get a good thrashing, hung up their boots and retired from the game. They invariably commented, 'I decided I didn't need to be knocked about any more.'

We also found that in young players with acne, often a staph infection, Arnica MM caused them to get fewer blows, and also improved their acne!

Taking Arnica converts the fear of not being or looking strong and tough into self confidence and knowledge. The eyes are opened to a new way of looking at life. Boasting of one's strength or admirable musculature is forgotten and the mind is free to allow true strength through the whole body.

Researchers published, in 2002, their investigation into the long-term effects of head injury. In one study[65], old soldiers who had been hospitalised for a range of injuries were reviewed. The researchers found that the risk of depression remained elevated for decades following head injury. The risk was highest in those who had a severe head injury.

A second study[66] reported a strong correlation between head injuries as a young adult and the development of Altzheimer's disease fifty years later. Those who had experienced a loss of consciousness or amnesia for less than 24 hours after the injury were twice as likely as the general population to suffer Altzheimer's; for those who stayed out for a count of 24 hours or more, the risk was quadrupled. The study involved over 1700 veterans, and the time between the injury and the onset of Altzheimer's was about fifty years.

We know in homeopathy that Arnica, when used immediately after a head injury, prevents brain damage, strokes and even paralysis and epileptic seizures, clears the thought processes and prevents the memory loss that often sets in if Arnica is not given. Its use is so commonly excellent that very often, no other remedies need be considered; however, we have a number of excellent remedies for the adverse effects that can follow head injuries, including Conium, Hydrastis, Hypericum, Staphisagria and Symphytum, and also Opium, Cannabis, Calendula, Helleborus, Veratrum Album and more. In the megapotencies, such conditions can be improved or cleared even many years after the injury.

Many people believe that every sign of physical ill-health or hurt is a sign of weakness, of softness that must not be tolerated or acknowledged. 'I am not sick,' they protest, 'Only wimps take time off to coddle themselves. Everyone gets a bit of pain sometimes, that's normal. I'm not going to any doctor. I'll be right in a few minutes, I'm OK, really.'

A lot of these people are real softies underneath, but their belief in the necessity for toughness hardens them to the core of their being, the heart. So they are inclined to feel very guilty at any display of love or gentleness, grief or shock. No hugs or touching, please! No tears, no comforting, we must be tough in all emotional situations. Yet it is the very guilt of not feeling tough enough that causes them to toughen up the muscular structures of the body - particularly the heart muscle, the home of love in the body. The heart, quite literally, becomes toughened, as well as the blood vessel walls, creating inflexibility of the arteries and high blood pressure.

How can it do otherwise? Your subconscious mind, the silent master of all the functions of your body cells, takes your instructions literally, without reason. It can only obey, it has no capacity to rationalise that you do not really mean it physically, when you tell yourself 'I must be tough'. It just obeys, taking every word literally, believing and acting upon everything you say as if it were a ruling from God - which, of course, it is, in a way. So never tell it things you do not really mean!

Lots of heart patients strive for toughness in the belief that it is the way to behave when they get pain in the heart. It is often this guilt of not giving in that kills them. Contrast the Arnica person, who strives to avoid letting anyone know he has pain, with the Aconite heart attack sufferer who feels a great deal of fear for his very survival. His fear infects those around him and he is raced to emergency care at top speed. Arnica tries his best to continue whatever he was doing, resting only if forced to by his condition, his bravery over-riding any fear he might have for his life. Indeed, he does not feel real fear but knows that his life is at risk; he is not stupid, after all, though he may be a bit thick. He simply believes, as with every other circumstance of his life, that only the tough survive, and he deserves to die if he is not tough enough. He often risks not only his own life but that of others, by insisting he is OK to drive his car.

Speaking of thick between the ears, Arnica is also the primary remedy for boxers, for chronic concussion, and for being 'punch-drunk'. But you do not need to have been punched out frequently to feel a bit woolly in the head. As we have seen, there are many Arnica reasons for this.

I had occasion to appreciate Arnica myself some years ago, when I took a coach trip with my mother. We were away for four days, travelling each day, and I began to get symptoms of reeling in the head on rising from lying down, and on hitting the pillow while turning over in bed - a jarring effect, as if from a hard pillow, although it is of feathers. (Arnica has the symptom, 'bed feels too hard.') Conium also has vertigo in these situations, but I did not have any other Conium features. After three weeks of wondering what it was all about, I realized that it must have come from the passive jarring of being on the road all day, albeit in a super-smooth cruising coach.

I took Arnica 10M that night, and awoke next morning with even more severe reeling and had to sit back on the bed until it stopped. Old Arnica sorenesses resurfaced - a sure sign of being on the right remedy. My thumbs felt very 'bruised', the same soreness I had had for two years after massaging at a triathlon years ago, which had put me off massage for that time. Also my vision was somewhat blurrier than usual. (Eye muscles are also affected by Arnica. My myopia had come on at age 12 after falling on my neck while

163

trying to do cartwheels.) The next day the reeling began to vanish, the pain went out of the thumbs again and the vision returned to usual. If I had thought to take MM Arnica, perhaps my myopia would have been more significantly reversed! Must try it. Perhaps it is because 'I'm OK' that I have not done so yet.

A woman came in 2001 with poor circulation. She had had several operations over the years, and after one of them she had taken eight hours to regain consciousness. Now, she was having broken sleeps at night and was sleepy in the afternoons, but found that if she slept, she found it 'hard to get back to reality.' This information was enough to indicate that Arnica would help her circulation, and I gave her Arnica MM with great benefit.

Fear of being approached when injured or suffering gout, in case of being knocked and hurt, is a commonly known Arnica symptom. This relates also to the fear of close physical contact from an emotional standpoint. The mental habit of avoiding the embarrassment of loving touch crosses over to avoiding all touch, as all too often, the main reason for touch in their earlier life has been as a punishment or in rough play. The sore Arnica person expects touch to hurt.

We were amused to find, as time went on in this research, that the Arnica people not only expected touch to hurt, but they even demanded pain. A massage was not going to do them any good if it was not hard and painful. Frequently, a fairly gentle massage student was told to 'get in as hard as you like, love, the harder the better for me.' We have a heavy duty thumping massage machine that only comes out infrequently, and I found it excellent for getting relaxation to occur in deep muscles where I would have destroyed my hand joints, trying to relax tension in the tough outer muscles of many Arnica people. They are hard work! And they really love heavy, thumping, percussive massage, against which their tough, tight muscles cannot maintain resistence for very long, and must, inevitably, relax. Their skin and muscle tension is stronger than the usual person's - part of their defense against the tough world. It often is associated with bulkiness, overweight, as if fat, but it is simply thick, toughened muscles.

Muscle disorders needing Arnica are sometimes of a different kind - chronic, inflammatory degeneration such as the following:

A woman of sixty, a nursing sister, came to see me about her mysterious condition, which had been given the diagnosis of 'auto-immune disease'. She had developed inflammatory muscular degeneration in the shoulder and pelvic girdles. She had been told the only treatment on offer was cortisone for the rest of her life, which she refused to consider. The doctors had been unable to give a prognosis. It had begun around eighteen months previously with loss of strength in the legs after kneeling to weed the garden - she was unable to rise normally. After twelve months, chest pain caused her to have an ECG, which was erratic, and her enzymes were elevated suggesting ischemia. A bruise at the deltoid muscle insertion on the right arm arose at the time of this

164

heart turn. A biopsy was done on the flesh at this site, and the diagnosis of 'auto-immune' was made. Two blocked cardiac arteries were found. Her energy had been down since the chest pain, four months ago.

Her history was of whooping cough as an infant (Arnica works on whooping cough); a chubby baby, always a heavy child. She had an unusual feature, in that she had never spoken until the age of ten or eleven, she would only point at everything. No cause was ever found for this.

The major Arnica shock cause was a car accident 20 years before, in which she was 'not injured', but she was caught upside down in her safety belt, could not undo it and felt bruised all over. Her blood pressure went very high after this (probably an Aconite fright effect).

I asked, as I always do, what her main feeling had been at the time of the accident, and she simply felt embarrassed at being in such a position. It was not her fault, the steering gave way on her new car and the manufacturers replaced the car. She could have said shocked, scared, angry, OK, vindictive, but no - only embarrassed, which suggests Staphisagria. I gave her Staphisagria, also for the grief of having lost her mother and her sister in the last two years, both sudden and unexpected deaths that still mystified her. The chest pain had come on after a period of long working hours with a very frustrating supervisor. Her blood pressure was still too high despite taking two drugs for it. Staphisagria works well on blood pressure and frustration, and the immune system.

The following month, her movement was not as stiff as previously but there was more muscular pain in the neck and shoulder blades. Her husband was very pleased with her improvement, though she was not very aware of it herself. This is typical of Arnica people, they feel OK and are unobservant of changes. She said the Staphisagria did not show any difference at the time of taking it, and she was getting a bit of angina still. A bruise on her arm had faded with the Staphisagria but returned on finishing the 3-day remedy. I gave Arnica 10MM.

Next visit, six weeks later, she was going very well. Her blood pressure had never been so low, down to 117/65, a few days earlier. She was still getting pain between the shoulder blades and in the neck, a dull ache not helped by pain-killers; and a few heart flutters - 'used to that'. This time I gave her Staphisagria M and Arnica M, to be alternated weekly for twelve weeks. I kept up the Staphisagria because it seemed to suit part of her attitude/belief patterns, and because it handles immune system disturbances, though I was not convinced about that diagnosis. She became genuinely OK, the muscle weakness, blood vessels and heart returning to normal.

Notice that this person had had high blood pressure ever since the car accident 20 years ago, yet had failed to register this as any problem until the muscles finally lost their integrity. A loss of awareness of being less than well is always a sign of Arnica.

When the guilt of not being tough enough to take life's kicks and blows without being affected emotionally dominates a person's attitude to life, extra energy is drawn from the spine at the second and fourth thoracic vertebrae to create the required toughness of the heart muscle. Softness guilt stores up in the spinal muscles at these vertebrae causing tension that creates a lordosis or loss of curve of the spine at that point. This is often visible and palpatable, and this subluxation of the spine then allows less nerve force through to the heart. This is a defense against having too much nerve energy drawn from the central nervous system. As a result, one is more prone to heart disease.

Furthermore, the mental energy involved in suppressing the shock effects of blows or jarring is great and affects the flexibility of the cranial sutures, through 'toughening' tension in the fascia of the scalp and of the whole body musculature. This tough fascia develops as an armour against the outside world. You can see how massage works so well for Arnica people, as it softens up the armourplate.

The effects of such toughening are lack of sympathy (for self or others), hard-heartedness, unawareness of the existence of a problem, and quite a lot of heart and circulatory disorders like hardening of the arteries, particularly those that appear to have come on without warning. The Arnica person, typically, ignores the early signs of the disorder, says nothing because he registers nothing, and he and everyone else is utterly surprised at the severity of the complaint once it can no longer be ignored.

We find that we can predict the likelihood of Arnica heart problems and take steps to prevent them, when we find this anterior shift of the thoracic vertebrae T2 and T4, or the area T2-4. Using Arnica MM releases the guilt of softness from the mind-heart, then from the spinal muscles which allows the spine to realign and the heart and blood vessels to revert to strength and flexibility.

And here is something wonderful to add the icing to the cake: Because of Arnica's wondrous ability to break down clots and coagulated blood into their raw components and send them back to the long bones' red blood cell factory for recycling, it is the main remedy for thromboses, cerebro-vascular and cardio-vascular disease, both as prevention and as treatment. Arnica has long been used for the paralysis following strokes, in any potencies. It should be thought of in any condition where blood supply to the brain has been restricted or cut off and unconsciousness or coma result. Any surgical work can be done if necessary (to heart or blood vessel rupturing) and the Arnica M or 10M should be administered as soon as possible after the incident occurs, to give the best possible chance.

I missed an opportunity earlier this year to save a young man's life in such a situation. Unfortunately, so did the doctors who operated on him, in their ignorance of this wonderful medicine. They fixed the tear in the heart but failed to address the shock, the brain trauma and coma. By the time I learned about the situation, nearly a week had gone by. I think Arnica at that point might have saved him, still, though the word was being given out that if he lived now, he would be a vegetable. The life support was withdrawn after another week as he was then considered 'brain-dead.'

Now that I look back, it was a typical situation of a really nice, soft-hearted lad toughening up his heart to the point where the heart wall tore away at the aortic outlet, causing a haemorrhage of great magnitude. Needless to say, medical knowledge had no such concept, nor any other, as to why it had happened, though his partner, my niece, said he had had one or two chest pains over the previous couple of years *after muscle exertion, i.e. shifting furniture*, and had risen above them, in typically Arnica attitude.

Of course, Arnica is only one of several excellent heart remedies. Another that I have found excellent in children is Ipecacuanha. Yes, Ipecac, the stuff that is given by chemists in a yukky syrup to make you vomit, after taking some kinds of poisons. Ipecac was proven homeopathically and found to be an excellent remedy for haemorrhage from the lungs or heart, where frothy, bright red blood was being coughed up. My use for it has been in children with heart defects such as 'hole in the heart', and also for surgery to any kind of heart/lung problem. It normalises the 'hole' situation, and in the other cases, prevents unnecessary blood loss during essential corrective surgery. I have even used Ipecac to stop years of morning sickness (four pregnancies) in a woman who had been a 'blue baby.'

'Hole in the heart' (or 'blue baby') occurs when the hole in the central wall of the heart, essential for circulation in the unborn, fails to close over at birth when the lungs begin to take in air. Normally, this is a spontaneous event that goes unnoticed, unless it does not happen! Such babies are fragile until such time as, hopefully, the message clicks in and the heart corrects itself, or an operation is done to seal the hole. Megapotency Ipecac, I have found on several occasions, causes the spontaneous correction to the heart, and health rapidly strengthens.

It does this because it has the ability to release tension in the musculature of the neck that is squeezing the atlas or first vertebra of the neck up against the skull. When this happens, not enough nerve supply can get through along the vagus or tenth cranial nerve that serves to energise the face, throat, heart, lungs and stomach. Birth trauma can cause this tension in the neck. Chiropractors and osteopaths know this and adjust the neck of the newborns when they get the chance, and the problems subside rapidly. But if Ipecac, Arnica and other remedies were used in hospitals, precious time would not be lost, and many problems would cease to be.

I have had occasion, now and then, to treat elderly people with Arnica because it had been needed all their lives, well indicated by the range of conditions they had experienced, since being severely bruised and battered by forceps during birth. By using the megapotencies, it is possible to deal with such trauma shock and resolve it, even after so many years.

CHAPTER 9

There is no dependence that can be sure but a dependence on oneself.
- John Gay

CONIUM - 'WHO WILL PROVIDE FOR ME?'

Mrs Grieve describes Conium (conium maculatum, *Poison Hemlock*, N.O. Umbelliferae) as 'sedative and antispasmodic, and in sufficient doses, acts as a paralyser to the centres of motion. In its action it is, therefore, directly antagonistic to that of Strychnine, and hence it has been recommended as an antidote to Strychnine poisoning, and other poisons of the same class, and in tetanus, hydrophobia etc.' The fresh juice, in drop doses, was used 'in cases of undue nervous motor excitability, such as teething in children, epilepsy from dentition, cramp, in the early stages of paralysis agitans, in spasms of the larynx and gullet, in acute mania, etc. As an inhalation, it is said to relieve cough in bronchitis, whooping cough, asthma.'

Most of these uses are homeopathic - the uses match the poisoning symptoms - and the very microscopic, non-toxic potencies can be used without risk. Mrs Grieve also adds: 'In poisonous doses it produces complete paralysis with loss of speech, the respiratory function is at first depressed and ultimately ceases altogether and death results from asphyxia.' In the past, less commonly today, Conium was all too often mistaken for aniseed or coriander by the gatherers of those herbs.

The Greeks and the Romans used it for the cure of tumours, swellings and pains of joints as well as for skin affections. We find mention of it in the writings of Dioscorides, Pliny and Avicenna. It is said to be the poison with which Socrates was killed, as it is notorious as an ingredient in the State poison of Greece, frequently given to criminals. Linnaeus named it Conium after the Greek word *Konas,* meaning to whirl about, because the plant, when eaten, causes vertigo and death.

Its extreme toxicity has caused it to be withdrawn from use in modern herbal medicine, where the focus is on harmless, gentle correction. Matthew Wood[67] mentions it only once, for its use in homeopathic microdoses for the pitch black bruises sometimes found in old people. However, in modern medicine, its toxicity made it attractive and its main alkaloid, coniine, was extracted and used in pharmacy. Ellingwood describes it thus: 'When given in a sufficient dose, conium causes complete relaxation of the whole nervous system; the eyes close, the movements of the eyeballs are sluggish, mastication and swallowing are difficult, speech is slow and maintained by an effort, the voice is hoarse, while the heart and the intelligence are not disturbed. In a fatal dose, the lower limbs become paralysed, the effect gradually ascending to the upper part of the body, intelligence being retained to the last.'

He then goes on to describe its usefulness in relieving the pain of cancers and ulcers, particularly ulceration of the stomach and incipient gastric cancer, glandular enlargements, cancer of the pelvic organs or of the mammary glands. However, to get the desired benefit, it must be used in large doses, which then 'must be carefully watched' lest you cause poisoning and death. (Where did they get the notion that you must almost kill if you are to get any benefit? So wrong, so unnecessary.)

Dr Ellingwood also described its use in paralysis agitans, chorea, hysteria, delirium tremens and acute mania, trismus, laryngeal spasm, wry neck, whooping cough, asthma, emphysema, laryngitis, dry bronchial coughs and phthisis (pulmonary tuberculosis), chronic hepatitis, ulceration of the cervix uteri, rectal fissures and pelvic inflammation.

CONIUM IN HOMEOPATHY

In its homeopathic provings, Hahnemann found Conium to cause most of the above problems, but some rare and particularly peculiar symptoms were elicited. Dr N.M. Choudhuri[68] describes them: 'The indication that stands out most prominently in Conium is its dizziness. It is brought on and aggravated by turning the head sideways. There is a good bit of dispute as to whether this giddiness is worse lying down. Dr Nash is of the opinion that it is not so much the lying down as the turning of the head sidewise, whether in an upright or horizontal posture, that causes the vertigo ..... In my opinion too, as I have verified several times, the vertigo is distinctly worse, when the patient turns his head, however slightly ..... Dr Nash, on this indication, used Conium in a case of locomotor ataxia with great success ..... Not only locomotor ataxia but other complaints have been cured on this golden indication.'

Another significant, unusual symptom relates to perspiration: sweat, only after closing eyes or while sleeping - drenching, which stops as soon as she wakes up. This is sometimes a good clue for sufferers of pseudo-menopausal nightsweats. And the cough - dry, tickling in the chest, spasmodic coughing that starts on lying down and is relieved on sitting up again. The disease name matters not - it could be whooping cough, bronchitis or asthma, the name tells you little - it is the peculiarities of the individual that lead you to the cure. Conium has been successful in removing cataracts, impaired hearing from earwax clogging, disagreeable, fetid and persistent armpit odour, catarrh of the nose and post-nasal pharynx, numbness in the fingers and toes, weakness and trembling in the thighs on walking, skin cancers, morning sickness, ulceration and cancers of the oesophagus, lungs, stomach and even brain tumours - *in the Conium person*.

Dr Choudhuri also describes Conium as mostly adapted to the debility of old people, where mobility of all limbs is compromised and dependency on others is increased; to tumours caused by a blow or fall, and particularly to the bad effects of sexual excesses. Equally, it can be needed by those who have long suppressed their sexuality - denied husbands, 'old bachelors, old maids, widows who suffer from the ill effects of suppressed sexual instinct and non-gratification of sexual appetite. It is useful in impotency with constant nightly emissions. There is great sexual desire with partial or complete incapacity. The erection is insufficient, only lasting a short time. There is discharge of prostatic fluid on every change of emotion on the voluptuous line, or even while expelling faeces. The slightest stimulus, such as looking at women or being in their company, bringing on emission, is a very typical symptom, and it has been removed by Conium.'

We commonly use Conium for enlarged, hardened testicles with shrunken penile size and strength; for tumours of the breasts, where the first indication is a shooting, needle-like pain; for the uterus and cervix, after undesirable cells are found in PAP smears. Always consider these in conjunction with the emotional aspects, which will indicate the best remedy.

George Vithoulkas[69] describes Conium as characterised by the word 'gradual'. 'Over many years he will go into a gradual paralysis and weakness. This is happening so gradually that he does not understand the process himself. He looks back over many years and sees this gradual decline. Therefore this decline is not bound to be noticed by the people around him. Then, as he thinks about his state, there is a feeling that something serious is going on.

'This can be seen in chronic drug users - those that have been careful enough not to take large doses at once, but enjoy it little by little for many years - they will keep going into that state. This would be the first remedy to be thought of in big, chronic drug users. There is complete apathy. The mind cannot think at all. They are 'spaced out'. The mental abilities are lost completely. There is a kind of paralysis of the ideas. The same with chronic alcohol users - an alcohol user who does not use too much.' The deterioration is gradual over a long time, decades. Yet they react violently in catastrophe. The sudden loss of a husband, a loss of possessions or inheritance will cause a rapid hardening in a gland and cancer follows. They are materialistic, and any threat or harm to their wealth or possessions hits hard.

Vithoulkas lists weakness of the bladder, intermittent urination with or without prostate enlargement, hard and enlarged testes or uterus. 'He tries until he is sweating and he cannot urinate. Then he relaxes, the urge comes again and some of the urine is voided naturally.'

Clarke lists the following complaints as appropriate to Conium:

Clinical.- Asthma. Bladder, inflammation of. *Breast, affections of;* painful. *Bronchitis. Bruises. Cancer. Cataract.* Chorea. *Cough. Depression of spirits.* Diphtheritic paralysis. Dysmenia (membranous). *Erysipelas. Eyes, affections of.* Galactorrhœa (spontaneous discharge of milk from breast; inappropriate). Herpes. *Hypochondriasis.* Jaundice. Liver, enlarged. *Melancholia. Menstruation, disordered. Numbness. Ovaries, affections of. Paralysis;* Landry's paralysis. Peritonitis. Phthisis. *Pregnancy, painful breasts during.* Prostatitis. Ptoses. Scrophula. *Spermatorrhœa. Sterility.* Stomach, affections of. *Testicles, affections of.* Tetters. Trismus. Tumours. Ulcers. *Vertigo.* Vision, disordered. *Wens.*

To this I can add: Blows, tumours after. Constipation. Coccyx, jarring of. Diabetes. Digestion, disordered. Ears, affections of. Enuresis, nocturnal; or retention. Fatigue, chronic, with pain. Fever, chills, profuse sweats. Gums, teeth, affections of. Headache, stupefying. Impotence. Intellect, weak. Mammary / lymphatic gland tumours. Memory, weak. Mental feebleness. Mesenteric glands, swollen. Ribcage, paralysis of. Sleep, affections of. Tongue, affections of. Vulvadynia. Whooping cough.

CONIUM IN MEGAPOTENCY

The most important thing to understand about Conium is that the one who needs it has a great fear of having to be independent, even while manifesting an apparent spirit of independence. Conium thinks he needs help, in any or every field of life, hates to think of doing things alone, even though, in the majority of cases, he is quite able to succeed on his own. Financial dependency is the most obvious way this is evidenced. He or she fears he may never provide financially enough for his needs or desires, or feels a great guilt that he is not able to do so. You will never need to use Conium for people who are happily bringing in all the money they think they need, without thinking twice about it. On the other hand, Conium is needed in every case where any one of the following thoughts or states predominates:

- Helplessness in the face of job loss, inability to get work, inability to earn enough

- Bewilderment as to where the money is going to come from

- I can't think of anything to do that will bring in enough money (guilt over feeling under-educated, untrained, unable to do anything that will pay enough). Someone more skilled than I will have to bring in the money

- Someone else will have to provide for me. I've always been provided for, I don't know how to provide for myself. The Government must provide

171

for me. (Widows, school-leavers very commonly feel this way.) The Government does not give me enough

- There's never enough money. However much is coming in, it is never enough

- I have great plans for what I want to do, but it requires a lot more money than I can imagine myself earning - who's going to be inspired by my dream and put his money into it?

- I'd better buy more lottery tickets, gamble more

- I'm getting deeper and deeper into debt and don't know what to do to get out of it. Please pay my bills for me

- I want to marry, then I'll be provided for

- What will happen to me if my husband dies? Will my children provide for me? Who will look after me when I am old?

- Where are the customers who will buy from me? Where are the clients I need, to stay in business?

Fear of lack, and the profound sense of dependency associated with these fears and guilts causes the sufferer to spill it over into other areas of his life. We find that guilt finds ways of increasing itself, perpetuating itself; so the lack of enough money causes the victim to spend unwisely, particularly on things that he can become dependent on. Drugs, cigarettes, stimulants, medications, chocolate, alcohol, new clothes will all give a temporary boost to the depressing sense of lack, but do nothing to lift him out of his poverty fear. Addiction to gambling only makes it worse. Dependency also spreads to relying on family members, walking stick, crutches, wheelchair, government, doctors and nurses.

Many Conium people have a fear of, or reluctance to work. We find the symptom recorded, 'cannot be persuaded to work'. I find Conium an essential remedy for the growing hordes of drug-users, drop-outs and invalids in the community, but consider also Aconite, who has a fear of criticism, of not being thought perfect, which stymies his attempts to apply for a job, or to succeed; and Hypericum, who fears responsibility and commitment and will cut and run as soon as work is not fun. Hypericum wants to stay nineteen all his life, Conium remains, in some ways, a dependent child throughout life, though fiercely independent in spirit.

The most significant guilt he has is that he has little or no faith. He has no faith in the God within him to lead him always to his supply, and no faith in the universal laws of survival. He does not understand that if you walk forward in the knowledge that your needs will always be met, they are met; that if you fear, you create from the power of your thinking, the very thing you are fearing.

Thought is powerful, creative energy, and we always reap the results of our fearful thinking by manifesting the very thing we anticipate fearfully.

172

Even the most devoutly religious can fall into this trap and forget that as we sow, so shall we reap. Think fear, create the feared thing; think lack, create lack in your life; think limitation, create a limited supply; and if we once realize this and reverse our habits of thought, we begin to see the power of positive, confident, joyful faith beginning to create abundance and infinite supply in our lives. Conium in megapotency effects this change from fear and guilt to faith, and money becomes then a non-issue, somehow enough is always there.

Conium allows the intuitive knowingness that all is well, that our own inner Self is on duty at all times, that we do not need to depend on others for our support; that we are never in the wrong place at the wrong time. Conium gives us the ability to listen to our instincts and act on them, to heed our intuition - the voice of our inner tutor.

In trying to sort all this out, I was confused about whether to use Ignatia or Conium in lymphatic problems. I asked Gonjesil for clarification, and this is his reply:

'Loss of faith is often manifested in the lymphatics. Feelings are, great guilt makes some people steel themselves against thinking poor. I'm quite sure it is this that starts off the process of lymphatic congestion.

'I think love of money often starts off as fear of lack. Feelings are, losing the guilt of loving money mightily gives them the ability to loosen up this lymphatic congestion. This era, more than any other, depends on money. Knowing this, it will be easy to see why Conium gives so many, freedom from lymphatic gland breast lumps. It gives them back their inner knowingness that they are always provided for when they follow their intuition. Lack of faith in the intuition is the major guilt of Conium.'

'So how does this relate to the paralysis of Conium?' I asked.

'Feelings are, this is still lymphatic congestion; thinking lack gives this mighty silly idea that life is crippled, paralysed without money; just as Phosphorus people are paralysed by the belief that they are not intellectual enough for this intellect-dominated society. Lack of money gives them (Conium people) inability to stand on their own feet. Their steely great thinking is that some great provider must appear to support them.'

Ignatia, on the other hand, became clarified as time went on, as a remedy for fluid level (pituitary) hormones rather than lymphatics. The other major lymphatic remedy I had been watching was Thuja, which is a major remedy for removing accumulated toxins from the body's fluids.

Conium is a very deep-acting remedy, and the problems that require Conium may be found to have been developing for the whole of the patient's life. The basic belief in limited or non-existent supply is one which is inherent in our society. We have been so successfully indoctrinated with the belief that money is essential for survival, that the lack of money and the pursuit of money has become number one consideration in our thinking.

Do you realize that this is the first time in the history of mankind that man, all over the world, is dependent on money for his existence? Do you know that this is a belief created and fostered by those who want more and more money, and the power it brings to control us, to make slaves of us all? If it were the case that money was essential for survival, we would not be here today, mankind would have perished many thousands of years ago. But we survived by growing, hunting and gathering, and may have to do so again before the world brings itself back into balance.

It is the pursuit of money that has brought us - some as masters, most as slaves - to the present state of world chaos. We are ruled easily, because we have taken on the belief that we will not survive without money, and we are slaves to the concept of the limited income. All we need is to eliminate that thought-fear from our consciousness and the power-seekers no longer control us. It then becomes a matter of personal choice, that we live a life of freedom and independence, the money always arriving when needed, and frequently, needing a lot less than we thought.

Our money-oriented society, our industrialised way of life have created a generation (or several) of children who are growing up not knowing, not taught as people have been taught since time began, how to feed themselves. Particularly in the cities, children learn nothing about hunting for food, gathering or growing their own sustenance, and increasingly, nothing even about how to make their own fabrics, clothes, utensils, furniture - even how to cook or preserve the produce of the garden is lost to many families dependent on pre-cooked instant meals, sliced bread and fruit juice in plastic bottles. We cannot even go anywhere without getting out the car, and our muscles deteriorate from lack of use. Dependence on industry and mechanisation and the race against time has made us cripples.

This may be hard for many of us to come to terms with. Only the use of Conium in the guilt-freeing potencies will show you the difference between what you have become and what you healthily can be. All the guilt-releasing potencies (of whatever the needed remedy) give such wonderful freedom from weighty fears, despondency and hopelessness that one is able to live each day with great joy and confidence. Try it.

Conium lacks an acceptance of the concept of creation, he lacks an understanding or awareness of the existence of a master plan for the universe, a DNA blueprint of thought from which each and everything in existence obtains and retains its form. Further to this, he has lost contact with the all-pervading presence of the great, universal creative energy, Love, without which all would still be at the blueprint stage, non-manifest.

He is unaware that the Christ principle of Love is always there, within and outside himself, available to be tapped and felt and used at any time, in any quantity, ever-replenishing. He wants it to be given to him, thinks he is outside of and separated from it, feels cut off from it, fails to understand that this universal energy tends always to nurture and sustain all life through its normal life cycle.

Thirdly, he is unconscious that all that exists in the material world has been created from mind plus love, so he fails to see the essential unity of all things, all creatures, all mankind and man's products (even money!), all Nature herself as equally deserving of and receiving the universal life-sustaining energy of love. He disclaims responsibility by separating himself (in his belief) from this brotherhood of life, yet the attitude causes him to wither and die, cuts off his access to his energy source while it denies him his sources of financial supply.

He has a big, big guilt over loving, needing money - as if it is something filthy. He has been taught in childhood that money is the root of all evil, and he has never considered that, perhaps, it is the ruthless pursuit of money at the expense of others that is the evil. He cannot see that money is merely a vehicle for exchange, a tool we can all use for the betterment of our lives. He/she shuns money emotionally and it has no alternative but to be repelled from him/her by this attitude. Such people are often the ones who feel guilty about charging for their services, particularly in healing, as if this must be a free gift to mankind and it is OK for the healer to try to live on debt-saturated air. Money is 'not spiritual!' though the spirit of life pervades money as it does everything else.

Conium is a remedy that acts on the pituitary and pineal glands. In all Conium sufferers there is a lessening of energy to these glands, owing to the closing off through misbelief, disbelief, of the universal sustaining energies of life. This disbelief is the reason why injuries fail to heal, and why conditions of physical helplessness, hormonal issues and paralysis develop in the Conium person. Specific muscles hoard the emotions that result from this disbelief. Conium in the megapotencies not only frees up the muscle tensions, thus allowing the cranial bones to regain correct alignment and reshape the head, but also acts on the non-physical energies, opening up the crown chakra to allow more cosmic energy to enter.

Dependency, financially, often goes hand-in-hand with dependency on drugs, whether social or pharmaceutical, particularly for a lifelong health condition like diabetes, thyroid insufficiency or some of the less well known adrenal conditions requiring cortisone; wherever an endocrine gland is out of order. I have found Conium conditions developing in people with such dependencies, which may have been congenital, or genetically predisposed.

My own Aunt Joan was an interesting Conium person. At the age of only 13 she was witness to a car accident outside her home, and the shock affected her severely, leading to pituitary/pancreatic disturbance - diabetes mellitus set in quite rapidly. Her life became one of constant dietary control and regular injections of insulin, with frequent visits to the specialist. She met and married a wonderful man who took it all in his stride and gave her the same devoted care her mother did. Her social conditioning and the dependency on insulin injections for her survival caused Conium characteristics to continue to develop.

Born into an era when women were brought up to believe that they would marry and all their needs would be met by their husbands, my aunt and her two sisters were given training only in typing and stenography after leaving school, and left their jobs on marriage to become full-time wives and mothers, never to have a full income of their own again. They were taught that it was right to believe that men could be expected, and would be there, to support them. Easy to see why so many Conium problems develop in today's older women who outlive their husbands.

After living for fifteen years with her parents, the couple bought a beautiful home in a tree-studded suburb, and for some years all appeared to be going well. Though she had expensive tastes, she was very talented and made her own beautiful clothes and hats, as well as finding time for oil-painting.

The time came when my aunt began to manifest more of the physical signs of a Conium condition. Her husband's business took a downturn and he wound it up and took a job. Money in the latter part of her life was not as readily come by as in her youth, and it was a constant worry, though all the work she occupied herself with was voluntary. Forty years after the onset of the diabetic condition, problems began to arise with her toes, her eyesight deteriorated and she began to become more and more helpless. As time went on her condition worsened. Eventually, her husband, by this time retired, found he was unable to care for her alone and found a nursing home for her.

When I visited her a few months before her death at 69, she was barely able to stand, walked only with a weak, shuffling gait with assistance and spent all day in a wheelchair watching those around her, with only sluggish response to what was happening. She needed help with every physical act, large or small. Her thinking was slow, though still intelligent. She was insensitive to emotional and physical pain, apathetic and resigned to her situation. Her voice was very small and weak, and she was having trouble getting her tongue around the few words she wanted to say. She was like a very little child, mentally as well as physically. She was totally dependent, her arms too weak to lift a spoon or fork to her mouth or hold a cup. Finally, the paralysis reached her ribcage and she developed dyspnoea and pneumonia, was acutely ill for less than a week and died. A lifetime of diabetes and insulin injections, when the right shock resolution remedy, given at the time of the shock, would have prevented it from ever developing.

It is not easy to distinguish Conium in the young, though we must learn to do so, because this is where the Conium mentality begins. Childhood is the time when we are expected to be dependent. It is 'normal'. But as children grow and become physically skilled and capable, and as they reach their mental peak at the time of puberty, many children, because of western society's emphasis on intellectual and sporting endeavours from then on, fail to develop the third aspect of themselves, their spiritual/emotional maturity, which, Rudolph Steiner identified, takes place in the third seven-year period, between 14 and 21 years of age.

For these children, growing up and having to take full responsibility for their survival is incomprehensible, particularly if they are female, since women have been dependent on and subjected to the will of men for a thousand generations, it is well ingrained in the cell memory. Although they may go through the schooling that takes them into a good job, and although the money may come in, somehow the fear of not having enough coming in, through lack of confidence in the processes of life, holds them back in a degree of spiritual immaturity.

It is from this starting point that material greed and insecurity sets in. Everyone who feels the need for lots of money needs Conium. Everyone who despairs over not having the ability to attract lots of money needs Conium. And everyone who buys lottery tickets, investment property, stocks and shares, and who regularly outlays money in order to get a better return on his investment, needs Conium. It is part of the isolationism and separatism of our culture, that we have reached the point where it is every man for himself, and what I have is mine, I need to keep it for my future, or it may it run out. Financial security is seen as the be-all and end-all of existence for a lot of people.

We see all too frequently, dependency in the teenager manifesting in petty theft, from the belief that they must have what others have, though they cannot afford it, or from the need to find money to support another form of dependency, drugs.

Kids buy into the drug scene for many reasons. They may feel the need to prove themselves somehow, to their peers, by going along with what seems to be expected of them (Staphisagria) even against their better judgement, needing to be liked; they may feel that life is a great adventure and that all avenues need to be explored, even if it kills them (Hypericum); they may feel that life is too boring, and take drugs that challenge death itself, just to get a bit of a thrill (Hypericum); or too frightening, so they take drugs to escape reality (Aconite); they may feel so low in self-value that the behaviours, ideas and beliefs of their peers (of equally low self-worth) take precedence over their instincts of self-preservation (Hypericum); or they may have the common belief that 'it is OK, nothing could harm *me*, I'm tough and can take it' (Arnica), or the guilt of knowing they are harming themselves (Hydrastis) that locks them into a behaviour pattern they cannot rise above.

It is the Conium aspect that keeps them depending on supply. It is the Conium immaturity that pushes them into addiction. Often, they have materialistic, well-heeled parents who have subtly taught them the fear of

177

lack, bought them too much, paid out for them instead of teaching them independence and the superficiality of possessions.

There is a similar reliance on the medical profession and pharmaceutical drugs, which are all too often found to be feeding people's dependencies.

Most of the time, the medicines are not addictive in themselves, and as a number of researchers are finding nowadays, it is the personality that is addictive, rather than the substance. Many a doctor is guilty of writing a prescription simply because the patient says 'Give me something'; even, in some cases, telling the doctor what it is he must have. Some patients boast proudly about the fifteen or more different drugs they are taking, some of these turn up at the doctor's waiting room every week without fail, addicted to the little bit of attention they are given - for Conium also craves company and for some, this is the only way to get it. The sense of need for some sort of support is always Conium.

Support from the government is a common outcome of Conium dependency. We find teenagers in high school who believe they will never get a job; they may enrol in subsidised tertiary institutions, and having finished their certificate or degree, enrol in another, eventually finding themselves too well qualified for the jobs that are available, so they prefer to remain unemployed and the government still has to foot the bill for their lack of independence by giving them a dole or directing them into an obligatory job not of their own choice. Everything they do seems to lead to their having to be provided for, by parents and/or the state, and this is accepted because they cannot seem to see their way out of the situation, and expect the job to be found for them without their effort of seeking. The dependent mind cannot even see how to go about it. 'I can't' is the belief, and it creates a mental vacuum. The parent is often the one to do the job searching or provide the opportunity, or alternatively, support the offspring throughout life. Contrast this with Symphytum, who must be working, somehow, whatever the job, and will be happy to work his way up to a good income.

Fear of being expected to manage on your own, whatever the age, is Conium. It helps young people who have physical handicaps, not only by strengthening their self-confidence but also, often, by strengthening their legs. Paralytic weakness in the legs can come at any age from a variety of named conditions, and when Conium is needed, there is an accompanying tendency to revert to babyhood, with loss of stature, inability to walk, talk, care for one's own hygiene, to feed oneself or dress oneself. There are subtle levels occurring for years before, for in many cases, the development of these conditions can be very slow and scarcely noticeable for a long time. Or you may even have been born this way. It still remains to be seen how much Conium can restore order to such people, and I expect it would require the use of other guilt-release remedies as well, to fire up action in the nervous system and hormones.

Dependency in babies is regarded as a tiresome but normal and natural phenomenon. Not necessarily so. One of my regular patients who uses a lot of homeopathy at home, being in an isolated rural area, gave birth to her third child on September 5th, 2000. She weighed 5lb 4oz. The child was grizzly and demanded attention a lot, and she had the typical tilted Conium eyes, as her head had not regained its best shape after the birth. She could not be left alone and screamed if her mother left the room. The mother developed some symptoms that prompted me to give her Conium CM, on May 11, 2001, at which time she was still breastfeeding the baby. She rang a few days later with the news that 'Joy is really alive, active and alert. She has been having three-hour afternoon sleeps, rare for her. Her feeding has improved, too, she had a lot of digestive trouble. And as for me, Conium has cured my face, I can chew again, my sinus pain has gone, and numbness throughout the face has gone. I feel slightly worse in the left sacro-iliac joint, it is twingy.' And here is a continuation of the little girl's benefits, as told by her mother:

'When Joy was born, in the doctors' opinion she was underweight. From the beginning, the doctors always looked at her and felt her head. The fontanelles closed nicely but they still persisted in feeling her head. The top part of her head seemed narrower than the bottom half. As she grew, it became more and more obvious, so in August 2001, I spoke to Jill about it and asked if there was anything that could be done for it. At the same time, Joy was having problems with her feet turning in, and was falling over her feet all the time.

She was treated with Conium 10MM to release the muscles at the side of her skull and the muscles around her hips to allow her feet to straighten up, and Hypericum 10MM' (also helpful for domed craniums, and she was hyperactive). 'After a period of approximately two months, I started to have friends comment that 'Joy's head seems to be filling out' and had started to 'even up.' Even before then she had stopped falling over her feet, they had straightened up considerably. Eight months after her initial treatment with the Conium and Hypericum, it became obvious that she needed another dosing of both. The remedies were repeated, with further excellent results. These remedies had such an amazing result that I will continue to use them, if needed, as she grows up.' In my opinion, Joy was born needing Conium because it was the remedy her mother needed during pregnancy.

Conium helps youngsters and older people who fear to go it alone, feeling that they always need someone to fall back on, financially. It is great for those starting out in a small business, and for those whose enthusiastic start has settled back into a fluctuating level of income. It helps them not to feel that the money will dry up. It helps people to manage money better, so that they have no desire to indulge in unnecessary spending. It also makes people more generous, for the fear of lack vanishes out of their consciousness and enables them to spread their possessions and wealth around for the betterment of all, helping to level the monstrous gap between the haves and the have nots. A more humanitarian spirit sets in, and those who acquire wealth find it easier to finance projects that will help restore the world to a healthier state. Following up with Calc Fluor seals in the benefits.

A young man I began treating in 1990 for chronic fatigue associated with allergies, had developed his problems as a result of immunisations (mumps, measles and triple antigen) together with a period of 'massive antibiotics' for a squashed finger, following a period of extreme work stress six years earlier. He had suffered from eyestrain and a back injury from schooldays, of subluxation of the right sacro-iliac joint. He would wake every day feeling stiff and sore, with an upset stomach and headaches that felt 'as if after a night on the grog.' He had fallen and hit his head some months earlier, and had never felt well since. He had used marijuana in the past, LSD once.

All these problems could have fitted Hypericum or Staphisagria, but I did not know that at the time, and it was Opium that began to help him (it is a good head injury remedy). Candida symptoms were prominent, and I treated them with Nilstat 10M, after which he had a return of flu symptoms and low back soreness. LSD 10M cleared this and his energy picked up for a while. Many treatments gave temporary help but we never won out. Throughout this time and for another eighteen months, he was suffering guilt over not having a well-paid job. The best he could manage was short shifts as a waiter. He felt lacking in direction, not happy with his marriage, felt his wife had led him away from a good job on a farm in another area, and felt very guilty over lack of finance. His wife worked and supported the two children. He had other emotional issues as well. The tiredness and sleepiness relapses continued despite good remedies, until in May 1993, he felt he was 'wasting away' - full of guilts, could not get motivated to live how he'd like to, felt he could not earn or do a day's work. This time I gave Staphisagria MM, and Nat Mur 50M, CM and MM, his primary constitutional mineral remedy, in a straight run of three days each.

Finally, he felt better able to cope. He was going to Sydney to stay with his mother and find work as a labourer. He was suffering pins and needles in the legs and aching in the arms, with spasm in the muscles between the shoulder blades. By this time, I had learned more about Conium, and I gave him Conium CM. He rang from Sydney a month later, saying he had been given lots of get-up-and-go from the Conium, lots of confidence. He was enjoying getting paid, and was spending lots (another, sometimes unfortunate, quality of the Conium person). The benefit was lapsing a little, so I sent Conium MM. At the last report, he was still feeling a lot less stressed, much stronger and enjoying the outdoor work of labouring.

I have found Conium a very satisfactory remedy for some people with 'sleep apnoea.' The characteristic that indicates it is a tendency to lose muscle strength in the jaw as soon as asleep, so that the mouth drops open and the person wakes later with a very dry mouth from breathing through it, though the nose is clear. I have found this common in older people, and it always indicates Conium may be needed. There may not be true apnoea, but the Conium dependency allows them to accept a sleep apnoea machine that pumps oxygen through a face mask. Paralytic weakness in the jaw joint muscles, the muscles of chewing and of swallowing are part of the general flaccidity of Conium musculature. You do not have to be old, though.

A woman of forty consulted me in 2000 for sleep apnoea, asthma and what she called 'toxic overload'. She had been using a sleep apnoea machine for nearly three weeks. She had had chronic constipation since age 13 and was overweight as well; she smoked and was addicted to chocolate. She felt that it was time to grow up and clean up, a significant admission of having been childlike, I thought.

She had 15 years of recurrent headaches, on account of which she was addicted, she said, to painkillers. In addition she'd had endometriosis for some years, for which there had been years of a hormone pill which she had discontinued. She had a phobia about the sharp blades of knives. This all fitted Staphisagria, so she had Staphisagria MM. At the next visit, she felt she'd had fewer painkillers, fewer headaches, but still lots of pain with periods. She was no longer fearful of knives, felt happy, but was still addicted to chocs and the sleep machine. She had darkness under her eyes, often a sign of grief over father, so I asked her about grief issues. Father had died of a melanoma 11 years ago, and she had lost her older brother to motor neurone disease five years before that. She lived alone, said 'I'd kill if I lived with someone.' I gave her Sepia 10MM for three nights. Sepia is the primary remedy for griefs and disappointments relating to one's father.

Six weeks later, she was exercising a lot, losing weight, had more energy on the hot days, and chocolate was rare now. She had not tackled the smoking yet, but was less dark under the eyes and had less period pain. Still on the sleep apnoea machine. She felt 'tougher, lately - able to not be upset by others, and much more energy, coping well with city traffic, in a good relationship and wearing sexier clothes.' Headaches rarer. Felt she had lacked confidence all her life.

A couple of visits came and went with not much further benefit. Staphisagria reinstated the improvements, and after this, having just discovered Aconite's benefits for confidence, I also gave her Aconite 10MM.

Chocolate desires came back. I gave Conium 10M fortnightly for two months, after which she said, 'You've cured almost every problem!' Bowel motions daily, the first time in thirty years. Still using the sleep machine.

Conium 10MM brought on some discomforts including a week of the flu, followed by benefits. Later, Conium MM completed the jaw strengthening. She had been taping up her mouth to stop it from dropping open during sleep. She even felt ready to give up smoking, and was 'no longer worried about having not enough money,' which she had not mentioned before. 'No longer self-centred, full of confidence, feeling well, sleeping well, feeling in love with myself.'

A woman of fifty five had had benefits over a couple of years for various problems, and reached a point where she felt she was at the end of an era.

Staphisagria had improved her ability to take a stand for herself and not put up with other people's impositions on her life, but she was uncertain about her future, feeling quite financially lacking in independence. In the hope of greater financial opportunity, she was buying Lotto and lottery tickets. Physically, she had very painful lumps in the breasts, but no heat flushes or menopausal symptoms except low libido. A clairvoyant had told her she had repressed sexuality because of rape in prior times. Conium 10MM helped all aspects.

Brain tumours may be suffered by people who need Conium. One woman for whom I prescribed Conium MM in 1993 was a divorced mother of a teenage boy. She had found life difficult as the bread-winner, there was never enough money, and although she lived a fairly monastic life, the responsibility became too much for her. When the brain tumour was diagnosed, she began to spend long periods in a Buddhist retreat where she did not have to make decisions, even about what to prepare to eat, leaving the boy to fend for himself. I am told that, without operation, the brain tumour diminished with three treatments over several months, in conjunction with the meditations she employed, and she lived on.

A case of incipient cancer of the testicles was one of the first megapotency cases I treated, back in 1991. He had good spiritual understanding, but had allowed his own intuition to be undermined and over-ridden by a very demanding, materialistic and greedy wife, who was perpetually driving him to work harder and bring in more money (which she was good at hoarding away in her own bank account). I did not have the chance to treat the wife but was successful in correcting the husband. Staphisagria MM gave him the ability to take a stand for what he believed in, so that he was able to extricate himself from the destructive marital environment and begin to get himself well again.

Staphisagria was repeated over several months, along with Conium, for he had taken on the materialistic money fears of the wife and had developed enlarged, thickened testicles. These two magicians gradually began to restore his sexual strength, which had been lost for a year, and the thickening of the testicles softened up and gradually dispersed. Two years later, he admitted he had not expected to live for more than a couple of years. He is still going strong in 2012.

I have, myself, had good cause to thank Conium. In 1987, I had had a mammary cyst drained after a mammogram, and later developed the same cyst again and four others. For a few years, these would come and go under the influence of other homeopathic remedies (Phytolacca and Ignatia), until

182

finally, in 1992, only the original one remained, resistant to the previous treatments, and now very hard. I began to get sharp pains in the nipple which extended as a painful, drawing feeling, towards the armpit. This is a feature of Conium, so I took Conium MM and this pain ceased. Pleasingly, the lump also began to diminish. I needed to take the remedy again every couple of years, whenever I started worrying about where the money was going to come from. It is a true life-saver.

Looking back, I can see that all my Conium concern for money only arose in 1987 after my husband's business began to suffer badly when, as a result of government policies, Australia went through 'the recession we had to have' (according to the Federal Treasurer). Many small businesses suffered and many went to the wall at that time, as did his, almost. We sold up, he retired on an invalid pension with a heart problem and died two years later, owning nothing. I was denied return on his very high insurance premiums by a freak set of circumstances that gave me no redress. I was back to earning my own living, which was OK, but it did not allow me to continue with the rather great plans we had had for our land, and I knew that more money had to come from somewhere, if this was ever to happen! No wonder Conium was needed.

While writing this chapter in 2002, I took Conium 10MM again, the first in five years, to see what it would produce. Firstly, I woke in the night, 2.30 am, to urinate. The urine fell in a weak stream, a vertical drop with no expulsive power. On waking in the morning, my eyelids would not open. It took me a minute or so of blinking hard before they functioned properly. (This tense-and-relax repetition is effective for muscle problems anywhere in the body.)

I awoke that morning also with a thin, watery post-nasal drip that caused me to cough but was not solid enough to expectorate. Then, my eyes were dry and my mouth was dry for two days, with a tendency for my jaw to drop and my mouth to open as soon as I fell asleep. And on the first day, I experienced a sharp pain at the ziphoid process, the lowest point of the breastbone. My breathing was impeded, I had to keep taking deep breaths, and I could not stop belching, as if the diaphragm was affected by gas in the stomach; the belching did not help the breathing difficulty. My bowels were delayed, as if no nerve supply was coming from the spine. For two nights, my shoulders were sore to lie on, I had soreness in the sacro-iliac joints on lying on my back, which had gone by morning, and sore tension at the back of my head, all day, with unusual thirst for fresh water.

It showed me that Conium was working on both the sacrum and the occiput, as well as somehow influencing the fluid distribution into, through and out of the body. To cap it all off, I was conscious of wondering where the money was going to come from, to build the home I was planning. After three days the adverse effects had worn off and I stopped thinking about money.

I mention these to illustrate how Conium can be effective against such types of sufferings, as 'what it causes, it can cure'. Along with Staphisagria and Ignatia, Conium is a powerful cranial remedy and pituitary corrector.

A beautiful woman of 45 came in 1996 in a very teary state. She spent three quarters of the two-hour consultation in tears, had been crying all day every day for some time, wanting to die, to go to sleep and not wake up. She could not cope on her own, felt as if in a quicksand. Her mother was her strength, now mother was overseas, and she was living in the mother's home, which made the sense of missing her more acute. She feared being alone in the house, felt protected if someone was with her, even if not in the same room with her. What triggered all this?

She had built up a really good business importing furniture, but when it was still at the top, she had lost confidence. She had feared losing her pension, was frightened of being successful, as it would mean she was independent. She could not believe in independence. She feared going to gaol if she kept the pension after earning enough to do without it. What if she gave up the pension and the business collapsed?

'I didn't do the books properly,' she said. The business had grown too big, and she had panicked and handed it over to a brother, who had made a lot out of it and was not giving her any of it. 'Greed has taken over,' she said, woefully. Conium 10MM, without any follow-up, produced 'an excellent result', I was told in 2000.

The Conium lack of faith can also cause death by injury, such as a severe head injury. The talented US musician, Kevin McDowall, suffered a severe head injury in a motor vehicle accident, after which he became more and more child-like and finally died, paralysed, at the age of only 47. Knowing what we know about Conium, we expect that McDowall suffered the financial insecurity typical of musicians, with their erratic incomes.

Every plant remedy has correlations with remedies from the mineral kingdom. The most significant mineral companions to Conium, I found, were Silica and Phosphorus, and the mighty Calcarea Fluorica, which is also a great follow-up remedy after Hydrastis.

Calc Fluor, like Conium, acts to relieve fear of the future, financial insecurity and fear of lack, while on the physical plane it strengthens spinal discs and bone surfaces, reducing arthritis and giving space in the spine for compressed discs to fill out again. I had a wonderful experience with Calc Fluor when I began to suffer, in 1999, what appeared to be a relapse of a spondylisthesis (forward slip) of my fifth lumbar vertebra, which I had corrected with Hydrastis MM and 10MM many years earlier. Xray showed this was still holding, but the disc between L5 and the sacrum was severely compressed, cramping the nerves exiting the spine at that level. How to fix?

I thought about what I already knew. Over the years, I had had a lot of great use from the Schuessler Tissue Salts, and knew the benefit of Calc Fluor in replacing the vital chemistry of the discs, cartilage and tendons. Would this

184

do the job? Or was it a case of dehydration of the disc tissue, that Calc Fluor would not necessarily correct? I decided to give it a try, and took a dose of Calc Fluor MM. My back pain disappeared overnight. Six months later, the benefit lapsed a little, and I took Calc Fluor 10MM. This lasted for another year, when, after some heavy lifting, I began to suffer again. I took Calc Fluor 50M this time, and have had no trouble in well over a decade. I have since used this remedy on numerous occasions to repair compressed discs.

Unless we have faith, we cannot receive abundance. The belief in limitation of the Conium patient leads him to fear that there is only a limited supply and he may not get enough for himself or to fulfil his plans. He is not a hoarder necessarily, not a miser, does not want more than enough, but is secretly terrified of being without supply, and of being reliant on his own efforts to provide the supply. He does not know where to start. Conium removes this guilt and improves the weakness, paralysis, cancer, diabetes, and the reversion to emotional and physical immaturity that can stem from guilt over, and fear of, independence.

A belief in limitation is all that stands between man and his unlimited supply. Once you gain faith in yourself and your inner connection to the limitless All-that-is and realize that the universe is actually, really, supporting you and all your ambitions and ideas, you cease to fear to stand independently. You are free to stride forth in confidence, and this very change of faith allows all things to work together for your good.

CHAPTER 10

An evil act may not return to the evildoer but guilt will fester in his soul
and sooner or later make him suffer.
- Leo Tolstoy

HYDRASTIS AND RESPONSIBILITY

Hydrastis (hydrastis canadensis, *Golden Seal*, N.O. Ranunculaceae) is a native of Eastern USA but is fast becoming rare in the wild, at risk of extinction, because the part used medicinally, the bright yellow root, requires that the whole plant be harvested, and also because of deforestation of its habitats. It is very difficult to grow in cultivation. If only herbalists would use the micro-doses of homeopathy! There is no need for the guilt of overharvesting.

Herbally, Golden Seal was used by the North American natives as a healing remedy for their battle wounds, for digestive complaints, for cancer and for smallpox. It has antibiotic, soothing, healing benefit to eyes, mucous membranes, skin lesions and flesh wounds. The early settlers learned of its virtues from the indigenous people who used the root as a medicine and its yellow juice as a stain for their faces and a dye for their clothing.

In modern herbal use it is valuable in disordered digestion and has a special action on the mucous membranes, clearing various forms of catarrh. It is valued for its insulin in hyperglycemia, used with Licorice Root in hypoglycemia and as a liver enzyme support, assisting habitual constipation, nausea and vomiting. As a tea, it prevents and cures nightsweats and is used as a gargle for ulcerated mouth, as a wash for conjunctivitis and as a general cleanser of wounds.

It is a powerful herb with some detrimental effects in prolonged use: it can cause constipation, lumbar aching and immune system weakness similar to the effects of pharmaceutical antibiotics, predisposing to malignancies including tumours in the bowel and liver. Nevertheless, it was one of the most favoured herbs in American medical practice in the days before the 'wonder drugs', and in 1898 was written up by Finley Ellingwood M.D.

Ellingwood gave its benefits as imparting permanent improvement in tone to the muscular structure of the heart, and all the muscular structures everywhere, being 'most valuable in altered conditions of the heart muscle'; tonic, restorative and soothing to the gastrointestinal tract, promoting appetite, increasing secretion of the gastric juices to normal, increasing peristaltic action and muscular action in the intestines; 'it supersedes all known remedies' for conditions of catarrhal gastritis and ulceration, and he mentions its use for atonic dyspepsia and stagnant, inoperative liver, chronic constipation, hepatic congestion, catarrh of the gall ducts, chronic alcoholism, general debility and nerve prostration after protracted fevers or nervous breakdown from overwork. Its influence, he states, is on the nervous system, promoting normal circulation and increasing nutrition to the digestive organs and heart.

As if that is not enough, Ellingwood writes of doctors who have used it with great benefits for women's problems: disorders of the womb, removing excess growth; for uterine subinvolution, menorrhagia, metrorrhagia, 'it is the best remedy we have'; for thick, yellow leucorrhea; in swelling of the breasts during menstruation; in cancer and scirrhus of the breast, it was used where the tumour was hard and painful, as opposed to Conium where they are small, hard and painless, and Phytolacca, where the swelling is soft and undulated and painful on pressure, with pain extending to the axilla; and it was often used in conjunction with Conium or all three together, with synergistic benefits in non-malignant mammary tumours.

Furthermore, Ellingwood says, Hydrastis was recommended for all catarrhal conditions, inflammation of the eyes, diphtheria and tonsillitis, gonorrhoea, prostrating night-sweats, eczema of the anus and fissures of the rectum, bladder catarrh, gallstones and gallstone colic and goitre (cured better than iodine and thyroid extract).

Only the un-patentability of plants has caused this wonderful herb to be removed from medical practice in favour of big money-spinners.

HYDRASTIS IN HOMEOPATHY

Hydrastis has long been felt to have three major spheres of influence - the liver, the bowel and on mucous congestion, particularly in the throat. The mental symptoms are not specific, simply general words like despondency, moroseness, gloom, irritability. Hydrastis has not been recognised, in recent years, for the magnificent, broad-spectrum remedy it is. Clarke says, 'more cases of cancer have been cured by it than with any other single remedy. In very many cancer cases there is what has been termed "a pre-cancerous stage," a period of undefined ill-health without any discernable new growth. This stage is generally marked by symptoms of dyspepsia, and this frequently takes the Hydrastis type,' with appetite bad, digestion poor for bread and vegetables, and an empty, 'gone' feeling. Conium dyspepsia is also a cancer precursor.

Hildegard of Bingen[70] regarded chronic dyspepsia as a sure indicator of cancer. She described her ideas for its prevention and treatment, which are being applied now by various doctors in Germany and elsewhere.

Clarke lists the following conditions as applicable to Hydrastis:

Clinical.- Alcoholism. Asthma. *Cancer. Catarrh.* Chancroids. *Constipation. Corns. Dyspepsia.* Eczema impetiginoides. *Ears, affections of. Faintness.* Fistula. Gastric catarrh. Gonorrhœa. Haemorroids. Jaundice. *Leucorrhœa. Lip, cancer of. Liver, affections of. Lumbago. Lupus.* Menorrhagia. Metrorrhagia. Mouth, sore. *Nails, affections of.* Nipples, sore. *Noises in the head.* Nursing women, sore mouth of. *Ozœna.* Placenta, adherent. Post-nasal catarrh. *Rectum, affections of.* Sciatica. Seborrhœa. *Stomach, affections of.* Syphilis. Taste, disordered. *Throat-deafness. Throat, sore. Tongue, affections of.* Typhus. *Ulcers.* Uterus, affections of.

To this I can add: Antibiotics, chronic effects of. Hyperglycemia. Injuries, all tissues. Skin, cancer of. Spondylolisthesis.

HYDRASTIS IN MEGAPOTENCY

Our remarkable experience with Hydrastis in megapotency showed it to be a most remarkable injury remedy and led us to many great adventures in the healing of stubborn chiropractic cases. Pelvic cancers following lumbar spinal conditions are common, and we need to consider both Hydrastis and Ruta whenever such cases present. I have observed that the Hydrastis cases usually have some liver involvement in their history, whether from alcohol, hepatitis, or too many antibiotics or other drugs, but this is not always the case.

The primary emotional hangup of Hydrastis, we found, is over-responsibility, with guilt. The Hydrastis person willingly carries the weight of responsibility and the loads of others, to his own detriment. He feels responsible for others' health and welfare, responsible or guilty for things done or not done in the past, guilty over things that are not his fault or responsibility, where he has a sense of 'It's up to me to fix this situation', or worse, responsible for the death of someone. Hydrastis sufferers range from the extremely helpful and generous, the Mr Fixits to the hard-hearted businessman, to the crime-boss, to the murderer, with many types under its umbrella.

In very high potencies, we found Hydrastis to have a profound benefit in treating the residual effects of old injuries. The critical attitude has always been 'It was my own fault', or 'It is my responsibility to fix the problem'. You need to look back on the injury and consider who you thought was to blame at the time, and if you felt responsible (rightly or wrongly), then Hydrastis could help you. Other feelings could be significant too, whether felt before or at the time, and these could suggest another remedy in this book.

A profound use for megapotency Hydrastis is in conditions that are directly related to the adverse effects of too many antibiotics. Relating to this is the guilt resulting from trying too many drugs in an attempt to get well.

The immune system and the liver are greatly benefited by Hydrastis in these cases. The patient will try persistently for year after year to find the solution to her health problem, using one medicine after another without permanent results, except that the liver becomes overloaded and unable to cleanse the body of the residues, and the immune system is impaired by the drugs. This can lead into liver cancer, which Hydrastis also helps.

The remedy works particularly well on bone and joint damage, both in the spine and limbs, and has a specific affinity for the load-bearing joints of L4-5 and L5-Sacrum and the lower limbs. These spinal segments govern the supply of nerves to the bowel and legs, thus when nerve supply is reduced over long years after spinal injury or too much guilt load, bowel cancer can result; or knees will give out from old cartilage injury or prolonged load bearing, mental or physical.

The weight of responsibility affects the lumbar spine by weakening the ligaments and allowing spondylolisthesis (disc slippage) to occur, even without any injury trauma. Weakness in the anterior spinal ligaments from L4 to the sacrum, caused by physically or psychologically carrying too great a load, causes the whole spine to shift forward from its stable position on the sacral platform.

Hydrastis in megapotencies strengthens these ligaments and in doing so, brings overnight correction of the spondylolisthesis and the lumbar curve is pulled back to normal, allowing full nerve supply to be restored to the legs and the bowels.

Where calcification of cartilage has occurred, the body is attempting to strengthen the damaged joint by solidifying the connecting tissues. We are finding that Hydrastis also reduces this calcification as it heals the damaged cartilage. Hydrastis also heals ruptured spinal discs when the mental picture matches. (See Calc Fluor in the Conium chapter, for disc compression.)

Hydrastis-responsible people carry the loads of others because they feel stronger and more capable of doing so, rather in a parental manner.

With Hydrastis the load is centrally carried, but too weighty for the ligaments and discs at L4 - S1 to maintain integrity. Hydrastis pain is felt as a persistent ache, evenly across the lower lumbars and out to the iliac crests. There is a weighty feeling in the legs. In extreme cases they are unable to stand up from sitting, or take their weight for more than a moment - indeed, this can be dangerous and lead to a ruptured disc. Lying on the back helps as this relaxation allows the vertebrae to sink back towards their normal position. Walking with crutches helps, as this takes the body's weight to the shoulders and allows the lumbars space to realign, a form of passive traction. This applies also to cases of knee damage. These measures are impermanent without strengthening the ligaments and cartilage through guilt release.

189

Weight-lifters typically get Hydrastis backs. The Hydrastis type of spondylolisthesis (the most common kind) is both palpable and usually visible in a prone patient. The lumbar curve dips at L5 or at L4 and L5 to form a straight line with L3, while the sacrum has remained in its rightful place. There is a definite step up to the sacrum from L5, as you feel it on the spine. There is no rotation - both left and right sides of the lumbar muscles and vertebrae feel alike. (Rotation indicates Ruta.)

At the top of the spine, the first cervical vertebra, C1, is similarly anterior to its normal position - not easily palpated if you are not trained to find it. C1 feeds nerve supply to the brain and particularly the vagus nerve, which innervates the face, eyes, nose, mouth, throat and all the digestive area. Because Hydrastis is an ascending problem, when we fix the lower spine the head end often fixes itself immediately, without any attention, and the cranial nerves are freed up to work at their best. These impaired nerves are related to the feelings of moroseness, heavy spirit, despondency and grumpiness that often are present with Hydrastis, and which lift off when the remedy is used. The 10th cranial nerve, the vagus, also supplies energy to the digestive organs, accounting for the solar plexus involvement in some Hydrastis problems, and the intellectualising of many life situations, the clamping down of intuitive and instinctive knowledge.

Whether or not you realize that carrying too much for others or holding on to guilt is part of your makeup, if you have any of the above patterns this is the cause for them. It is the body's way of saying 'enough', time to let up and take care of yourself rather than everyone else. It is also saying 'forgive yourself', everyone makes mistakes, everyone has weaknesses and that's OK, it is all part of our learning. Our chief responsibility, every one of us, is to attend to this learning ourselves and leave others to attend to theirs. Indeed, we are not helping others if we take on their responsibilities for them, unless they are totally unable to help themselves.

After our initial experience with Hydrastis (described in Chapter 1) we began to look at spines and other injuries more carefully. We had a very enlightening experience with one patient. We had initially thought that the guilt with Hydrastis was only over harm caused to oneself. Thanks to the sensitivity of this one lady, we now understand that it incorporates guilt over harm done to others. This is very important knowledge, as it makes the use of Hydrastis even more widely needed than we believed. So many people have guilt over something they did or didn't do, that led to someone else's being disadvantaged, maimed or killed. Here's what happened to this over-responsible, guilty patient, a woman in her fifties.

I chose Hydrastis on July 13, 1992 for this person as she kept coming in for chiropractic treatment for recurrent injuries sustained by falling off her horse, which she persistently rode bareback over rough, hilly country. Surely a case of 'This is all my own fault!' Her symptom that week had been distressing, asthma-like difficulty getting her breath. I asked her to write down her reactions, and they were as follows:

'Dose: *Hydrastis MM, on 3 consecutive nights:*

'Days 2, 3: Some improvement; still distressed.

'Day 5: I didn't like my husband's criticism of my tone of voice, verbally flared up and started crying, couldn't stop for at least 30 minutes (unusual for me). I knew the tears had nothing to do with him. I came to remembering the death of our dog, how I'd felt responsible because in trying to push her clear of the car when she was jumping out, I just complicated things - she lost balance, went under the car and broke her neck. Died in my arms. (I'd had a dream two days earlier where I had seen her lying dead - had suppressed it.)

'Then came thoughts of Prince's death. I was fifteen, and had felt guilt and grief that I had gone to school when he showed signs of being sick. He died of poisoning. I can now see that I did not know what else to do; I was able to forgive myself and let the guilt go. I felt some immediate improvement in breathing. Over the next few days breathing returned to normal.'

The guilt over *not having been able to do what was necessary to save* these animals that she loved was related to the bareback riding. She loves the horse very much and felt guilty that she might be harming the horse if she continued to ride it without a saddle, yet enjoyed doing so so much that she was reluctant to stop. She has stopped falling off now that the guilt has been released.

This same interesting aspect of Hydrastis was shown up in a woman of 61 who had nursed her elderly mother for six years before her death, and who had then found herself with bowel cancer. She came to me having had surgery seven months before and was still on chemotherapy for one more month. It seemed to me that the main guilt feeling contributing to the cancer was the feeling that she had been unable to do enough to relieve the pain her mother had suffered.

The old lady had had severe shingles which gave her agonising pain in the face for the next six years; she also had had to have one leg amputated during that time, which made her very dependent on the daughter. It had been a long six years, watching mother suffer such pain and gradually deteriorate. Her death was a welcome peace for both, but the guilt of not having been able to do enough to lessen the pain now threatened to become the killer of the daughter. The choice of Hydrastis was standard therapy from repertorising, its use in very high potency cleared the guilt. Ten years later, she developed a Conium abdominal tumour (a virgin and a spinster all her life) but she couldn't ask her brother to bring her to me, had given up driving herself, and she finally succumbed after five years.

Injuries of long-standing, where the feeling at the time was of 'my own fault', always respond well to Hydrastis. Here's another example:

This man's problem began in 1972 when he slipped on some stairs and damaged his right knee. The knee was locked into a bent position. At a major Sydney teaching hospital, they tried to straighten the knee forcefully, wrapped it up and gave him crutches to keep him going until three weeks later, he had a cartilage operation. After two months of physiotherapy, he could still not straighten his knee normally, and this condition remained the same until 1979, when he slipped again and felt severe pain in the lower back. This time the doctor recommended rest, pain-killers and a back brace. He sought help from a chiropractor and was back at work in two weeks.

Between 1979 and 1996, his back 'went out' numerous times and he always had benefit from either massage or chiropractic. In July 1996, walking up some steps, he felt something go in his right knee and was in constant severe pain until an arthroscope was done and extraneous cartilage fragments were removed. This produced very little change, and he discovered Bryan and began to get chiropractic care again.

Bryan found the right calf and foot were in extreme pain still, he suffered back aches still, and migraines. His fifth lumbar vertebra was anterior to the lumbar curve, his pelvis was left rotated and his right sacroiliac joint was posterior to the left one. There was heavy spasm in the right calf muscles and to a lesser extent, in the hamstrings. The right leg could not be fully extended nor could it flex. Bryan gave his usual deep tissue massage to the legs and full spine, and adjusted the spine, but gave no remedies. At the next visit a week later, there had been no improvements, the leg was still in extreme pain. Bryan found the tibia/fibula joint was jammed. Twice-weekly visits gradually began to show a little improvement, but not much - heat improved, sitting was terrible, he could not sit down long enough to have a meal. By September 19th, applying pressure to the soleus trigger point had given a lot of relief, but this was still painful. To help himself, he was cycling two kilometres a day and was able to sleep without the back brace.

At this point Bryan thought of Hydrastis but did not give it yet. Because of the rotation of the pelvis he was unsure whether to use Ruta instead. The calf and ankle 'still gives me heaps', our client said in November. On 12th November, Bryan bit the bullet and gave him Hydrastis MM and followed this up with Ruta MM for the rotation. These gave great relief, and at the next week's visit, he confessed to having felt so good, he did a lot of cleaning work over the weekend and had given himself a touch of sciatica (probably a Return of Old Symptoms from the earlier back injury). After the session the knee was able to bend to 90°, the best so far. Bryan gave him Hydrastis 200 for three days but not more Ruta.

Leg pain persisted and our client lined up for another arthroscope in December that year, this time with a different surgeon, where he was found to have a piece of broken bone loose in the knee area. He returned to Bryan in March 97, May 97 and January 98 without a repeat of the remedies, somewhat better than in 1996 but still a long way to go. In March 98, I intervened and gave him Hydrastis MM, and in July 1998, 10MM.

Improvements would lapse after a couple of months. We never gave him Ruta again, which, looking back, I think would have completed the job more rapidly and totally. Hydrastis 50M followed, in January 99. In April 99, he told us the right calf muscle, that had for so long been in constant pain, was now 'hardly there,' only felt with deep tissue massage. In June 99, he reviewed the two years of homeopathic and chiropractic treatment, saying 'Results good and getting better.' I gave him Hydrastis MM again in November that year, for a repeat of the spondylolisthesis of the lumbars. He continues to have regular massage and mobilisation and is pleased to have his thirty-year-old knee problem well under control.

Never believe that a problem you have had for many years cannot be resolved. It just takes a little longer.

In a similar case, an ex-footballer in his mid forties walked around the end of his bed one day and fell straight to the floor. One of his knees (both were damaged several times twenty years before, in football injuries) had given way on him as he took his weight on it at an unusual angle. He went to the Casualty department at the hospital and they X-rayed and sent him home on crutches, well strapped up. Pain was severe and he could take none of his considerable weight on it. He took the X-rays and report to the orthopædic specialist who told him the knee was too badly damaged to be operable, there were too many fragments of bone and cartilage floating about, he was too young for a knee replacement for at least ten years and he would be in a wheelchair within months.

Our man was not going to take that lying down, and began to give himself regular massage and a course of mineral tablets suited to joint repair. He had struggled around on crutches for four weeks when I saw him. I had already given him Hydrastis MM four years prior for his spondylolisthesis, which had given benefit at that time, so remembering this, I immediately gave him Hydrastis MM again and we put him on to sedentary office work.

Benefit began almost immediately. Within one week he had replaced the crutches with two walking sticks, and three weeks later had gone down to one stick. After Hydrastis 10MM this stick was abandoned as well. It was about six months before he was able to work on his feet for long, but he does not intend to ever see the surgeon again.

This case also shows you how healing takes place in specific directions. Have another look in Chapter Four at Hering's Laws of Direction of Cure. Healing takes place from above downwards and problems go in the reverse order of their arrival. After strengthening up the lumbar spine the older picture of the knee injuries came up to be healed properly. The funny thing was, 'This was my good knee!' Evidently this had been the worst knee at one stage but the body had managed to compensate for this and the other had given trouble over more recent years. The body brought up the worst injury and both knees benefited from the treatment.

A young man of 19 fell from his cycle during a training run, landing on his right shoulder and his chin, and grazing the full right side of his right calf. The shoulder was immobile and stiff and it was hard to write. The handlebars had rammed into his right ribcage, and his jaw and teeth were sore. 'My own fault,' he told me, 'I was riding two abreast with another cyclist, and swerved to miss a rock on the road. We were going downhill at over 70kph, and we both went down.' Hydrastis 10MM saw him recovered in very quick time.

Another young man of 25 had had a back problem for over five years when he found me. He had an L5 vertebra that was sitting anterior to the rest of the lumbar curve, causing pain in the lumbars and buttocks. Pain was bad in unsupported seats, and at its worst, in any position, but lying on his back and drawing his knees up towards the chest relieved. It was hard to rise without using his arms to pull his weight up, and hard to bend forward, the spinal muscles were trying so hard to maintain the fragile integrity of the spine by keeping his centre of gravity vertical. These are all good indicators for Hydrastis, and MM fixed.

In cases of extreme guilt, it is often the liver that is carrying the 'my fault' or 'it's up to me' load. Using Hydrastis will improve the temperament and lower cholesterol and calcium in the blood vessels, repair alcohol damage, cleanse the blood, abolish anaemia and set the stage for the reversal of serious degenerative disease.

The way it helps anaemia is this. In the liver are cells called Kuppfer cells which normally break down old red blood cells (after 120 days of use) into their components, which are either re-used or discharged. In the sluggish liver, this process can be slowed down so that components are not as quickly available to the bone marrow as they normally are, and red blood cells can only be made at a slower rate of production, causing a depleted situation to develop in the blood. By stimulating better liver function, Hydrastis and numerous other homeopathic remedies restore order to red blood cells. Many anaemic people have normal iron intake.

I have often used Hydrastis for people who have been heavy drinkers, who carry a lot of guilt over their former behaviour. I remember one particular man who had been a very heavy drinker through most of his long marriage, who had behaved unforgivably toward his wife and was so saturated with guilt, although he'd dried out and tried to make good, that he developed, firstly, bowel cancer which was operated on, and later, liver cancer. Unfortunately for him, he was beyond physical help by the time he found me, though I think he cleared out a lot of guilt before he died. That is healing, too. On this level the healing stands you in good stead for the future even if this body is beyond help. Cancer patients need to keep in mind that it can take twenty years or more for a cancer to develop from one cell to a tiny tumour of a square centimetre. By the time many are detected, they are likely to be irreversible.

If you are a heavy drinker, you could also try Hydrastis in the megapotencies to help give up alcohol - clear the guilt and the problem ceases to be perpetuated. If the whole idea of giving up alcohol is frightening to you, take Aconite MM first.

Hydrastis promises to be mighty in its guilt-freeing of our Australian aboriginal population. Massive guilt cripples these people over losing their land, much of their population and their personal sovereignty when the whites moved in. This great guilt has caused them to become prone to eye diseases, to abuse alcohol, to abuse their families (both sexually and by bashing and verbal abuse) and engage in anti-social activities like smash-and-grab robberies, fist fights, petty thieving, destruction of property and generally, to be picked on and picked up by police far more than anyone needs. It has contributed to our significant mistreatment of their race generally - Hydrastis needed all around.

Our over-refined diet has also weakened the aboriginal population. Refer back to Chapter 3 for the diabetes experiment on aboriginal men in Sydney, in which a return to a natural diet eliminated their diabetes. This is also a case of guilty lost intuition causing racial abandonment of their healthy diet in favour of the 'desirable' or enforced modern one that kills.

Another example in Chapter 3 was of Dr Archie Kalokorinos, who made a name for himself some decades ago by treating aboriginal populations in central New South Wales with large doses of Vitamin C, which was very deficient in the inland modern diet of the day. Dr Kalokorinos achieved great benefits to their eye conditions and general resistance to the white man's diseases of measles, colds and flus, not to mention immunisation injection effects, from which many children were dying. At the time, medical opinion ridiculed him greatly, in their arrogant ignorance.

Risk of infection from poor living conditions is always Hydrastis. Overcrowding and water contamination from lack of sanitation, causing risk of food poisoning gives many westerners fear of contracting hepatitis, typhoid, 'Bali belly' dysentery, gastroenteritis, giardia lamblia, helicobacter pyloris and guilt conditions of many other names. 'Mighty loss of interest in historical lessons is the reason. It is thinking you are beyond great, guilty responsibility - I think this is the reason that poverty still exists in overcrowded countries. Put the leaders of such countries and cities on to Hydrastis and they will begin to put resources towards lifting the poverty line. Slow progress, but it will happen,' Gonjesil advised.

When we westerners go to impoverished countries and find ourselves assailed by beggars, the guilt of being better off and yet being unable to improve their lot, whatever we may hand out, causes us to come down with dysenteric bowel complaints ('Bali Belly' we Aussies call it) that always respond well to Hydrastis in medium potencies.

Mucus is one of the conditions common in Hydrastis people. Mucus production is the body's mighty way of flushing away the residues of the lymphocytes' battles against invading foreign substances, toxins and bacteria. When this mucus clearance is slowed by sluggish lymph and liver functions, such residues remain in the tissues too long and may cause clogging of organ functions. White, yellow and old, brown or greenish mucus indicate this sluggishness. The mucus eliminating via the mucous membranes is grinding out slowly into the nasal passages because the liver is sluggishly overloaded and the lymphatic system is unable to dump its loads into the liver for elimination via the bowel. As the skin can be used as a safety-valve eliminatory organ, so too the inner skin of the nose and throat.

The contribution Hydrastis makes to assist this process is to stimulate the liver and bowel functions and speed up elimination of the old hoards of toxins, thus making it unnecessary to use the mucous linings for this purpose. It is of no benefit to take antibiotics under these conditions, they only add to the accumulated rubbish waiting to be eliminated, while undermining the cleansing functions of the immune system. Fix the guilt of not knowing how to loosen off the problem and it starts to fix itself.

Hydrastis in megapotency is a remedy of profound and far-reaching benefits to all practitioners of the healing arts. If that means you, consider it for yourself. It will break the impasse if you have a problem that is resisting full clearance. Clear away the guilt that you are unable to fix or help everyone, or even just one person, and your own problem may dissipate into thin air.

The usual chronic problem of the Hydrastis type is one of obstinate determination to remain, which gives the sufferer a growing feeling of guilt that whatever is tried, nothing seems to work, or not permanently. The patient begins to accept that he will never be any better. Even the use of Hydrastis in medium-high potencies will not shift the problem permanently. Hydrastis MM will sometimes break the block, whatever the indicated remedy may have been that had failed to act, and the symptom picture will rapidly shift (overnight perhaps) to that of the next remedy, which will then work well (I speak only of chronic, not acute complaints). So Hydrastis in MM is a prime remedy for those who have arrived at a despondent belief in, and guilt over the hopelessness of their complaint - whatever it may be - when not for the want of trying all avenues. This is just another way of saying 'guilt over not knowing how to save oneself'.

It may be that several other remedies will be needed as well - for Bryan we had used Staphisagria earlier, and later he benefited from Silica (which established the bowel action that Hydrastis had failed to touch). The animal-lover had previously had great benefit from Staphisagria and later Ignatia before arriving at the Hydrastis symptom picture.

' There is a reflex link between the lower spine and the upper. Spinal ligaments attach like long ropes to the sacrum and to the occiput, so that problems in the lower spine often flow along the rope like whiplash, appearing in the upper neck. In particular, L5 Hydrastis problems become C1 problems that inhibit or restrict thinking processes quite a lot, guiltily producing quite loveless thoughts of life, even to suicide.

Parents of teenagers who go their own way and have to learn from getting into scrapes need to realize, through Hydrastis, that they do not have to carry blame on that account; likewise, those who feel great guilt when youngsters overdose on drugs or commit suicide. While freeing the guilt-feeling of failing in your responsibility as a parent, Hydrastis opens the mind to new ways of overcoming these social problems.

Guilt over harm done to others covers a very broad field, including that of suppressed guilt. Many people continue to cause harm, one way or another, because they refuse to acknowledge that any harm is being caused. Into this category come alcoholics, fast food operators, people who enjoy blood sports, people who practice western medicine, farmers using herbicides and pesticides, veterinarians, all exploiters of the earth and the forests, wildlife and the oceans, sexual exploiters, unscrupulous business people, dole-bludgers, malingerers, litigators, con-men, parents, teachers and clergy, and more.

In the latter half of the nineteenth century, John D. Rockefeller was a young man with a strict religious upbringing and a strong, disciplined code of social ethics and morals - the typically wholesome, all-American boy. He was a generous man with a strong sense of responsibility to assist those less fortunate wherever he could. He had, he believed, a God-given gift to make money, which became a mission for him. Everything he handled turned to gold. By the time he was twenty five he was already a multimillionaire, which was big money back in those days, even before he discovered the potential for oil. Once his oil wells were flowing, he cornered the market in rail transportation and refinement of the crude, and distribution of the petroleum, buying out the lesser companies and thus setting up the first major monopoly in the world, Standard Oil.

Guilt of making too much money set in, and to offset this, the well-meaning Rockefeller set up the Rockefeller Institute, a funding organisation for welfare and charitable bodies, schools and universities. Misguidedly, under persuasion from drug companies, he also put fortunes behind drug 'research', thus establishing the perpetuated ignorance of the old chemistry-based medicine as the primary option for Americans. The newer homeopathy, which at the turn of the twentieth century had about equal numbers of practitioners to the 'old school' (as it was called then, now called 'modern'!), and which was enjoying great popularity on account of its successes in epidemics, was gradually forced into a long hibernation from which it is only lately emerging.

So, you see, Hydrastis carries benefits for both the Goodies and the Baddies of this world. Think of it always for people who feel responsible for seeing to the correction of harmful situations, most doctors, nurses, carers, social workers and health practitioners, teachers, help-yourself organisations, gaols and correction centres, fund-raising supporters of charitable organisations, even fund-raisers for cancer 'research' and other heart-string-pulling exploitations, Greenies, many small business operators and countless more. There are lots of good people out there battling to overcome a lot of damage. Many need Staphisagria as well.

Gonjesil says 'Great guilt is one thing that is crippling the princely cleanup of this lovely planet. Put lots of people on to Hydrastis who think it is not doing any harm to log mighty forests bare. Feelings are, filthy greed is the main reason (Conium). Love for the planet must be put before the fear of not enough money. Funny thing is, it is the same Hydrastis guilt that is driving the push to halt logging. Such people are feeling it is their responsibility, up to them to force the companies to wake up and ease off. It is up to all the guilty to get free of their guilt and balance would be restored.

'Fear of lots of things doing harm to the planet gives in to Hydrastis. Fill lots of people with Hydrastis who go to great lengths to do no harm. It is this that is giving greater loss of integrity of their immune systems. Love for this very lovely planet is the driving force. This will not be killed out by the remedy, instead princely new ideas to look into will give them great joy. Guilty loss of energy is depleting their efforts, with guilty fear that their efforts will be in vain.'

But how do we get it into people like loggers and multinationalists?

'It is easier than you think. Give knowledge to most professionals and sooner or later, these people will turn up wanting help for their maladies.

It is estimated that in fifty years, unless there is a turnaround in 'progress', half of all the plants existing today will be extinct. Flora and fauna are becoming extinct at the rate of fifty species a day. Great work is being done in seed storage and wildlife protection, but it requires a massive shift in the consciousness of those causing the degradation as well as all of us who buy their products.

You will have noticed earlier in the chapter, that a century ago, doctors were using Hydrastis as a herbal medicine with greater success than they now get from the new wonder drugs they continually abandon in favour of newer, greater ones that also prove harmful in time. Since Rockefeller's time, the western world has been hooked into the delusion of greatness of monopoly medicine and its twin brother, the oil industry which forms the basis of most of the drugs they produce. This delusion has fed the growth of international banking, broad-acre farming, chemical fertilizers, pesticides and herbicides that have killed forested areas and devitalized soils in every continent, as well as exploitation of the resources of almost every country in the world, affecting every individual, every animal and every plant. And, contrary to the initial vision of Rockefeller, wealth is in the hands of the greedy and unscrupulous.

We are wallowing in the filthy guilt of over-industrialisation pollution. Let us shake it off, once and for all, and get our planet back to clean. Hydrastis enables instant knowledge of how to get into cleaner transportation, cleaner power, a better balance of trade and the abandonment of fear-based greed that causes stockpiling of resources while many starve. Let us follow the lead of organic and biodynamic growers, who use harmless methods including radionic energy fields to defend their crops and stock against harm, and recycling of compostible materials to replenish the soil. Lift the Hydrastis guilt and the Conium greed and we can be driving the already-invented cars that run on water, using already existing technology that extracts electricity from the air and ground - stored lightning - that requires no extraction of coal, gas or oil from the depths of the earth and contributes no waste to our air and water environment; lift the Hydrastis guilt and we can discover that money is a resource that can be used for the benefit of all, rather than fleeced from every individual for the pockets of the infinitely greedy. All our answers are already known and available to us. Let us get back to the good intent of Rockefeller - for our own survival depends on it.

CHAPTER 11

If I die in War you remember me. If I live in Peace you don't.
- Spike Milligan

HYPERICUM - 'LIVE FAST, DIE YOUNG AND HAVE A GOOD-LOOKING CORPSE'

Hypericum (hypericum perforatum, *St John's Wort*, N.O. Hypericaceae) is a plant that is native to Europe and Britain, and widely naturalised to the point of becoming a noxious weed, in North America and Australia, where it causes cattle grazing on it to become light-sensitive and die. Farmers hold meetings specifically to consider and decide upon methods to eradicate it. We found this extraordinary once we found the greater homeopathic uses of the plant, as it proved to be a great remedy for those with a killer attitude. The plant, as often happens, is growing exactly where it is needed.

Mrs Grieve mentions that the Greek name for this plant was *hypericon*, meaning 'over an apparition', seeing this as 'a reference to the belief that the herb was so obnoxious to evil spirits that a whiff of it would cause them to fly.' The name St John's Wort refers to its beginning to flower on St John's Day in mid-summer. Mrs Grieve notes its historical use in all pulmonary complaints, bladder troubles, in suppression of urine, dysentery, worms, diarrhoea, hysteria and nervous depression, haemoptysis and other haemorrhages, and jaundice. As a tea, she says, it can be given at night to children with nocturnal incontinence. It was also useful in pulmonary consumption (TB), chronic catarrh of the lungs, bowels or urinary passages; and externally in fomentations to dispel hard tumours, caked breasts and blue-black bruising.

The Elizabethan herbalist John Gerard recommended an olive oil infusion of the leaves, flowers and seeds as 'a most precious remedy for deep wounds and those that are through the body, for the sinews that are pricked, or any wound made with a venomed weapon.'

The modern American herbalist Matthew Wood says 'Hypericum was largely ignored by the eclectic and physio-medical doctors of nineteenth century America. They seem to have identified it closely with 'the enemy', i.e.

homeopathy. However, it slowly crept into American usage, probably from European immigrants.' Wood waxes lyrical in its praises: 'It is hard to imagine that this herb could ever have been abandoned by herbalists. It has the most beautiful, warm, balsamic, healing taste. I sometimes think of it as the archetypal medicinal herb. Father Sebastian Kneipp called it the "perfume of God"and the "flower of the Fairies."'

In his modern scientific compendium 'Herbal Drugs', Max Wichtl gives its indications as 'For milder forms of neurotic depression, e.g. during the menopause and in nervous exhaustion. The only side effect noted is photosensitivity (from high or prolonged doses) but no cases of phototoxicity have been reported in humans.' The German Standard License gives its uses as 'in supportive treatment of nervous excitement and disturbances of sleep.' There have been recent trials applying it in the form of high doses of hypericin against retroviruses. Hypericin is the main active constituent and is believed to be a monoamineoxidase inhibitor. According to recent reports, St John's Wort has become Europe's number one antidepressant. About three million prescriptions are written annually for it, in Germany alone - that is about twenty five times the number written for Prozac.

In modern native American herbal medicine, according to Matthew Wood, Hypericum is used extensively 'for most of the medical problems known to traditional European practitioners, for physical and metaphysical problems.

'Hypericum has been used in homeopathy and herbalism externally as a soothing anti-inflammatory for fresh, bleeding wounds, sores, burns (in all degrees), bedsores, chaps, folliculitis, abrasions and injuries from work or cleaning agents, bumps, boils, furuncles, dry and wet eczemas and insect stings. It is also useful as a cosmetic skin-care cream for scaly, dry or unclean skin and very effective as a massage oil for muscle spasm, cramps, stiffness, ache, overuse, sprains, bruises, articular aches and backache, rheumatism, gout, sciatica, neuralgia, and poor circulation to the extremities.'

Hypericum is used herbally, internally, for chronic illnesses that relate to nerve depletion - chronic pain, nervous exhaustion, emotional depression, mental and physical weakness, in association with stress and fear. Originally, those who succumbed to Hypericum conditions were people of high nervous energy who had become burned out through stress, overwork, overtraining - all prolonged draining of Vitamin B1. It has a great affinity for the solar plexus, benefiting the acid levels of the stomach and soothing ulcers, heartburn and bloating through its energising of the nerves to these areas. It assists all the digestive processes in this way.

As a Flower Essence, St. John's Wort is used to bring emotions and thoughts into synchronicity. It deals with an over-expanded state leading to psychic and physical vulnerability, lack of groundedness, dream disturbances and weak or distorted connections between the physical, etheric and astral bodies and the ego. This gives us the lead-in to understanding Hypericum in its megapotency homeopathic uses.

HYPERICUM IN HOMEOPATHY

Hypericum is widely used in homeopathy for injuries to nerves, such as spinal jarring, falls on the coccyx or blows to the top of the head, and as a treatment and preventive of tetanus. It is renowned for its benefits in the treatment of insect stings, bites and other puncture wounds from, for example, barbed wire, nails and knife-stabs - wherever the flesh is penetrated and closes over again, leaving potential for anaerobic infection to develop. There are sharp, shooting pains along the nerves, and Hypericum is one of the all-time greats for pain relief after surgery, dental work, violent injuries and spinal damage. We refer to it as 'the homeopathic morphine'. All in all, a very useful remedy for today's frequent violent injuries from aggression, speed and recklessness. But that is not all.

A patient on chemotherapy asked for something to help her with the side-effects, which she found wiped her out of activities for days at a time. She handed me a small square of paper on which, in microscopic print, was listed the effects she could expect from the treatment. I read them and said to her, 'This all looks like Hypericum to me.' I checked up the symptoms and they were all listed under Hypericum in Clarke's Materia Medica. I gave it in 10M, and she ceased to suffer. Many others since have been enjoying freedom from chemo effects, which has gone a long way to speeding up their recovery from cancer treatments.

Clarke lists the following conditions as appropriate to the use of Hypericum in potency:

Clinical.- After-pains. Asthma. Bites. Brachial neuralgia. Breast, affections of. Brain, concussion of. *Bruises*. Bunions. Compound fractures. Corns. Coxalgia (hip pain). Diarrhoea. Gunshot wounds. Haemorrhoids. Headache. Hydrophobia. Hypersensitiveness. *Impotence*. Labour, effects of. Meningitis. Mind, affections of. Neuralgia. Operations, effects of. Panaritium (inflammation of the fingernail). *Paralysis*. Rheumatism. Scars. Sciatica. Spastic paralysis. Spinal concussion. Spinal irritation. Stiff-neck. Tetanus. Ulceration. Whooping cough. *Wounds*.

To this I can add: Alopecia, traumatic. Bronchiolitis. Chemotherapy, effects of. Fevers. Herpes. Hypodermic injections, effects of (including epidural spinal blocks). Laparoscopy, effects of. Pain, hypersensitivity to. Scoliosis, structural distortions. Shock. Ultrasound, effects of. Viruses.

HYPERICUM IN MEGAPOTENCY

I was treating several people for several years, noticing their commonality of injury history and apparent super ego, before I connected the two and understood the mental to be associated with their old Hypericum injuries. Once I noticed the common factor of *low self value*, often masked by an overbearing ego, the remedy took on a whole new complexion. It was this previously unknown relationship that was causing Hypericum injuries or complaints to remain unresolved for many years, and indeed it is this belief that causes people to have these particular injuries or diseases in the first place. The following factors were found to be common in people who benefited from Hypericum in megapotencies.

A sense of worthlessness is at the core of all chronic Hypericum problems: low self-value, unimportance, extreme humility, feeling small, ridiculed or treated with contempt. The only way he can prove his worth is to become better than everyone else, to get to the top so they cannot treat him as worthless. We found several causes for this low self-worth belief.

He or she feels abandoned, or did at one time in the past: rejected, adopted as an infant (can't be worth much when even your own mother doesn't want you), made redundant, deserted, ignored or left out; or perhaps, a parent has died. Having felt abandoned, he finds it easy to abandon someone else; and is likely to be abandoned again. Hypericum not only frees up the guilt/hurt of being abandoned but also of having hurt someone else in this way. The guilt of abandoning or treating someone as of low value is enough to create an imbalance disease such as haemochromatosis or leukemia.

Hypericum is always out of balance and struggling to find balance in life: he uses the word 'balance' frequently. He or she goes to extremes, goes overboard, can never find the point of balance or the middle path.

Think of a tall-masted sailing ship. There she stands, gently swaying from side to side, stay wires firmly running from points up the mast to the bulkhead. Think of how these wires are maintaining the stability of the mast, to strengthen it against the forces of wind and sea. Tension must be fine-tuned in each wire to prevent the mast from breaking and going overboard.

Now think of the human backbone, held vertically above the pelvis by muscles that must maintain even tension on both sides, to prevent the straightness of the spine from turning into something of a snake-like curvature.

Hypericum is the remedy that is needed when these torsion muscles (all the diagonal muscles - trapezius, rhomboids, latissimus dorsi, teres groups and others) get out of balance in their tension, pulling the spine out of alignment in this diagonal manner. Other balance muscles are also affected, such as sartorius and gastrocnemius in the legs and the sternocleidomastoids in the neck. When the Hypericum person's nervous system is shocked, the spine itself gets out of balance, and many other imbalances follow.

The Hypericum person's language uses extreme words of violence such as smash, blitz, bomb, wild, kill, boring, screwing, shoot up, wipe out, all or nothing. He feels devastated, crushed, wounded, stabbed to the heart, violated, blown apart, shattered. Extreme words of any kind - 'far out' to mean excellent; or words whose meaning is at the opposite extreme from the one you mean, e.g. wicked, to mean excellent. Accurate use of words is 'boring', normal boundaries of speech and behaviour are 'straight' and 'boring'. Life must be full of change and excitement, new is always better, to remain in the one spot, steady, is intolerable.

The Hypericum type misses the point, talks a lot about the point, 'The point is...'; he bores you to tears trying to get his point across long after you got it, even boring into your chest or your air-space with his pointed finger; he suffers from pointed instruments (daggers, hypodermics, bees, dogbites, keyhole surgery), gets viruses from stinging insects or from injections, indulges in self-mutilation or destruction by pointed instruments (pierced ears and other parts, tattoos, injected drugs). He loves pointed, spiky things like gelled hair, cactus, star-shapes, sharp weapons, studded belts.

The 'hyper' words all apply: hyperactive, hyperglycemic, hypertensive, hypersensitive, hyperreactive - all forms of imbalances and excesses. Excess cholesterol, excess calcium, excess iron, excess sodium, excess sugar, bulimia... The Hypericum type goes to extremes in every aspect of his life.

The nervous system is shocked out of balance by violence, speed injuries, puncture wounds, becomes traumatised and is unable to rebalance itself. Speed and violent sports are indulged in because of the low self-preservation instinct. Our current medical practices add to this by treating people like pincushions, with no respect for their bodies as temples of their immaculate souls. Babies feel this, and many babies believe the message they are getting, that they are not worthy of respect.

Life has no point so he devotes himself to filling it with fun. Fun is the criteria by which all activities are judged. Fun comes from speed, racing sports, driving to win in business, fast, racing vehicles, playing with younger, smaller people who look up to him instead of disparaging him. Fun and work are at opposite ends of the spectrum of life, so 'work cannot be fun'. If there is no fun he is likely to walk out of the job and go looking for fun. The only fun in work comes from competition, so you need to give these people someone to pit themselves against who is not too much smarter or more skilled.

Hypericum fears responsibility and always denies responsibility for injuries, accidents or anything going wrong. It is never his fault, he is a hapless victim of other people. For this reason, he finds it easy to sue others for compensation, the amount of which is always way over the top, beyond reason. A typical example of the refusal to accept personal responsibility came when, in August 2002, 'a 123kg man sued McDonald's and three other fast food chains, alleging they were responsible for his obesity.'[71] No-one forced him to buy their food. Hypericums are very smart at finding ways to get money for nothing, and if they can get vengeance at the same time, well and good.

Hypericum would like to stay nineteen all his life, and avoid the responsibilities of adulthood and marriage, so the spouse carries the load.

Those who accept the responsibilities of management in their work do so only to get the extra money for the weekend's fun activities or the opportunity of going one better than the neighbours in visible assets or power. You do not find many Hypericum types owning and running their own businesses, this implies too much sole responsibility, duty and long hours of work, unless they can manage to get others doing all the work while they have fun. But they are to be found at the top of the corporate ladder, or in top army positions or political leadership where they can be seen to be above the rest of the population. They will heartlessly kick everyone else off the ladder in their determination to get to the top.

You may remember in 2001, former Serbian Prime Minister Slobodan Milosevic, when facing charges of genocide in the United Nations HQ in The Hague, was addressed by the judge: 'You have the right to have the indictment read out to you at this point. You also have the right to waive this reading. Now, do you want to have the indictment read out?' Milosevic: 'That's your problem.' No responsibility taken, even for that.

Retired GE chairman Jack Welch, in his autobiography, *Jack*,[72] described how he felt about being at the top. 'Being a CEO is the nuts! A whole jumble of thoughts come to mind: Over the top. Wild fun. Outrageous. Crazy. Passion. Perpetual motion. The give and take. Meetings into the night. Incredible friendships. Fine wine. Celebrations. Great golf courses. Big decisions in the real game. Crises and pressure. Lots of swings. A few home runs. The thrill of winning. The pain of losing. It's as good as it gets! You get paid a lot, but the real pay-off is the fun.' Jack says it all - Hypericum to the back teeth.

Competition is believed to be essential, necessary and healthy. You cannot get to the top without a competitive spirit, and getting to the top is essential. In sport or in business, competition is a cut-throat sport. The competitor becomes the enemy to be conquered. He thinks it is OK that competition means there is always a loser, he has never thought that all might be winners, there is only enough room at the top for one. Social competition is high, too - he must have the biggest and latest car, the biggest boat, the biggest and loudest sound system, the biggest house on the highest hill with the best view and preferably a high wall and wide lawns to keep the neighbours at a distance. People can't be trusted.

Ha! as I wrote this, the morning paper (SMH Weekend, June 29-30, 2002) brought the story of the collapse of WorldCom, following the discovery of 'the greatest fraud ever on Wall Street - wrong, illegal and also cruel because, while WorldCom lurches toward what could be the world's largest-ever bankruptcy, it threatens not only to derail a shaky economic recovery in the United States, and to force share prices down in a market that is already badly depressed, but also to disintegrate the savings of a band of loyal, God-fearing folk in a small college town called Clinton, in the state of Mississippi' (the home of WorldCom). WorldCom, of course, had a most sensational Hypericum-style rocket to the top, rising from its foundation in 1983, by buying up many other companies, to a multi-billion dollar public company with, at this point, over US$6billion of debt. President George W. Bush called for American businesses to have more responsibility than to 'fudge the numbers.'

There is often enemy-consciousness. Distrust of others stems from earlier hurtful experiences. Territorial rights are very important. Hypericum needs plenty of his own space around him, and likes to protect himself by owning weapons of violence, and/or vicious dogs (he goes in for bull terriers particularly, intuitively choosing a dog of similar qualities). He suffers from claustrophobia in close areas, and gets panicky if he feels he may be unable to escape quickly. He prefers the policy of 'strike first, ask questions later', of 'I must get you before you get me.' Another typical Hypericum belief is 'an eye for an eye, a tooth for a tooth' - literally. Vengeance is important, and the Hypericum person can be swift and ruthless.

Swift cruelty is often Hypericum, as is the escalation of weapons of total and absolute destruction, for the murder of individuals, races and nations by annihilation. Who cares, when all are worthless? Who cares if I tie a bomb to my body and blow myself up trying to kill others? Who cares if I fly my planeload of passengers into a building and kill thousands? All are worthless, and they all think I am, even my God has abandoned me, so I must be. Who cares? I'd rather be a dead hero than a living nobody. (Fame and notoriety are equally attractive.)

Ex-soldier Chris Moon, working in Mozambique supervising mine-clearance work, was blown up by a mine in a supposedly clear area, and lost his right leg and right arm. Undeterred, Chris, a positive, determined man with a strong Nat Mur chin, decided to run in the London Marathon, managing to do so less than a year after his release from hospital. At the time of publishing his book[73], Chris had run in fifteen marathons raising money for charities assisting the disabled, including land-mine victims.

In the book, Moon mentions a story of Hypericum significance: 'A friend of mine who was clearing up after the Gulf War told me about an American EOD team that had a run of bad luck; in a series of unconnected incidents, the section were killed until there was just one left. He committed suicide. Perhaps it's harder for the ones who are left behind.' To be the only one left behind, in charge, responsible, is Hypericum abandonment, devastating, particularly in soldiers.

All historically knife-wielding peoples need Hypericum or Ledum - Hypericum for the swift retaliators, Ledum for those who grimly hold on to grudges for years. Hypericums believe in quick revenge and sneak up from behind to put a knife in your back, or a plane through your tower; they get used by the Ledums. Ledum types will plot and plan for long years to get their revenge, never relenting, never forgiving - the Osama bin Ladens and the George W. Bushes of the world stage; they despise as weak, those who turn the other cheek. While ever vengeance is practised in the world there can be no peace.

Hypericum lifts people's self esteem so they no longer feel the need to cut others down, and closes the wide space between one person and the next, allowing closer harmonious, trusting relationships. One woman, four weeks after one dose of Hypericum 10MM, said to me, 'Is it just me? People seem to be a lot nicer than I used to think they were.' And this sentiment was often stated.

It also goes a long way towards bridging the gap between male and female. The Hypericum races treat male children very leniently, while women and female children are shown great cruelty, treated as worthless. Once Hypericum lifts the men of these races out of their guilt of feeling such disrespect for life, all this will change.

Strangely, perhaps, the opposite polarity of great sympathy and love for people also is a strong quality of Hypericum and shows its great potential for world peace. Hypericum people act from the heart, impulsively.

Hypericum has big distrust of intellectually smart people, if he feels he cannot beat them at their game. At the same time, he worships the halls of learning that others attended to gain important-looking pieces of paper for their walls. Many Hypericum people have been under-educated and believe that the only way to the top is via the bit of paper. If this does not discourage them totally, they push themselves through one course after another, getting every possible certificate, diploma and degree in their chosen profession or trade, regardless of its value or relevance. It is the only way they can prove they are as good as anyone else - but being as good is not enough, they must exceed all others or they are failing.

Distrust of others stems also from distrust in himself. Because of his great distrust of what his ears have heard, he twists what you have said to something that sounds similar but means something quite different. No matter how illogical this may be, he does not register his interpretation as different from what you meant, and thinks you are the illogical and strange one for having said what he thinks you said. Consequently, he frequently misses the point of what is being told him, and life is one long misunderstanding. The invented version is based on the belief that you are really more against him than for him.

One of my patients demonstrated this twisting very clearly. She was a young woman with a lot of emotional trauma of a Hypericum kind, and when I gave her the remedy I wrote on the little envelope, 'Suck two pills going to bed for three days.' 'I can't do that,' she said, firmly. Puzzled, I asked why not? 'I can't go to bed for three days,' she said belligerently. I made sure I put a comma, then 'for three nights,' after that, though I doubt it would matter to the Hypericum types, who are not interested in spelling and punctuation, anyway, it slows you down too much, having to be accurate in things like that.

Enemy consciousness creates the distrust in what others say. It is this distrust that prevents many adopted children from ever believing in their new parents' love. We found that many people who had been adopted as children needed Hypericum. We also found many Hypericum people had a history of having been put into hospital and left with strangers, a terrifying thing for baby or child, especially when the strangers keep sticking needles into you. Others had been put into children's homes or foster homes and left, their parent(s) unable to get together a home for them for a long time. Invariably, they had been promised that it would not be for long. If you can't trust your own parent, why trust anyone? People lie to you and treat you falsely, so how can I believe my new parents really love me?

In spite of distrust and twisting what you say to mean something else, the Hypericum person is inherently honest. Unless he has a strong Staphisagria overlay (fairly rare), it does not occur to him to be hypocritical. He speaks his own mind. Even though his ideas may be based on misunderstandings, he does not hold his words back except in consideration for the underdog, whom he will not hurt. He will never say one thing and mean another and lets you know exactly how he feels, particularly when he is trying to cut down someone who, he believes, thinks he is a cut above him, or someone whom he perceives to be trying to cheat him somehow. His competitive spirit brings out an 'anything goes' set of rules, and he will try every trick in the book to outsmart that one.

Hypericum must win, at any price. But where to go once you have reached the top? Life is cyclic, no-one stays at the pinnacle forever, sooner or later it is someone else's turn. With his belief that second place is unacceptable, depression and even suicide may follow a downturn.

Many Hypericum people have a great fear of aging, and cannot imagine themselves as old, age means you are 'over the top' and they would rather die young. The great US orchestra conductor/composer Leonard Bernstein's son described Bernstein as 'always a young guy, in his mind. He declined rapidly, once he realized he was old. Even then, he was still at the top - 'I am at the zenith, the absolute peak of my decline,' he said in his final year. Leonard's father had never accepted that music was a worthwhile profession for his son. Leonard always felt unaccepted by his father, on this account and also because he was bi-sexual, another Hypericum swinger state. He never really thought he was good enough, could never quite accept that he was the most loved, felt to be the greatest conductor/composer America had ever had.

Worthless to the father translates to worthless to God, and there is often distrust of God in the extreme. Distrust of his inner Self, his intuition and instincts, denial that he is a piece of the universal God-consciousness that pervades all forms. His life is lived totally by the standards he perceives society is finding acceptable. His deepest inner craving is to be recognised and accepted, beyond the normal. His belief is that he is distantly removed from, even abandoned by the God out there somewhere who did not save him from his earlier experiences. This is the ultimate proof of his worthlessness.

Hypericum, used in the guilt-releasing potencies, imparts a sense of satisfaction with life and gives the ability to trust others and value oneself. It can be a slow and painful lesson, for some, needing repeated doses over several years (many have tens of thousands of years of Hypericumness in the cell memory, since the 'fall from grace' in the Garden of Eden, when we forgot we were our own god). For others, the quick, early results are permanent, changing their lives totally. Social misfits find their place in the community, and the undesirable Hypericum qualities are converted into their opposite, positive polarity of love, trust, joy, confidence, faith and the ability to live in and enjoy the present moment without racing into the future. They find the straight and middle-of-the-road path they have always sought but failed to find, and become powerful, energetic forces for good in their community.

The range of conditions I have seen improve with Hypericum never ceases to amaze me. It is a most exciting remedy and one which still reveals its mysteries. We have used it for young and old, for dogs and horses, people from all walks of life and with mild and kindly or violently distrusting dispositions. We have given it to the newborn, to restless, hyped up children of school age, to teenagers with socialising problems, drugs, tattoos and pierced bodies, petty thieves, young parents with relationship difficulties or broken marriages, people devastated by the grief of abandonment or redundancy, by motor vehicle accidents, by the violent death of another. We have learned to recognise them as they come in the door. Here is a typical story:

A young man in his twenties came for chiropractic treatment one day, having just hurt his back while holidaying. He was a motor cyclist, with short, spiky hair and many piercings in his ears. His leather jacket had pointed studs around the waistband, his belt was the same and it sported a 10cm sheath knife. When he stripped, Bryan saw that he had tattoos all over his arms, chest and legs - vicious images of animals with their teeth bared, and birds of prey. His speech was violent, and punctuated with words like skewer, spear, prod. His back was very sensitive, almost too sore to touch, but he responded to what Bryan calls his 'boring' technique, a one-finger deep-tissue massage using very small circular motions. Putting all this together, Bryan gave him Hypericum 10M, three daily doses, plus some spinal adjustment, and he continued on his holiday. Ten days later, he rang in. 'No pain, free movement, never been better.'

Ours is a Hypericum society nowadays. Not as many elderly people need it as young ones. It is a remedy of the present age, for the extremes of electronic technology, the competitive edge, fast foods, killer weapons, 'kill and devastate' computer games, fast cars and Harley Davidsons, the youth cult, spiky hair, shaved heads, rebellion against all the old traditions, the desire to break down customs, institutions and regulations, shift the education emphasis away from the historical foundations of intellectual knowledge to exploring the arts and impulsive, spontaneous creativity and sport. Hypericum is all about change and creating the new, abandoning the old.

The famous Canadian professor, Marshall McLuhan (1911-1980), analysed the effects of the communication media on people and society. He identified the age of print, 1700 to mid 1900s, as encouraging individualism, nationalism, democracy, the desire for privacy, specialisation in work and the separation of work and leisure. The electronic age, he found, speeds communication so greatly that people in all parts of the world become deeply involved in the lives of everyone else. As a result, he said, electronics leads to the end of individualism and nationalism and to the growth of new international communities. We are already seeing this.

Despite many shifts towards egalitarianism, lack of respect for the individual is a feature of society on most levels from the top of the clerical tree and the government educational institutions to the lowest rung of the ladder, the poverty-stricken and infirm; from the heights of the infinitely greedy insurance companies, banks, legal firms, medical profession, private hospitals, pharmaceutical industry and public health facilities to the struggling small businesses, now unable to afford to employ the many they would happily have given work to in another time and place. The individual has fewer and fewer freedoms, and more and more of his earnings are grabbed up by those mentioned above. All are being brought into a conformity that makes it easier for those at the top to keep power over the rest of us dangerous unknowns. We have a new set of Gods.

Extremes of income - of housing values - of lifestyle. We no longer have a middle class, either you are up with the winners or down with the losers, there are few in between. Hypericum's desire to win at any price, countered with the opposite extreme of cutting down the tall poppies who dare try to make it to the top on their own individuality, courage and skill, is bringing our country to an extreme condition from which, eventually, the pendulum must swing.

Not that this is all bad. Revolution must be extreme in order to create the opposite swing that eventually balances life out in a return to a middle path, always a new middle position and hopefully, this time, one which will redress a lot of the injustices of the previously Staphisagria society we have been built upon. Change is in the air, Hypericum thinks he is in the forefront of it, but he will find the new age will incorporate the best qualities of humanity, from whichever historical viewpoint we come. The world no longer tolerates its former cruelties, and little by little, people power is beginning to find its voice in creating the new, classless, nurturing, humane world.

And speaking of cruelties, modern medicine is the absolute tops. I have shown you many examples in Chapter 3. Many of their ruthless practices of disrespect for the individual as a human being come from the Hypericum mind-set, and have adversely affected the lives of countless families. It is no wonder our doctors and surgeons panicked and refused to work when told their insurance company had gone to the wall. Panic over litigation, and indeed, the litigation-crazy mentality of recent years, stems from the Hypericum consciousness, always expecting the enemy, the public whom they despise as ignorant fools while knowing or fearing that they are not, to rise up and stab them in the back with a law suit. What goes around comes around, they say. What you put out, you get back, sometime, somehow.

In the meantime, the duty-conscious Staphisagria doctors went on doing their good; over-loaded, well-intentioned, albeit poorly equipped to heal. Typical of Hypericum to refuse responsibility and demand that the government cover their insurance. (Coming up to elections, the NSW Government was promising them exactly this!) Hypericums are always happy for the free ride, and it is never their fault. The government cannot bail them out for long, nor can the phenomenal blowout in pharmaceutical costs be sustained. It remains to be seen how many doctors will see the writing on the wall and begin to seek training in harmless, inexpensive methods of genuine healing.

If you are a person practising within the establishment, have a long, hard look at Hypericum, Hydrastis, Ledum and Staphisagria and please, treat yourself to whichever applies to you. You will love your new self. The freedom they bring is invigorating!

The after-effects of injections, of whatever substance, can be far reaching and long lasting. Immunisation, particularly the Pertussin (whooping cough) inoculation, has been implicated in thousands of mild and very severe reactions. A vast amount of research has been done into medical records and statistics covering many years, in many countries, and there is no longer any question about it - immunising can kill or maim, and does, frequently.

Back in 1990, before I set off along this research pathway, I was taken to an institutional home in Canberra for severely handicapped children. I was shown - I can hardly say 'introduced to' - some children whose medical records stated that their brain damage had been caused by immunisation. The worst of these was a little boy called Danny, aged twelve, who had been mentally and physically stopped at the age of three months, when he had his first triple antigen shot. Danny was by this time the length of a four-year-old, and his only interests in life were eating and bathing. While in the bath, he was quiet and passive, outside it he was wild and difficult to manage, so the staff kept him in the bath for long periods of the day, to keep him happy. He had no capacity to run about, to enjoy toys or people or any interaction with the world. Totally autistic, constrained by an undeveloped brain and body, he lived in an isolated world beyond our imagination. Had I known Hypericum then I would have given it to him, he needed it.

Four years before my meeting Danny and his housemates, a mother in her sixties had brought me her daughter to see if I could do anything to help her. The daughter was now aged twenty nine, but had a mental age of eighteen months, the age she had been when she had her third triple antigen injection. Although she had been walking and talking at that time, it was seven years before she walked again, and her speech had never returned. She jabbered like a year-old baby. This giant toddler was just as she had always been, into everything, inquisitive, friendly, but unable to develop beyond this point. She was physically normal in adult height, though overweight, with an enlarged abdomen resulting from an obstructed bowel, her reason for seeing me. Her poor mother was tiring and worried about who would look after the girl once she was too old to cope. The nuclear family model of living, most prevalent in the western world and particularly in Australia, had isolated this woman and her daughter from all the family assistance that would have been theirs automatically, in a closer community.

How can anyone believe that this kind of life-time damage, common enough after immunisations, is lesser in magnitude than the risk of suffering death or after-effects from contracting whooping cough, a complaint quite successfully treatable, no after-effects, using homeopathy? Wake up, parents, and start demanding healing medicines for your children's complaints. And wake up, doctors. The time is now.

A fourteen year-old girl was brought by her mother in 1994 with kidney problems. She had been 'borderline hyperactive' when little. Since having a measles/mumps inoculation at 18 months of age, which gave a bad reaction, she had been getting recurrences of 'parotid blockage', a hard gland under her left chin would develop; the last one had been a couple of months ago, and they were able to massage it out. (The mumps serum was still affecting her 'mumps' glands.) She had had a severe scald on her chest from boiling oil, some time before the vaccine, which had been very traumatic and required six weeks of constant care. She had been in hospital for three days for this, and her mother had been told to leave her and go home, feeling guilt that she was abandoning the child to unknown people.

Kidney problems are not uncommonly related to burns, but this one was not discovered until the child was ten, when she had fallen off her bike and hit her head (at the occiput). Hospitalised again, she had been concussed and delerious, took a seizure and was kept in for a couple of days for observation. There, they took tests and found blood was coming into the urine from the kidneys. Her kidneys on this day felt sore and stressed.

She is a child who enjoys sports, plays soccer and basketball, and loves the winning. At this first visit, she had yellowish discolouration around the eyes. I gave her Hypericum 10MM followed by Parotidinum 10M, the nosode for parotid gland infections. At the next visit, two months later, mother told me the jaundiced look had gone away within two weeks, the parotid blockages had gone, and there had been a return this week of kidney soreness in the region of the lower ribs, on both sides of her back. I gave her Hypericum 10MM again.

Seven weeks later, at the next visit, I was told that after the last dose, one night the lass had woken a couple of hours into sleep, with pain on the chest, burning in the skin. She had gone to her mother, who had rubbed cream on it and she went back to bed, not remembering a thing about it in the morning. Since then she had been well, the colouring around the eyes was light, her face was a good colour. Her periods had become less heavy and were free of pain. She said she always felt pretty happy after the pills, more so than prior to coming to me. She was due for a urine test in two weeks, and would return if the problem had not fully cleared yet. It must have, for I did not hear again.

So many problems are suffered these days that are never related to immunisation, much less to abandonment. Yet Hypericum is a first-aid kit remedy that could be preventing many of them, if given at the time of the injury (needle) or accident.

You do not need to be a practitioner to be successful in treating your family with homeopathy. Years before I had the chance to attend classes, one of my sons, at fifteen months old, developed a cough that became very persistent. Several of my friends became a bit panicky when this cough continued, despite my using one after another of the common cough remedies. He was seemingly quite all right during the day, just one or two bouts of cough, but during the night, the cough was frequent, in groups of three. After six weeks, the pattern changed to many more coughs ending with a long, strangulated gasp for air, several times a night, and I took the clue and searched among the whooping cough remedies in the materia medica. Mephitis was the one that seemed right, but I had to ring the city and have it sent to me, eighty miles away, and it was two days before it arrived.

Mephitis 3X, three times a day, conquered the whooping cough in three days, with not a trace of residual effects. Faith and determination always win. If I had had a homeopathic doctor who knew better than I what to do, it would not have taken so long to find the remedy. Since such doctors are not trained in any Australian medical schools, and they were very thin on the ground in the seventies, I knew none. I had no alternative but to study the subject myself as soon as the opportunity arose, and become my family's practitioner. Both my sons are, and have always been, very healthy as a result, unlike the many poor kids we see these days, victims of fearful, brainwashed parents and congestive, destructive drugs and serums, scarcely able and often, scarcely daring to breathe.

Chronic allergies and asthma, hypersensitivities of all kinds can be helped in the Hypericum type, and these are often initiated by a Hypericum trauma such as immunisation. In an instance typical of many I see, a ten-year old girl was brought to me with persistent 'colds'. She would wake every day with sniffling, sometimes sneezing and having to clear her throat of mucus. She had runny eyes and often a blocked nose. A cortisone spray had been used but it damaged the linings of her nose. Asthma attacks aggravated the situation.

Her temperament was irritable over everything, and she was relieved by Nux Vomica, our great 'cranky' remedy. As a baby, she had had gastric reflux and screamed all the time. She had had asthma since age two, and by age six was on tablets and puffers including steroids. Ventolin made her shake. A pediatrician had weaned her off all the drugs and she now used only an occasional steroid or nebulizer. She had recurrences of a rash of vesicles on the insteps of her feet. She had had the whole routine immunisation program. Hypericum 10MM for three nights, then once a month for six months, completely cleared the symptoms, the effects of the immunisation needle shock of many years before, and she reached a level of health never before experienced.

In 1993, an eleven-year-old boy had had severe, frequent headaches for four or five years, getting worse lately. He had had his tonsils and adenoids out nearly two years previously, which had stopped his snoring and heavy breathing but did nothing for the headaches. The symptoms were of frontal pain, behind the eyes, lasting up to four days, when his face would bloat, he flushed easily, and dark circles would come under the eyes. He was hypersensitive to touch, and sensitive to heat and bright light, which often triggered the attacks. In addition, he was claustrophobic, needing an open window with a breeze on his face when travelling by car. The headaches would also come after travelling or going to the movies, and also from doing his customary art work and watching a TV screen.

His history prior to the onset of the attacks was all I was interested in, as I was not going to get anywhere if I did not find the cause. He had had the full immunisation program from two months to five years, and had reacted very badly to the second shot at four months old, with high fever, so the Pertussin serum was not included thereafter. He had had further tetanus shots, the last at age ten. At age two, he had woken from a nap and could not find his mother in the home, so set off to walk a long distance to the neighbours'. He was found an hour later, in great panic and distress. One can only imagine his feeling of abandonment. He had also had numerous falls, including a fall on to his head from a branch three metres above the ground. He was ambitious, wanted to do well at school in order to build a big business in graphics and get lots of money. Every inch a Hypericum. I gave him the usual three nights of Hypericum 10MM. Three months later, word came that he had had no more headaches. I met his father nine years later, and he thanked me again for curing his son.

By the perversity characteristic of polarity we find that many Hypericum types believe that when in they are pain, nothing is going to help except the most extreme painkiller, and they tell me that only a pethidine or morphine injection does them any good. Some ask for a bullet.

Injections of any kind offer a complexity of Hypericum links, from introduced and difficult to eliminate viruses (AIDS, herpes, many others) from other animal tissue or cultures (similar to the way insects transfer viruses with their stings) to tetanic shock effects resulting in low-grade tetanus, believed to be a significant cause of cot-death in those babies who die mysteriously, several weeks after an injection. Effects can be swift in showing, when babies receive skin pricks immediately after birth, and range from skin rashes to bronchiolitis to respiratory distress to kidney failure.

Hyperactivity, labelled with many names, responds well in a number of cases - the nervous system has been sped up by the shock of a needle. Often they are simply delightful little children who are into everything, wearing out their mother's energy, but so quick-minded that they learn rapidly, talk fast and get bored quickly with others who are slower. One such funny little two-year-old was so keen to get into the next moment that often he could not, his mum told me, stand long enough at the toilet to finish urinating. His excitement and joy in living whipped him back into his play, still trickling! Hypericum 10MM brought him back to concentrating on the present moment rather than racing into the future.

Another typical Hypericum child and youth is reckless, devil-may-care, and respects no-one's life or property, much less his own. He craves fun and can be very disruptive in class, has trouble concentrating and therefore gets behind in his learning, which only adds to his low self-value. He reaches a point where school is so boring he must leave at the earliest opportunity, cannot get a good job, cannot consider further education, so turns to stealing to get what everyone else has - the money to have fun. He believes, somehow, that the world owes him a living, it is no fault of his that he is a loser, and to some extent that is true, society has created him this way from the day of his birth or even before. Having been taught very early in life that it is OK and good for you to inject, he is happy to inject his own flesh with heroin, and OK to steal the money for the drug. He will carry pointed weapons like knives, stillettos, hyperdermics filled with blood, and does not hesitate to threaten or even to use them, people are all as worthless as he is, so what does it matter? Furthermore, he attracts to himself knife wounds, gunshot wounds and similar violence.

Not everyone who needs Hypericum gets to this point, thank heavens, but the remedy is all the more remarkable for the way it swings people back from these depths. The majority of youngsters needing Hypericum are sped up, interested in things that move fast, bored by things that make them wait, and have an imagination filled with thoughts of stabbing, killing, bombing, shooting or winning, as seen in the computer games of the last decades. One of my friends worried about her nephew's obsessive love of his air rifle. 'He's shooting everything in sight,' she said. She gave him Hypericum 10M in a composite remedy, four doses over a couple of months, and after the last, he told his mother he wanted to sell his air-rifle, he was no longer interested in shooting, and they sold it. (This combination remedy, containing also Belladonna M, Chamomilla M and Staphisagria 10M, is amazing for a wide range of problems, for some people. I call it Pain Mix, but it goes far beyond pain relief.)

In Tedd Koren's on-line chiropractic newsletter, January 2003, is the story of 'Matthew Smith, 14, who dropped dead of a heart attack while skateboarding. The 9th-grader had been on Ritalin (methylphenidate) since the first grade. Lawrence Smith, father of the boy, testified that he and his wife were forced by Michigan Social Services to put their child on Ritalin or else be charged for neglecting their son's educational and emotional needs.

'No long-range studies have been made of the effects of Ritalin on children who take it over a number of years. However, since 1986 it was known that Ritalin causes shrinkage of the brain. Psychiatric Research (Vol. 17, 1986) noted: "Mild cerebral atrophy in those who had received stimulant drug treatment for a period of time." (Stimulant drugs like Ritalin are given to children to calm them, they have a homeopathic effect on over-stimulated children.) A July 1996 study in the Archives of General Psychiatry revealed that "Subjects with ADHD had a 4.7% smaller total cerebral volume."

'Nearly 6 million children take Ritalin or one of a number of other stimulants in order to attend school.'[75]

Many people with a Hypericum overlay come to me after they have realized it is time to get their act together. While they are sinking into the worst aspects of Hypericum characteristics, they have not the trust or self-value to consider seeking real help. But once they see the need for change, it comes rapidly with the speedy Hypericum.

A mother of a teenage boy came a few years ago, saying she was 'out of balance' and wanted to get straight again. She had been a sole parent for four years. Prior to this she had used heroin, alcohol, marijuana and tobacco to excess, and she was now working hard to give her son a good home life and get him diet-conscious. Her father had had two brushes with death lately and she now felt very close to him, having had some distance between them before.

She still had many Hypericum characteristics hanging on, slowing up her personal growth. There was a bad scoliosis, with pain in the sacro-iliac joints and back of hips; the sacrum and pelvis looked level, but the spine from the sacrum to T8 was scoliosing with a right anterior rotation. She had had four terminations of pregnancies, had a very hyperactive nervous system and was very impatient with the daily grind of living.

This lady had begun early in life with alcohol and marijuana. She had dropped out of university, met inappropriate males unacceptable to her parents and 'had to escape'. She had been a chain smoker, still smoked, and was hooked on coffee after giving up the alcohol and heroin. She still used a little marijuana as it helped her feel 'more centred' when tense. (The Hypericum extremists are always trying to become centred, move towards the straight and narrow midline.) She had never injected the heroin herself, her boyfriend did it ('I couldn't do it to myself.') Finally, she had hit rock-bottom and had kicked him out and begun to get her life in order.

This confirmed the evidence of her face, which had a Staphisagria chin and a semi-Hypericum (Ledum) line running from one eyebrow to the centreline of her forehead, saying that her Hypericum characteristics were always battling with her strong Staphisagrian upbringing. (See Chapter 6 for visual indicators for the remedies.) She knew she was not so worthless as many true Hypericum types think they are.

True to Hypericum form, she went into a great panic before taking the remedy, yet she did take it. After Hypericum 10MM, a fever came on which lasted for three days, and was accompanied by delerious dreams of the heroin kind, in which she had overcome and conquered harmful entities. She felt very humbled and introspective after this, and when I next saw her, felt she had made a great breakthrough. Back and hips felt good, periods were better. She felt free and detached, able to experience the moment without fearing effects from it. The next Hypericum caused her to go a bit 'overboard' at first, but more benefits followed, her stomach felt as though it had let go of stress and she stopped feeling nervy and racy. She shifted into Staphisagria symptoms after this, with misaligned jaw and memories of having been treated unfairly and unjustly, and that mighty remedy completed her getting back on track.

Bruce Lipton describes what happens when we are under stress. Firstly, the viscera shut down, and the heart and limbs take all the blood for flight or fight; secondly, the immune system shuts down, as this requires too much energy that could be used for fight or flight; then, the thinking brain shuts down, because only the limbic brain is needed for flight or fight. Lipton says that because of the stresses children are placed under today, they are living in fight or flight mode all the time, unable to think intelligently but more inclined to fight. 'We are creating a dumber and dumber society,' he says. Such is the Hypericum world. Recently, I spoke to a woman who is working in paediatric care, who said "I am so worried by what I am seeing! All the babies are in 'fight or flight' mode from birth! It's really scary."

A young man came to me a few years ago, suffering from depression. He had had an extremely troubled childhood, with an uncle who sexually abused him constantly ('I can't get him out of my mind - so much pain from one man') and an alcoholic father of whom he was terrified. ('I don't know what a normal life is.') He had become a bit of a rebel, getting into drugs and alcohol. At the time I saw him, he had a girlfriend and a lovely baby, and they rented a flat in a seaside town. He feared now that he might abuse his own baby daughter, and could not allow himself to bath her or change her nappy. Because of this difficulty in being a normal father, the young mother had just left him, taken the baby and returned to her parents.

He was constantly thinking of the pain inflicted by his uncle, and 'would be happy to kill the man if I caught him'. He had fear of being hurt, but also of hurting himself - so many bad memories he could not get out of his head. He had always been told he was useless, and now he felt he was - but indignant, very distressed that he had lost pride and dignity of living. He had been abandoned by his mother and stepfather, and struggled from age sixteen, living in a caravan - always on his own, not trusting many, surviving on a very low wage. 'A living Hell,' he said. He was hypersensitive, 'very touchy if someone looks sideways at me, exploding in anger, over nothing, they think.' He had never wanted to turn out like his father, with a broken family. He had hurt many people who had been close, did not want to continue in this pattern.

Sitting before me was a man with numerous tattoos, looking totally devastated. He wanted help to get his life and family together again, and was prepared to work at it. I gave him Staphisagria 10MM (indignant, lost dignity, inner rage bubbling out, sexual abuse, fear of sexually abusing another, lower teeth cramped together, and because he knew, in his heart, that he was worth more than his family had ever thought he was). The next morning, he woke feeling a lot better, and went to talk with his girl. She agreed to get back with him once he had proven he had turned over a new leaf.

He found a new job but did not lose his erratic temperament quickly, and he remained estranged from mother and baby. After three weeks, he came again and was given Hypericum 10MM (abandonment, sensitivity, distrust of others) and Staphisagria 10MM again. I lost sight of him then, and heard six months later, that all was going very well for him. The family was re-united in another home, his job was going well and he was a new man. His best self had emerged, and he gave all the credit to the remedies.

Some 'worthless' children become social rebels, some take the path towards highest social credit, via business or education. They do tend to take the extreme path, whether up or down. There is no middle road for Hypericum.

Take the case of Jim Clark,[76] the founder of Netscape, and a true Hypericum. Jim had been abandoned by his father when small, and had grown up in extreme poverty. Rebelliousness caused him to be expelled from high school after he told his English teacher to go to Hell, having previously been guilty of exploding a bomb on a school bus, and setting off firecrackers inside another student's locker. Once expelled, he abandoned home and joined the Navy, vowing to show them all what he was made of. Within eight years, Jim had achieved an MSc in Physics through the University of New Orleans, and a PhD from the University of Utah, in Computer Science.

Jim Clark is extremely hyperactive and a typical Hypericum swinger, from one extreme to another. His second wife left him because she wanted a more settled life. This abandonment caused him eighteen months of dark depression. Counselling was no good, and he finally decided, at age thirty eight, to start achieving something. He re-invented his life, revolutionising everything he could, and determined to make a $100 million (which grew into billions) or consider himself a failure. First he created Silicon Graphics, then Netscape, which opened up the Internet to the home computer, and then Healtheon, his master plan for computerising the trillion dollar US health industry.

Clark never looked at yesterday, only tomorrow. Once it became today, he lost interest. He had to be at the top and always a step ahead of everyone else. He put phenomenal mental energy into his IT ideas and expected his employees to do likewise. Wanting lots of fun and needing to have the biggest and the best, he designed and had built the world's first totally computerised sailing yacht, the largest single-masted vessel in the world. Full of ideas, he had many enemies trying to tear him down and disparaged everyone who took an opposing stance to his. Nothing less than the absolute pinnacle of success was ever enough. He was every inch a Hypericum archetype, and, true to form, was racing himself to extinction.

Insomnia in the Hypericum person takes the form of a racy, logically thinking brain going along in beta mode throughout the night, while the body sleeps. The Hypericum person swears he has not slept, yet he does not suffer from lack of sleep. One patient told me she had not slept for fifteen years. The thinking brain just never shifts out of beta waves into the slower waves normal to sleep, though the rest of the brain and body are getting their rest. Many great ideas are thought out during the small hours, and are remembered next day because the brain carries on all night as if it were day anyway, there is no dreaming. The Hypericum person's brain is racy and alert, quick to respond to any trigger for physical action.

Dyslexia occurs when the Hypericum mind races too fast for concentration and words are misread or twisted about. The fact that this is an imbalance problem is demonstrated by the success achieved by those who get such children crawling about on the floor. The action of co-ordinating the arm and leg actions using alternate limbs - 'cross-crawling', often difficult for these kids - somehow co-ordinates left and right sides of the frontal cortex.

Brain and spinal injuries frequently need Hypericum, though it is not the only remedy for such injuries. Using the remedy at the time of injury, though, can prevent a lifetime of Hypericum extremes from developing. Here is an extreme example, and I don't say we would have saved him, but who knows?

In the 1850s, a man called Phineas P. Gage[77] was the foreman of a gang of railway workers near the town of Cavendish in Vermont. He was levelling the ground for a new piece of track when an unplanned explosion blew a three foot iron bar clean through his skull, like an arrow. Gage was thrown on to his back, his body convulsing and jerking, and was swiftly carried to his hotel, where he was attended by a Dr John Harlow. Amazingly, Gage was sufficiently aware to explain what had happened, even pointing to the hole and saying 'The iron bar entered here and passed through my head.' He then became feverish and lost consciousness.

'In the days immediately following the incident, the prognosis did not look good. Fungus started growing from the hole in Gage's head; his friends implored Dr Harlow to let him die. But the doctor continued to bathe his fevered patient, anxious to save his life and fascinated, despite himself, to see what would happen if he did. For the iron bar had torn right through the front of Gage's head, while leaving the deeper parts completely intact.

'Slowly, Gage began to recover, and after a month of non-stop nursing, Harlow released him, anxious to see the result. He did not have to wait long. Gage was dismissed from his job because 'the equilibrium ... between his intellectual faculties and animal propensities seems to have been destroyed.' He became wilful, obstinate and unrealistic, dreaming up escapades and adventures that were no sooner devised than abandoned. He turned to drinking and brawling. He ran away from his wife, embarked on a string of unsuccessful affairs, fell in and out of brothels and finally died in 1861 after a series of epileptic convulsions. At first Gage's story had seemed like a miracle but it turned out to be a tragedy. Without the controlling influences of the frontal cortex, his instinctual impulses had been unleashed - and they combined brute sexual desire with urgent, often hostile, impetuosity.'

This story gives us an extreme and graphic idea of how damage to the frontal part of the brain removes the controls of common sense and rationality.

Spinal injury of the Hypericum kind ranges from partial or complete paraplegia from violent accidents to very painful nervous system trauma from lumbar punctures, injected dyes for X-ray, and from epidural anaesthetics, as well as the lifetime after-effects of surgery such as the removal of the coccyx bone, the tail bone. This is a bone that is often displaced from its normal position at the base of the sacrum by falls, or through inflexibility of the pelvic joints in childbirth. Many people have had their 'broken' coccyx removed by surgery instead of corrected by manipulation back to its true alignment. The result can be, often is, a lifetime of pain at the top of the head. My Aunt Jess was one such sufferer. Her life, to 95 years, had been lived for many decades, with constant head pain that would come and go in intensity, often curtailing her activities of the day.

Jarring to the coccyx sends a whip-like wave through the spine to the skull. This results in trauma to the dura mater or inner lining membrane of the skull as the energy wave hits the occiput and passes on to the sphenoid bone and the crown. When the coccyx remains out of position after such a jar, permanent trauma is produced unless the displacement is corrected. A slower, but similar trauma continues to reach the head through surgical removal of the coccyx, via the damaged spinal ligaments and the internal dura mater that extend all the way up the spine. Shock effects to the brain tissue and the pituitary and other glands in the brain area can result in some mighty major adverse effects developing in the long term.

A woman of 69 came in 1994 with 'arthritis'. She had 'broken' her coccyx

27 years prior, falling on a cement path, had been put into traction for a few hours, then on a board. She had forced herself to get up and walk. Now it was starting to catch up with her. She had had pleurisy for two months. She ached all over, was hypersensitive to the weight of blankets, and had been diabetic, on insulin, for 32 years, which was affecting her nervous system. She had a little psoriasis, and had had a triple by-pass heart op seven months ago. She had had vitiligo since age 21, had curvature of the spine after the birth of her daughter, and was lately getting giddiness, losing her balance. The first Hypericum experience was after her own birth, when the doctor thought she would die, 'gave up on me,' because of respiratory congestion. Her father was advised by a gypsy to take her to the top of a hill and expose her to the sun's rays at sunrise, which he did for a couple of days, and improvement set in.

In addition, she had always felt she could not grasp intellectual things well enough, it was always a struggle. She put herself down a lot and disliked accepting gifts and tributes, 'not worthy.'

One week after Hypericum 10M, she felt 'very well! Better than I can remember for many a long day.' Pleurisy went, sugar readings came down somewhat. Still in a lot of pain. Hypericum 10MM was given nine weeks later, after which 'sugar has been excellent.' One night a month before, she had woken feeling nauseous at 1am, then 'half-filled a two gallon bucket with watery fluid via the mouth.' This had happened once again, after which 'sugar has been down ever since.' She had had a similar thing happen once previously, when in hospital for a carpal tunnel operation, and had covered the doctor and nurses with this watery fluid. (Shock effect, the old symptom returning after the remedy.) The skin changed to hives, which went away, and the body soreness settled down.

A lady came in in 1997 with a continuous niggling, nagging ache in her back. She had broken the end off her tailbone by falling over on the beach, 18 years previously, 'the most painful thing that's ever happened to me.'

She had many Hypericum characteristics - a slight scoliosis, and the right shoulder and right hip were higher than on the left side. She ached from the shoulder blades up to the vertex, the top of her head; 'it tries to pull the skull apart.' Her teeth had felt tender on the left side of her mouth, for a couple of days. When young, she had had a severe virus flu which left her with pins and needles in the arms and legs, no strength in them, and caused 'nervous tension', and a neurologist had given her shock treatment. She used to drink a lot of coffee and was now down to three cups a day; she had no desire for fruit or vegetables or wholegrains, so was not getting much nutrition for her nerves. Her sleep was poor.

Furthermore, her father had died four years ago, which left her 'devastated,' a good Hypericum description.

After Hypericum 10MM, she was really amazed, her back had been excellent since the second day of the three doses. She had slept better than for years. We repeated Hypericum 10MM twice for minor lapses, and two years later, Staphisagria symptoms came to the fore to be dealt with. She remains well.

Many people suffer Hypericum trauma from lumbar punctures and epidural spinal injections. Only recently, a woman of 28 came in with great difficulty, leaning on her partner's arm, hardly able to put one foot in front of the other. She had woken one morning with generalised pins and needles and had had massage and physiotherapy with no benefit. The problem had come on a month after she had fallen and hit her head on tiles, an epileptiform fit after going overboard drinking and having fun at a party. She said she was 'a bit hyper,' often goes overboard on fun. A few petit mal attacks had occurred at long intervals over fifteen years, since her grandfather had died when she was 13, but tests for epilepsy had proven negative. She had married a man who frightened her somewhat, and she left him, after which he poisoned and killed himself in 2000, and the police finally tracked her down two weeks later, at 4am, at a party where she had been out having fun. Unfortunately, they were ill-informed and told her her father had died, not her former husband, which was a bad shock.

She was losing strength rapidly, so the physio sent her to a doctor who suspected Guillain-Barré syndrome, an acute inflammation of the nervous system that usually burns itself out in a couple of months. The doctor sent her to hospital Outpatients for a lumbar puncture, which confirmed the G-B. She was admitted and spent two nights in hospital from the lumbar puncture, during which she said she had been able to feel the needle hitting something in the spinal cord. After this, her walking had become worse and worse, as she had no strength in the lower spine. The arms and legs were getting better, but not the spine. She needed help to walk and could hardly get out of a chair without something to hold, to pull herself up.

A good few years of Hypericumness there, and because the injection had been so recent, I just used 10M for a few days. Four days later, she rang to say, 'Thanks for all you've done for me.' I saw her a week later, when she walked in unassisted. She still needed megapotencies, I'd say, later on, but I did not see her again.

Have you heard about the new psychological disorder, 'Pain Avoidance Behaviour'? This is the name given nowadays to the condition of 'cowering or flinching away from the doctor,' whether or not he is about to inflict pain. No wonder; and no wonder children run for their lives from men in white coats. I'd be more inclined to see it as a healthy self-preservation instinct.

Skin rashes of a Hypericum kind start as clusters of tiny, burning, itching vesicles that turn dry and flaky, lifting off after a few weeks, but appearing in all stages at once, spreading and shifting location en masse. Herpes of all kinds can be of Hypericum causes. In a typical case, a 21-year-old girl consulted me in 1994 about genital herpes she had had for six months, which was under control mostly but 'loves to rear its ugly head the second I begin to worry.' Many antibiotics for this had given her thrush and bleeding gums. I gave her a run of Hypericum in strengths of 200, M, 10M and CM, three days each, and asked her to keep a record.

Here is her response: 'The remedies certainly brought up a lot of emotional issues for me. On the first night I felt frustrated and anxious, hyper energetic and also short of breath. I also experienced a fuzziness with my sight - sometimes it would be clear, sometimes not. Second day, I had a sore throat, anxiety, then a range of emotions: sadness, frustration, lethargy, confusion. As the week went on, these feelings intensified and by the end I had a very bad flu, where I couldn't move for about two weeks. I had severe anxiety attacks where my heart would 'hurt'. I wouldn't be able to breathe, and I just cried, non-stop for the whole time. This finally took me back to an event in my life a year ago, where I had been raped - although I didn't want to believe it at the time. I've finally been forced to deal with it and have sought counselling. It is great because I feel like a huge weight has been lifted. The anxiety has gone and I finally almost feel human again. The herpes is gone, though I still have thrush, some days worse than others, but I feel it is slowly going. Thank you for all your help.'

Notice how the demeaning assault of rape had manifested its devaluing effect on this young woman as a herpes virus, and the Hypericum had released this and activated and shifted other flu-like viruses from her body. I chose Hypericum for this girl because I had just begun my own proving of Hypericum, in which I had developed herpes-like vesicles on one foot.

My esteemed teacher, Alan Jones had pointed out, years before, the anti-social nature of Herpes Simplex II sufferers when he described, at a talk he gave in Sydney, how he had given the HSV II nosode to a group of young men who had been irresponsibly damaging property and generally treating their local community with no respect. After he had neutralised the genital herpes virus, these young men became responsible citizens. When I learned about the sources and similar effects of Hypericum injury-shock on society, it was obvious where the HS II virus was coming from - being treated as worthless. Hypericum does the same job of socialising those on the fringe, who treat others and others' property as worthless until they realise they are no longer worthless themselves.

Viruses of many forms are the special domain of Hypericum. It particularly suits those who come down with severe illnesses like Lyme's disease, from ticks, or any of the many kinds of mosquito-borne viruses. Stinging insects, with their puncturing of the skin, shock the body into virus manufacture when they catch the Hypericum people. They can also transfer viruses from other animals or people through the sting. There seems to be a correlation between susceptibility to insect bites and a deficiency of Vitamin B1, which is one of the features of a Hypericum nervous system.

The other predominant factor in virus sufferers is the great fear of the infinitely small. I have noticed that whenever there is an epidemic of any sort, the Hypericum people around me get very panicky about catching it, and run for their lives away from range. It is part of their enemy consciousness, their victim consciousness - they must kill the enemies before they are killed by them, but the unseen enemy is so hard to keep on top of! For the same reason, many people become over-diligent in trying to protect against the spread of infection, and their fear and their ignorance of how to discipline the power of their own mind for healing the cells of the body creates the feeling of need to bring out the big guns. We know now, that the big antiseptics and sterilizers are indiscriminate as to who and what they are killing. Also, mighty great focusing on infection creates infection to occur. People who fear enough undermine their immunity.

Fear of the infinitely small is also the reason why Hypericum people are very often afraid to get close to homeopathy. They do not understand how tiny can be powerful, or how such power for good is not also power to harm them. Because they expect harm from all sides, not knowing anyone they can trust, they are slow to accept remedies. My patients, on occasions, dose such people in their families surreptitiously until the benefits of trust set in enough that they can be told.

The Hypericum world is always trying to get in with some kind of defense before the unseen enemy gets its claws in. Babies in Australia are routinely injected with Vitamin K into the heel, immediately they are born, unless the mother knows to expect this and makes it known loudly that she refuses it. (Apparently one newborn in 30,000 may suffer from insufficient Vitamin K, the blood-clotting factor.) Mothers sign a consent on entering hospital on which this procedure is not specified. They think they are signing to allow any emergency procedures to be done that may be needed, not this routine, non-emergency needle. Consequently, most babies are jabbed before their mother knows what is going on, and indeed, this is usually done beyond her view. All too many babies suffer needle shock from this first day. Here's one typical case:

A baby boy of four months was brought to me after getting no results elsewhere, for bronchiolitis, which he had had since not long after getting his DPT inoculation around 2 months of age. He had had the Vitamin K needle at birth, and had reacted by developing sleep apnoea. He would stop breathing (as of cot death), and the parents had had to use a sensory mat to tell them by alarm when the breathing had stopped. After the DPT, the bronchiolitis had begun, and at three months, he had been taken to the major Children's Hospital for a sleep study. Of course, the doctors there put him on to antibiotics and a Ventolin nebulizer, and whenever the course of antibiotics ended, back would come the bronchiolitis - three times, over one month. His chest was full of mucus and his breathing was noisy.

This baby was the fourth in the family, and the second and third were hyperactive and 'getting out of control', mum said. The third, a boy of 5, had been three months premature and had still some problem with immaturity in his lungs. Mother has facial evidence for Hypericum as well, and I gave her Hypericum 10MM for all the family. Four days later, the baby was breathing (awake and asleep) very much better.

Extremes are a feature of the Hypericum person's life. He is first racy and hyped up, (needing very high potencies of the remedy to bring him into normal) but eventually the nervous energy burns out and he sinks into an opposite extreme. Blood sugar swings between high and low, blood pressure may do the same, and one strange thing I have noticed is that one side of the body is at variance from the other. Even the blood pressure readings vary by as many as twenty points from one arm to the other.

A lovely lady of 69 consulted me in 1993, not long after I had had the bolt of Hypericum enlightenment hit me (see Chapter 1). Her complaints were late-onset diabetes of two years standing, controlled by tablets, and recurrent urinary tract infections. She also had been on blood pressure treatment for 14 years. Her husband had had a paralysing stroke three years earlier, and she had had a lot of stress, helping him to regain some mobility; furthermore, during that time, two brothers had died suddenly, a year apart, no apparent preceding illnesses for either of them. Her mother had long had heart problems, yet lived to 90 with angina and high blood pressure. My client had had a hysterectomy at age 41 and was still hooked on Premarin, the oestrogen from mares' urine. She had had pneumonia five times in the last five or six years and was fearful of bronchial or throat infections as a result.

She had been vaccinated against smallpox, typhoid and cholera 45 years ago, and the smallpox vaccine made her very ill, she felt it affected her spine and head. Since then, a lot of back trouble, the L4-5 disc was 'almost non-existent; throws the neck out, too.' Once, her leg had been numb for a long time after a bad period of back pain. She would get pain in the groin if the spine went out again. She had recently come up under a hanging plant and banged her head, had a sore neck and needed chiropractic. She had fallen on the back doormat and torn the ligaments in her ankle, chipping the bone; then an operation for a second cyst on a buttock, followed by a bout of pneumonia, and later a tick attached itself to her head at the mastoid process and caused a rash and burning itch down her neck. She was very susceptible to March flies, bee stings and bull-ant bites, which led to severe swellings. To top it off, her blood sugar would go up and down a lot, and she 'gets a bit of imbalance when the blood pressure goes up.' All these physical conditions could suit Hypericum.

When I asked about her reactions to life's events, from an emotional point of view, her response was classic Hypericum: 'I was devastated by the shock of my husband's paralysed condition. It was even worse when they told me he would have to come home from the hospital over the Christmas period (only three weeks later), it sent me into further panic and fear of not being able to cope with the responsibility of him. A nurse was coming but did not come for four days over Christmas, and I had to change the perspiration-soaked sheets by myself.' This man had been in and out of hospital for the previous nine years, with by-pass surgery, three prostate operations, haemorrhoids. She had already had a lot to cope with; Hypericum hates to have to take on responsibility for others, but is kind enough to do so.

I gave her Hypericum M, CM and 10MM, one dose of each on successive days. She developed first a severe reaction to her head and the whole body, as she had had at the time of the smallpox vaccine: sleeplessness, alert mind, high odour to scant urine. Finally, severe cold shivering set in, as had happened, she said now, at the time of the hysterectomy. (Wonderful signs of the correct choice of remedy, when you get a Return of Old Symptoms!) A week after the first dose, the symptoms were expanding. there was fever after the chill; everything eaten was brought up within the hour. She felt exceedingly weak and remained in bed, her nights full of wakefulness, spent doing crosswords in her head - a daytime leisure pursuit. Cold sweats alternated with hot sweats every four hours, and she had persistent aching of the head, still as of the post-hysterectomy time, which she thought had been caused by a reaction to the pre-med given at that time. I was visiting or talking by phone every day at this stage. 'My son is a doctor,' she told me. 'I can't tell him what we are doing, he will only think I'm sick and want to give me antibiotics, but I know I am getting better. I have used homeopathy for thirty years and I know you sometimes feel worse before you get better.'

After nine days, she began to feel she was turning the corner. Looking back on all she had been through over the years, she commented, 'I just couldn't seem to win.' She remembered having had the same alternating fevers and chills after her third child was born, when she had had to be kept in hospital for three weeks, 'they couldn't get the fever down.' She also remembered a time when, 44 years earlier, she had had kidney trouble and was given a sulfa drug which caused terrible heads, hot and cold flushes and pains down her back. A dose of the same drug many years later gave the same bad reaction, similar to what had been coming up this week. On this day she also experienced a return of old pain in the hip, groin and left leg, and also pain in the right leg where she had been hit by a car as a child.

On day 14, she reported a return of the bearing down feeling she often got with cystitis. The blood sugar was up and down, mainly down, though she had stopped taking the drug. On day 16, she was very excited with her progress. Sugar readings had come down greatly, and blood pressure was normal, 124/84, and it continued to get lower yet, with the strange feature common to Hypericum, of different readings from both arms.

Knowing that a remedy brings up old symptoms for which that remedy should have been used years ago, it was quite an education to see the extent of Hypericum features in this woman's life. As the Hypericum benefits set in, other symptoms of drug toxicities came up and were dealt with with other remedies, and gradually, the back strengthened, the cystitis and bronchitis ceased to recur, the sugar and blood pressure stayed in reasonable limits and at the last contact in 1999, at 75, she was swimming sixty laps of the pool every day, in her retirement village. Her lifetime of 'medical victim' effects had been cleared away, leaving her healthier than she could remember, a winner at last.

In order to clarify my ideas on this remedy I began to do a proving of it on myself. The first dose, MM, was taken going to bed on 23rd June, 1993. It caused my brain to be on full alert all night, thinking in beta mode as though I was awake - very clear, sequential, logical thoughts until 5am, when I finally drifted into unconsciousness. The amazing thing was that I had actually been asleep, physically, only the brain would not switch down to a lower speed. I was unaware of surroundings while these thoughts were happening so clearly. It was as though the body and consciousness slept while the frontal cortex worked on. On waking next morning, I found that my right foot had broken out in a few herpes-like vesicles in the centre of the sole, at the junction of the soft instep skin and the tougher pad, but only on the softer skin. This was intensely itchy if scratched, with a burning, caustic feeling if a vesicle was broken by scratching - very painful, and worse for the warmth of bed or shoes.

More clarity of thought persisted throughout the day. I also felt 'sped up' - I'm usually slow-thinking and fairly sedentary. That night, alert brain all night again. I was losing my usual caution - forgot to buckle up my safety belt in the car, and when I realized, talked myself out of doing so, as if ridiculing those who consider it wise or necessary. This sense of recklessness persisted and was intensified, along with the tendency to disparage others, whenever I took Hypericum over the ensuing years. The wide-awake brain slowed down the next night and I felt I had slept well.

I developed a strong desire for red meat. As I had been mainly vegetarian for three decades and had rarely eaten red meat this was very significant. I began buying meat pies and sausages, and enjoyed these greatly until the Hypericum began to wear off. My vegetarian mind would not allow me to go to the extent of eating beef steak, but I could understand now why some people really crave red meat. (Magnesium carb. sufferers also have a desire for red meat, and magnesium is a strong component of the Hypericum plant.)

No other symptoms arose and all but the foot symptoms faded out. The vesicles on the foot had begun to spread into a patch, running together, blistering, new ones coming while the first were drying and flaking off. The patch remained after all other symptoms had subsided, spreading down the instep and eventually towards the dorsum of the foot over the course of a year or more. Every dose of Hypericum intensified the pain, burning, itching and heat sensitivity, worse for scratching.

I took my second dose, 10MM, on 4th August, 1993 at 10.30pm. Again, mental alertness as before, all through the night - yet I knew I had been asleep. I began to understand how people could come to me complaining adamantly that they hadn't slept for years, yet were still able to carry on with life without flagging. It is an illusion of being awake. The desire for meat arose again. On the following night I 'awoke' at 3 am with the image clearly in my vision of a see-saw balance. I contemplated this aspect of Hypericum for several hours, mentally chewing over the ramifications of imbalance, its causes in our society and the many ways that imbalances manifest in the body and mind and spread over into social, political and governmental attitudes.

The mental alertness and clarity of thought experienced during sleep was present during the day, particularly for the first few days after each dose of Hypericum. During these days and for the duration of the proving, I felt restless and racy, wanting to move quickly especially while driving, and often found myself speeding and darting in and out of traffic. It was like the effect I would get from having a cup of coffee prior to or during the four-hour drive home from Sydney at night - without which I usually found sleep would take over. Unlike coffee though, Hypericum gave recklessness and a sense that it wouldn't really matter if I took risks, which was, fortunately, usually corrected by my natural inclination towards caution and self-preservation. (Bryan says otherwise!) Like hypnotherapy, provings will not create you to be different from your true self, except at a superficial level. They are merely signposts to the similar conditions that the remedy can cure.

I hated Hypericum for what it caused to me, and realized how much worse it would feel, to be someone really needing this remedy. People really had the most encouraging, exciting benefits from it. Many suddenly realized that the people they had thought to be unfriendly were really nice. 'Is it just me? People seem to be a lot nicer than I used to think they were.' Their enemy-consciousness went out the window along with their sense of being a wounded victim of life.

Four subsequent doses of very high potencies were taken at intervals over the next eighteen months, with similar effects each time. The vesicles on the foot would appear also on toes at times. It was three years before there was any respite in this phenomenon, when there was a brief period without any and then they arose, instead, on the left foot and began the same pattern, to a much lesser degree. The desire for red meat returned with each repeat dose, together with recklessness, mental and physical raciness and low self value, each time lasting only a short time.

Over the initial period, and intensified by the second dose, I experienced a growing conviction that no-one would ever believe what I was learning about Hypericum. I came to believe that others would disparage what I was learning or worse still, totally ignore me because I was a mere woman, a sole practitioner working in a small country town, not worth considering. It was mind-boggling to me, so how much more unbelievable would it be for anyone else! This is a typically Hypericum way of thinking. Many Hypericum men fear and disparage women, often, and all Hypericum people expect to be dismissed as of no account.

No-one was going to believe that Hypericum would be a primary remedy for the viral infections following injections, or for the iatrogenic conditions consequent upon so many medical procedures. The more I used Hypericum for such conditions, so successfully, the more secretive I became about it, believing somehow that my findings were bound to be ridiculed and treated as worthless. It became such an ingrained belief that it was not until November 1995, when the Hypericum effects had all but worn off, that I first talked about it to the Sydney AHA meeting - and even on that occasion, when half the meeting got up and went home before my talk, I almost went with them, 'abandoning' the remainder. Fortunately, I was encouraged to stay and talk.

Who was ever going to accept that the major trends in society today - the desire for ever increasing speed in every part of life (computers, computer games, fast motor vehicles, fast food, acronyms to save us using so many words, microwaves to speed up cooking, drugs to speed the brain), the increase in violent crime, drug problems in youth, victim consciousness, over-the-top litigation, medical abuses, family breakdowns and many lesser changes away from stability - all relate to the personality picture of this remedy? Could it be that this trend, begun in America and now equally severe in Australia, is purely the result of the spread of one deeply held belief? And could it really be that this one deeply held but erroneous belief is being spread to virtually every young person born in recent decades, by a simple medical procedure regarded by most as a harmless but necessary event, the jab?

The plain truth is that our orthodox medical model comes largely from a Hypericum mentality. The whole standpoint of most medical treatments today involves lack of respect for the integrity of the human body, the psyche and the spiritual nature of man; a belief that only violent means will be of any advantage, that if there is no risk of death, there is no hope of killing out the problem. Harmlessness, as it always is for the unenlightened Hypericum type, is regarded as useless and ineffectual.

There is a belief in hopelessness that is a natural consequence of knowing they have nothing healing to offer; a great fear of the microscopically small, the unseen enemy, the virus and the germ; a belief that the public are out to sue, to seek financial compensation, the medicos understandably expecting this, knowing they deserve such retribution for their actions (Hypericum believes in an eye for an eye); an absolute disbelief in anything based on the all-powerful natural creative healing force of love, and most strange of all, a *preference* for abusive, killer-mentality treatments. This is a really sick standpoint from which to run one's life and work, and cannot possibly result in healing. [Look into Hydrastis (guilt of harm done to others), Staphisagria ('I know what's best for you') and Ledum (fear of not being in control) also, in relation to the medical profession.]

As you, the public, demonstrate a greater preference for harmless, non-invasive healing methods, the Hypericum-minded profession, fearing the loss of its long-held, God-like position at the top of the ladder, fights dirty. In the USA and in Australia, natural therapies based on wholism, particularly homeopathy, are constantly having to defend themselves against the disparaging tactics of the 'old school'. We can expect this for some time to come. They do not know how to come down, and panic over where they might end up if forced off the top perch. Their fear, distrust and ignorance of life will be their own downfall, as understanding gains a stronger foothold amongst the public.

We do no need to buy into their battle, there is no battle. Knowledge gets around, and we who recognise and respect the Vital Force, the Innate intelligence, have already won, it only remains to manifest on the physical plane. Should we abandon them to their fate, as Hypericum expects?

CHAPTER 12

When you realize the value of all life, you dwell less on what is past and concentrate
more on the preservation of the future.
- Dian Fossey (1932-1985), US Primatologist

IGNATIA - 'WHERE DO I GO FROM HERE?'

The seeds of the large, woody, climbing shrub, Ignatia (ignatia amara, '*St. Ignatius' Bean*', N.O. Loganiaceae) were, historically, used in tea form as a remedy against cholera, and certain forms of heart trouble. A native of the Philippines, where the people were in the habit of wearing the seeds as amulets for the prevention and cure of all kinds of diseases, it was highly esteemed in Cochin China. It attracted the attention of the Jesuits, who named the tree after the founder of their order, Ignatius Loyola, and took the seeds wherever they travelled for medicinal use.

According to Dorothy Shepherd, 'it is a beautiful tree, with long, twining, smooth branches, and its flowers are very long, drooping, white in colour and scented like jasmine. The fruits are the size and shape of a medium-sized pear, and the seeds are about one inch long and extremely bitter.'

Ignatia is not used in modern western herbal medicine, and is not listed in Max Wichtl's Herbal Drugs and Phytopharmaceuticals, the modern, scientific compendium of plant medicines. The beans contain strychnine and have a tonic, stimulating action to the heart, but must be used carefully, as they are quite poisonous. Symptoms of overdose produced by it include palpitations, tachycardia, muscle spasm and tremors, and faintness, a keyed-up, distraught, even hysterical condition, with sobbing, inability to speak, racing breathing and heaving chest, fever alternating with thirsty chills, stopped menstruation, dysmenorrhoea, diarrhoea and indigestion.

Nevertheless, American doctors early last century saw fit to use the fluid extract or the tincture in 5 - 12 drop doses, as an efficient nerve tonic. Harvey Ellingwood's recommendations for the people and situations requiring Ignatia come directly from homeopathic provings. He recommends it for melancholy, hysteria, sleeplessness, suffocative grief symptoms, sighing and weeping, alternate laughing and crying, puberty, amenorrhoea, menopause, leucorrhoea, persistent uterine disorders, dysmenorrhoea, sexual apathy, intercostal neuralgia, aphonia, congestive headache, burning soles, nervous depression; and uses phrases like 'Will be found an important remedy' and 'an excellent remedy.' These doctors used Ignatia homeopathically, by the Law of Similars, from the homeopathic provings, while publicly decrying Homeopathy.

IGNATIA IN HOMEOPATHY

Ignatia was proven as a remedy in Hahnemann's days, and it was he who pointed out the characteristics of this great nerve remedy. Long before psychology was thought of, the mental peculiarity, or psychology of each remedy, proven on healthy people, was studied and carefully documented, and 'nerves' (as 'nervously keyed up') were treated successfully by Hahnemann and his followers, while they still remain a problem to modern medicine and psychiatry, who can only palliate by drugging.

Ignatia patients exhibit three features that are readily apparent:

- Constant sighing, needing to take a deep breath now and then
- Frequent yawning, again trying to get more air into the body
- Intolerance of cigarette smoke.

In the acute phases of Ignatia problems, you see extreme instability and sensitivity of the nervous system, changeability of moods, being contradictory and quite paradoxical, and full of extreme anguish and excitability. A typical situation requiring Ignatia is the shock of a sudden death. The Ignatia sufferer becomes extremely emotional, even hysterical, one minute laughing and the next back in the depths of great grief and despair, with uncontrollable sobbing and eyes pouring tears.

In addition to extreme emotional sensitivity, there are pains that are acute and extremely sharp; any pain is unbearable, and they occur in small areas - neuralgia, fleeting pains that come and go rapidly, erratic and changing location. The complaints that develop are always the result of nervous tension, the nerves are strung tight as piano wires, and produce some very strange, unexpected effects. Abdominal pain and bloating, for example, could disappear after what, to another, would be an indigestible meal, while simple foods normally easy to digest, such as milk, will aggravate the condition.

Shock also gives the Ignatia person a sensation of a lump or ball in the throat, or rising from the stomach to the throat; a sore throat which feels worse for empty swallowing than swallowing of food or drink; an irritating, spasmodic cough that gets worse the more she coughs; nausea and vomiting at the start of eating, which then is followed by eating a full meal without trouble; diarrhoea; palpitations of the heart, unstable and variable pulse. The pains are relieved by heat, warm atmosphere, hot drinks, hot applications, walking and keeping the mind occupied so there is no time to dwell on the upsetting events.

Clarke lists the following conditions that pertain to Ignatia:

Clinical. - *Abdomen, distended. Anger, effects of. Anus, affections of. Anxiety. Appetite, disordered.* Back, weakness of. Catalepsy. *Change of life. Chorea. Clavus* (c. hystericus: a painful sensation as if a nail were being driven into the head; affecting hysterical patients). Convulsions. *Croup. Debility.* Dentition. *Depression of spirits.* Diphtheria. Dysmennorrhœa. *Epilepsy. Fainting. Fear, effects of.* Flatulence; obstructed. Glands, enlargement of. *Haemorrhoids. Headache. Heart, affections of. Hiccough. Hysteria. Hysterical-joint.* Intermittent fever. *Locomotor ataxy. Melancholia. Numbness. Oesophagitis. Paralysis.* Phlyctenular ophthalmia. Proctalgia (pain in the anus or lower rectum, of no physical explanation). Rectum, prolapse of. Rheumatic fever. Sciatica. *Sensitiveness. Sinking. Sleep, disordered. Spinal irritation. Tenesmus. Throat, sore.* Toothache. *Tremors. Urine, abnormal. Vagina, spasm of. Voice, lost. Yawning.*

To these I might add: Anorexia. 'Dry eye'. Fluid retention. Metrorrhagia. Wasting disorders.

Clarke gives as causation: Grief. Fright. Worry. Disappointed love. Jealousy. Old spinal injuries.

What is not brought out fully enough in our standard texts is that many of the above complaints occur in people who are not outwardly excitable or emotional. Many Ignatia sufferers are people who are very good at suppressing grief, so that all they display to the outside world is a kind of numbness of the senses, something of a blank space. These people retreat from the world, are unable to be coaxed out to social events, in effect become reclusive and uncommunicative.

Or in many cases, they are not consciously unhappy, and just go about their day doing what they most enjoy, be it writing, gardening, reading, sewing - minding their own business and not participating in the outer world if they can avoid it. It is easier to live this way than to expose oneself to further opportunities for sadness and grief. They have had their fill. They eat sparsely and sporadically, are thin and become grey-haired and gaunt.

In such people, the Ignatia chronic conditions may develop, from the inner muscle tensions that continue to exert influence on the skull and spine. Homeopaths tend to give them Natrum Muriaticum, a wonderful remedy renowned for its benefits on the effects of suppressed grief. I use Ignatia first, as I like to use the plant remedy before the mineral, the plants cover more than one mineral picture. It seems to me that the acute Ignatia symptoms of very active, emotional hypersensitivity shift into an opposite polarity of emotional shut-down if unresolved by this remarkable remedy.

233

IGNATIA IN MEGAPOTENCY

There are common situations where the need for Ignatia in megapotencies develops. It is exceptionally wonderful where a person has had an sudden, unexpected change of circumstances beyond his control or choice, causing life to be thrown into a different pathway. This change of life-path may later appear to be advantageous in itself, and be happy; yet a sense of having been thwarted, stymied in some way, sets in, consciously or unconsciously. A plan for the future has been destroyed, hopes lost, ideas foiled, a door has been closed, and such hopes or intentions never get the chance to materialise, being thrust to the back of the mind and left, seemingly hopeless, below awareness. Life goes on in a new way and the old plan gets discounted, leaving a degree of grief symptoms that do not appear relevant to the person's present life.

This person may have no sense of inner tension of a physical nature. The tensions that are causing the physical symptoms may be set in and tolerable, affecting more the cranial structure and the internal head - the brain and the pituitary gland, and altering the function of various body processes as a result. The person may or may not have coped reasonably well at the time of the sudden change (which may have been related to a great grief), but unbeknown to herself, has remained inwardly strung up, so that years after the event, nervous tension reaches the point where the nerves 'snap' and the person has a nervous breakdown.

I remember such a person from forty years ago, who had a sudden nervous collapse that totally amazed her. She found it very hard to understand how she could be so emotionally out of control, so suddenly, it seemed to her, when the grief that she had had was experienced five years prior, and she had reached a place, she thought, where everything seemed to be going right for her. If I remember rightly, her husband had been killed in a freak accident, and she was, by this time, happily remarried. This woman had moved on, into a new beginning, before her grief shock had been resolved, so the shock tensions remained, locking in the old emotions of lost hopes and plans, together with the grief that her children had lost their father, their futures had also been affected indelibly, in a way not totally erased by getting a new father.

Ignatia would have worked on every aspect of this person's problems, as it does also on grief held on a much broader scale, when whole communities are altered by large scale traumae beyond their ability to control. It is brilliant for people traumatised by war, by natural disasters such as flood, earthquake or fire, by loss through deaths from any cause, through loss of business, of job or any position, whether social, work-related, educational, marital, or any other relationship, wherever the reason or cause was beyond the sufferer's control and life could not be set back on to the previous track.

The tendency to repeatedly incur such griefs and collapsed ambitions can instill a fear of a grim future, and will be cleared by Ignatia. Recurrences only happen because of residual guilt holding the person in the same rut of thought energy frequencies. Once you clear the guilt, this all frees up and a completely new way of responding to life develops.

For many, this clearance opens up new opportunities that would not have occurred or been seen under the old thinking. When you need Ignatia, something from the past is still holding you back there, something inside you is still feeling stymied and denied opportunity for realisation. When you get Ignatia, suddenly, often overnight, thoughts open up and ideas come in as to what to do next, to start getting back into creating the dreams that had been lost. True, the lost loved ones may be irretrievable for this lifetime, but you are living your life, not theirs, and it is your life that must be put back on track to achieve your personal dreams for yourself, and your children's lives that must be de-grieved so they can achieve their best ideals for their lives.

Nervous tension held inwardly, below the conscious level, does specific things to the body.

- The act of suppressing grief and tears affects facial muscles in such a way as to cause the sphenoid/pituitary impairment to occur mainly at the posterior pituitary, or neurohypophysis, thus affecting the kidneys. Thus, suppression of the flow of tears causes disturbance to the flow of water through the body and out of it. Oxytocin release is also impaired, resulting in difficult labour and refusal of milk to flow post-natally. Painful engorgement of the breasts occurs owing to the failure of oxytocin to contract the milk ducts. Gonadotrophic hormones are also affected, causing irregularities with menstruation and menopause. Fluid filling the breasts occurs, with or without relationship to cycles. Grief stress can also be the cause of suppressed menstruation. Infertility may result; or the periods become erratic, excessive, painful, with tears and lamentations. Heat flushes also occur, with or years away from menopause.

- Suppression of urine is the accompaniment of retained grief tears. On the other hand, the anti-diuretic hormone can be affected, causing too much loss of body fluid, dehydration and weight loss. This dehydration is one of the reasons the lymphatic system becomes compromised and lymphoedema can set in. This can be a result of too much flow of tears after a death or loss, in people who did not stop crying for a long, long time - the opposite situation setting in as retention of tears.

- The production of eosinophils drops, causing a reduction of antihistamines and thereby fewer antigens are destroyed. Allergies may set in.

- With or without allergies, there can be a post-nasal, watery drip down the throat, on lying down at night, causing cough. As the denial of vocal expression of grief creates tensions that change the positioning of the

235

sphenoid and the ethmoid bones in the front of the head, the inwardly directed tears can build up in the facial cavities. Sinusitis, deafness and post-nasal catarrh are common, as is hay fever, which, in my opinion is, in these cases, simply a way of expressing those tears!

- Tremors, chronic muscle tensions, even spasticity may occur. There is an inner tension in suppressed grief sufferers that belies their outward calm, their control is great. Deep inner tension can result in heart palpitations, fibrillation, muscle spasms and Parkinsonian tremors, with painful, stiff neck, back, shoulder and chest muscles causing difficult respiration, heart symptoms and inflexibility.

- Constrictive tensions occur in the throat and oesophagus, causing dysphagia, chronic hoarseness, or just a lump in the throat feeling - sometimes affecting the swallowing of food, sometimes the larynx.

- Nervous 'asthma' can occur, the tense, locked up ribcage cannot move freely. There is a desire to take a deep breath frequently (frequent sighing), to consciously expand the ribcage as it is not moving freely enough of its own accord to get sufficient exchange of air. It is an illustration of the inner tension of one who has to work hard to hold himself/herself together.

Look into Ignatia for all long-term problems that originated in events that were beyond your control. Whereas Ledum people tend to want everything under control all the time, Ignatia types are more allowing, but when something happens for the worst that was beyond anyone's control, that is when Ignatia is needed. It is not the sense of helplessness that Staphisagria has in the face of authority, this is helplessness against fate and destiny itself.

You might think this would be more easily accepted, but this kind of shock numbs the brain into an inability to know where to go next, what to do to redress the situation, or what path to take next, that would put you back in the same previously chosen direction. This benumbed, vacant sense regarding the future leads to numerous physical complaints that set in and become chronic, unable to be resolved until the shock blocks have been cleared out of the non-physical you and energy flows have been restored to order.

An inability to see how one should act to create the next stage in life, once the mind becomes held up by events of the past, is one of the common indicators for Ignatia. Many patients have said to me, 'I feel at a crossroad, not knowing what to do for the best, but something must happen, I cannot stay like this forever, I am going nowhere.'

Many Ignatia problems develop in the same circumstances as Staphisagria problems, and I sometimes need to use both remedies to deal with the two aspects of one problem.

While Staphisagria deals with the anterior pituitary problems resulting from helpless indignation over offenses done, Ignatia deals with the posterior

236

pituitary effects of helplessness over grief. Here is an example of how these two occur side by side in the one person.

In September 2001, a woman of about my own age came in using a walking stick, having had a bad knee injury. Her complaint was osteoporosis, a condition caused by underfunctioning of the parathyroid glands, which then fail to send messages to direct the movement of calcium around the body.

Normally, as you will read in the Staphisagria chapter, calcium moves into and out of bones at different times of the day, according to where it is needed at the time, and if the parathyroids are not sending out enough parathormone, calcium gets deposited on the outside of bones or left in the muscles instead of going back into the bones. When the hormones demanding calcium from the bones outnumber the ones that say 'go back', a leaching effect occurs and the bones become depleted and weakened. It is the pituitary gland that needs correction to strengthen up the parathyroid glands and get them working normally again. It is purely a failing of the pituitary that causes the situation in the first place. Even when the pituitary has been compromised by injury to the skull, it is worth trying to get better function through freeing up the sphenoid bones and getting better nerve and blood supply to the damaged organ, by giving the patient Staphisagria and/or Ignatia.

This lady had had a massive Staphisagria-type assault on her thyroid in the 1960s, when she had been part of trials using radio-active iodine to determine whether a thyroid was under- or over-active. Her thyroid had been reduced to almost no function by the trial. This in itself would have placed an enormous load on her pituitary, the master gland that tries to make up the difference whenever an endocrine gland is not able to supply enough of its hormones. (The mind boggles at the ingenuity of medical bastardry, ever happy to come up with fresh ways to assault you, in trying to overcome their guilty ignorance.)

In 1978, at age 37, my patient had had a son by caesarian, her only child. The stitches after the op came undone and set her back a long and terrible time (more Staphisagria). There was a lot of grief dating back to her childhood with a violent and cruel father, a long-standing sense that she could not logic away, and because of which she was introspective and had not much humour in her life. She felt she should have been able to put it into the past, but could not. She disliked herself, and was suffering grief over having had to put her mother into a nursing home against her wishes, but dementia was setting in and mother was becoming unmanageable. Life had rarely been the way she had hoped it would at the start. This was a typical Ignatia scenario.

I gave her Staphisagria MM followed immediately by Ignatia MM. At her next visit five weeks later, she spoke more about the past, her father's violence and of her occasional migraines affecting the temples and eyes. This time, she told me how, all her life, she had had a tremor in her hands that sometimes affected her head as well, making it nod a little. She found it hard to let go of the past, felt she could never forgive her father for all the indignities he had inflicted on the family. 'I am annoyed with myself for not being able to do this,' she said, 'it gives me a twisted knot of emotion that I cannot let go of the past, can't get into tomorrow.'

More Staphisagria, 10MM, and Ignatia CM, and this time I followed these up with Ledum 10MM to speed up the letting go. Ignatia and Ledum are both needed for getting free of such stored tensions that cause tremors. The osteoporosis was fast becoming normalised.

Improvements set in in many ways, and time went on without another visit. Eventually, in September 2002, she approached me again about the tremors, the oldest of her problems. Healing was occurring in the reverse order of the problems' development, a positive sign. I gave another Ledum 10MM, intending to follow it up with Symphytum MM if this didn't finish the job, because I suspect the nerve damage is also part of a genetic predisposition. For many people, Symphytum is needed to reverse the trend into destruction of tissues.

Sometimes our relationships with others seem irreconcilable, especially when the other person refuses to have contact. This can be a great grief, with a real feeling of being helplessly stymied by the situation. My lovely friend Helena, who had been adopted as an infant, had just such an estranged relationship with her natural mother, who, after Helena had been through all the heartache of tracing her and contacting her in September 1996, refused to acknowledge her and would not allow any communication.

Such is the controlling power of guilt and fear, for this woman had been a strict Catholic and dominated by fear of punishment (Aconite) for her sin of having this child. Helena was further grief-stricken by this attitude, and it was a great delight to learn that after I had given Helena Ignatia CM in August 1998, within a week she had met the mother. (When we heal ourselves, people change towards us, even when they do not consciously know this is happening.)

Three months later, Ignatia symptoms were to the fore again, this time a sensation of a lump in the throat that could not be swallowed away and a suffocative feeling waking her in the night, choking her; or while eating or drinking, the throat seemed to close over as if she would choke. 10MM fixed this time, and CM two months later. 'Great calming benefit.'

The grief of foiled hopes and intentions frequently relates to failure to conceive despite repeated efforts, or failure to carry a child to term. One of my patients was a school teacher who had spent years waiting for such a happy event, having had three miscarriages when I began to treat her for this in 1990. Her main symptom apart from the grief was severe, very uncomfortable swelling of the breasts after ovulating. In those days I did not know that this would be fixed with Ignatia, I had not begun the megapotency research yet.

The remedies I used gave some benefits and she entered the IVF program in 1992. In December 1992, she felt she had a lot of built-up resentments and anger, including anger towards herself for not falling pregnant yet.

By now we had begun using megapotencies, and I gave her Staphisagria MM followed by Sepia CM, which both gave lots of physical benefits and 'great calm, nothing phasing me any more, and I am not getting irritated with my class, no more anger is rising up.' Pregnancy tests revealed that the IVF implants were not taking, and she became despairing of ever getting pregnant again. She felt obsessed, crying over anything (Ignatia), full of resentment (Ledum), frustration and indignation (Staphisagria), and felt it was 'all my own fault!' These remedies helped, but by September 1993, enlargements of the breasts began to set in again (Ignatia, but I still did not know this).

Time went on, and still no pregnancy. Time after time, disappointments. By February 1994, she was disillusioned with her husband and felt like leaving him, and had slumped after having been very hyped up the previous year, burning the candle at both ends to finish work for a uni degree. 'How come my prayers are not answered?' Having just learned about the 'abandoned by God' and 'desire to abandon' aspect of Hypericum, I gave her this next - it fitted the constant needle-jabbings of the IVF program requirements. After this, she was able to continue with great energy, very organized, capable and achieving well - but no pregnancy.

By December 1998, this determined lady was still trying to get a successful pregnancy. She had found her own eggs were not viable and had been given some from her sister, who had three children. The first two implants were unsuccessful, and she was due for the final one three weeks after I gave her Ignatia CM. The symptoms were 'constant sighing; tired, heavy eyelids.'

After the three nights of Ignatia, she awoke next morning with a great sense of release of a lot of old problems. The embryo implant failed, and she coped a lot better than previously, better than she had expected. She found she could let go of the dream and accept an alternative, if necessary. Some physical symptoms developed in the legs and feet, a good 'direction of cure.' In January, 1999, she had given up the IVF program and had accepted that it was OK to be childless. I gave her Ignatia 10MM to finish off the improvements. She and her husband had regained a good relationship and were developing a viable business breeding animals. She still looks and feels well and is in charge of her life, free of grief and guilt.

Suppressed griefs, or long-held feelings of grief or disappointment that have to be put to the back of your mind in order to keep your day-to-day life running normally, have a way of breaking out once the inner storage areas become too full. I had an enlightening experience of this in 1999 when the husband of a young friend of mine brought her to me one morning.

My friend, a young woman of 38 at the time, was in an hysterical state, quite out of mental control and her grief emotions had really taken centre stage. I had been treating her and her family for about six years at the time, and I remembered that at the time of her first visit in 1993, I had given her Hypericum 10MM for emotional sensitivity that had been aggravated by assisting her sister at her confinement. They had lost their father only two months prior, and their mother was getting heart symptoms (for which I advised Cactus grandiflora tincture, did wonders).

My friend had been suffering a lot of runny nose, sneezing, blocked nose and sinuses symptoms, and was also getting weak, shaky, with palpitations and panic feelings and sometimes, pain in the chest. The Hypericum had helped greatly, but over the years, she still took to heart too much of her sisters' family's problems, and was disappointed for a long while that they had not come for homeopathic treatment. She continued to get returns of the nasal and sinus congestion through holding back tears. By June '99, an horrific grief event in a friend's family, three days prior, had triggered off this attack of hysteria, which had rapidly worsened and had been very severe for thirty hours. She had not slept for three nights.

My friend was totally absorbed by thoughts of all the griefs she had suffered over years, and could not focus on what was happening outside of herself, and all day, she cried, screamed, muttered rapidly about old events, reliving her three daughters' births, her father's death, and the fear she felt for her mother's health since Mother had developed the heart problem. I put her on my bed and wrapped her up in the blankets. 'I just want my mum,' she kept saying through the tears, then would disappear from us again in a confusion of memories.

Her husband was not prepared to take her to hospital as he had had to do this once, years ago, and was not happy with the slowness of her recovery then or the drugs she had been given. He knew that the right homeopathic treatment would not only get to the bottom of the problem quickly, but would strengthen her against repeat episodes.

I gave her Ignatia M, Ignatia CM and Ignatia M again, one hour apart, keeping her with me all the day. Her husband and girls came to get her in the evening, by which time she was calmer and becoming more mentally coherent. Once home, she ate a meal and went to sleep, slept nine hours and woke feeling much better. She was still thinking and talking about old events, but now was much happier and quite lucid. Some months later, doses of 10MM sealed the improvement.

See the difference, between drugs and healing energies? Ignatia was able to release stored grief tensions, restore cranial alignment and repair fractures in the energy field of the astral (emotional) body to get the flow of spiritual life force moving evenly through her, all in one easy step. And the benefit was rapid, without trauma, smooth and definite. Drugs would have been given to sedate her, to 'supply the missing chemical in the brain, replace the body's own anti-depressant elements.' How unnecessary and forcefully palliative, not to mention somewhat long-term and even addictive, when all you need to do is supply the missing vibrational frequency and the non-physical self, now repaired, passes the benefit on to the physical body in an instant.

Take Ignatia,

- whenever life deals you a sudden change of plans or lifestyle, whether by death of a partner or family member, through a failed relationship, an accident or illness, loss of a job, being made redundant, or when, through failure of business, plans for your future are curtailed, leaving you disappointed and at the whim of fate.

If these things make you feel worthless or abandoned, take Hypericum;

or if you simply feel hotly indignant at the injustice of it all, take Staphisagria;

if you feel it was all your fault and you could have done things differently for a better outcome, take Hydrastis;

- when ideals fail to materialize, for any of the above reasons or from repeated disappointments, even from such idealistic dashed hopes as failed lottery tickets: whenever you feel inclined to say 'I never get the breaks, when will it be my turn?'

Take Conium as well, if you feel the financial deprivation badly;

- when you feel regret over a missed opportunity, lack of foresight causing you to miss the wave that would have carried you on to fortune;

- when you feel grief over the state of the planet, the suffering in starving nations and war-torn areas; Ignatia helps you get the strength to take some action towards changing the state of affairs. It is this that will raise the planet out of poverty and filth.

If you also have a helpless fear of authorities who will not listen, take Staphisagria as well;

if you suffer guilt of inaction over things that could have been done to help, through fear of retribution, take Aconite;

and if you find it hard to forgive the situations you encounter, take Ledum too. Ledum's ability to bring forgiveness is going to prove the greatest factor in speeding up world healing. I often use Ledum immediately after Ignatia for this forgiveness benefit;

- when you feel grief/guilt that you cannot afford the high cost of living in the expensive capital cities, yet do not know how to solve the dilemma - Ignatia helps you to see a solution and move into a new future with excitement and joy;

- when you cannot get your mind off the past: nostalgia, remembering how good things were at one time or another; dreaming of schooldays,

241

school friends, childhood experiences, earlier married days and such;

and look into Natrum Muriaticum as well, a long-respected remedy for suppressed griefs, and often the mineral follow-up to Ignatia;

if this retrospection makes you feel grumpy or resentful over how things are at present, take Ledum as well;

- when you feel grief over loss of youth and vitality, particularly when it seems impossible that they could ever be regained because of injury, chronic illness or aging.

I found out a lot about the physical symptoms applicable to Ignatia by taking Ignatia CM on 20th June, and 10MM on 22nd June, 1999. My reason for taking it was that I had been developing quite a lot of chest tension, with sighing, over several months, and it finally dawned that this was an Ignatia pattern. I had last taken Ignatia in 1997, as described in Chapter 1.

The first thing to happen, on the 21st June, was that fluid build-up in my breasts began to vanish, as urination increased in frequency. Excess water was shifting out, and it stayed away. In addition, water loosened off from the sinuses and I sneezed all day, as if I had hay fever. It made me think that perhaps, hay fever was sometimes the result of suppressing grief.

My notes of 25th June record pain as if the spine were breaking in two, in the small of the back, only on coughing, causing me to have to bring my knees to my chest to prevent pain with every cough. This was only happening at night, and each cough was accompanied by spurting of urine. I began to call this 'cough and leak syndrome.' I repertorised these symptoms and came up with Nux Vomica, a plant remedy similar to Ignatia, but took nothing.

In addition, there was post-nasal drip, thin, watery to frothy, catching on the larynx and causing cough or hemming. In the night this dripped further down and accumulated in the bronchi. Mucus was bland, tasteless, difficult to bring up or drag down from the posterior nares to the mouth; I needed to keep coughing in the evenings and mornings to shift enough. Continuous, since the first dose.

Muscle tensions, severe: upper trapezius, both shoulders; all abductor muscles of the thighs; the bladder meridian point at the top of the Achilles tendon was painful, as was the leg end of the foot flexors and extensors, especially laterally. Quadratus lumborum tension, both sides at the ribs and pelvis. Joint pain at the lower sacro-iliac joints, both tender to palpate, the left being anterior to the right, while the pelvis sat on a level sacrum. This did not improve with mobilisation of the pelvis.

By the 28th of June: Cough improved, with only occasional bouts of post-nasal drip causing coughing. The pain in the spine on coughing, the bladder weakness and the desire to bend forward to cough to prevent pain had gone. The muscle tensions of the upper trapezius, legs and lower back were not freed yet.

The 29th was as the 28th, with an addition - a severe stitch in the left ribs at 1am, anteriorly at the 5th and 6th intercostal muscle, while lying on that side for several minutes, and I had to shift position to relieve it. I was feeling a lot of grief over a situation with one of our staff who had a hostile attitude to me, failing to see the point of the work I had been doing and hostile to homeopathy generally. I wrote, 'Tending not to get anything done, although much to be finished, hardly knowing where to start - lacking fire.'

Next day: 'Improving. Thoughts getting into better order, knowing where to begin now and able to get on with it.' The next day, my friends Jackey and Phil expressed great confidence in my research, which, in true Ignatia contrariness, left me feeling more teary and depressed. I went to have my spine X-rayed and found an extraordinary reason for my breathing tension, which had not improved or altered with the Ignatia.

The effects of taking Ignatia eased off, including the depression, and I got on with the job of fixing the problems that had shown up in the X-ray. (See the Hydrastis chapter for the Calc Fluor experience.) On arriving back at the office with the plates, I showed Bryan. He immediately drew the anomaly to my attention. This was a 'black hole', a large, wide bubble of gas that extended from the fifth thoracic vertebra down to the stomach, creating a space between my spine and my lungs, and thus restricting the space available for the lungs' expansion. Bryan reached up to his books and pulled down an X-ray text, opening it at the right page - a photograph of a very similar blackness. The cause was described as being gaseous virus toxins generated by an old virus lodged in the tissues.

It was evident to me that this was coming from a virus that had entered via a smallpox vaccination I had had at age 24, as I had had health problems ever since that time as a result, although it has been only since studying homeopathy and learning of the effects of vaccination that I had made the connection. I had learned that Thuja Occidentalis was a remedy that could clear the lymphatics of viral toxins. Through iridology I was able to see that the toxicity was focused in the mesenteric lymph glands near the stomach. I took Thuja MM and later 10MM, 10M and again 10MM over the next twelve months, with benefit, though warts came out on my fingers. Better out than in! After trying for over twelve months to eliminate the most persistent of these warts, I cursed the dose of Thuja that had initiated them, and Gonjesil told me, 'Give love to Thuja, it has saved your life.'

In the meantime, I had a return of the severe pain on coughing that had been triggered off by the Ignatia, the need to jack-knife, the watery mucus, long bouts of sneezing, especially in the sunshine, and the cough-and-leak bladder. I tried several remedies for this symptom picture, and finally sought clarification from Gonjesil, who said, 'Knowingness is, this will often happen to Ignatia people after you free their guilt. It leaves the back unsupported for a while, and the suppressed tears must flow out until fully cleared, as sneezing and coryza.

You must be ready to come in with glowing doses of Nat Mur M.' I took Nat Mur M and later 10M, and my back is no longer troublesome in that way.

NATRUM MURIATICUM

It is fascinating to me to realize that while the first previously described case was typical of Ignatia textbook hysteria and Ignatia fixed the long-term aspects of it, homeopaths still hold to the idea that Ignatia is an acute-level remedy and will not cure the chronic complaint behind the acute episode. Certainly, this is the case if you only use low potencies and do not supply the remedy at the particular fineness of vibration needed to heal the subtle body in question, the astral body. Instead, many homeopaths believe that the remedy Natrum Muriaticum, given in M potency, must follow the Ignatia and finish the job of releasing the stored grief. As it often does - or it clears physical symptoms. The connection is that both remedies act on the body fluids, the nervous system and hormonal imbalance resulting from grief shocks.

Natrum Muriaticum, or Nat Mur, as we call it, is such a broad-spectrum remedy that it is worthy of some description. Not broad-spectrum in the medical sense, covering a multitude of problems, but in the sense that it is needed by a large number of the population in every western country. Natrum Muriaticum is the latinised, homeopathic name of common salt, sodium chloride, which is a substance that is used, not only as a table condiment, but in the manufacture of bread, the processing of butter and margarine, cheese, almost every food on your supermarket shelf. Mankind is over saturated with salt and it is not doing us any good to be so. Nat Mur in M and 10M has a wonderful ability to antidote the adverse effects, in terms of physical conditions, of taking too much salt into the body, while at the same time, curing many complaints that develop out of suppressing grief.

Grieving as a process is something that often needs to have its formalised ritual or ceremony. We should never underestimate the necessity of funerals, and their ability to bring a relationship to a sense of completion. The same applies to the ritual of 'viewing the body', whether this is a formalised event or simply being present when someone dies, or even having to identify someone at the morgue. Children, also, should not be denied the experience of seeing that the person they knew is no longer inhabiting the body. It makes it much easier to accept a death once this has taken place, which, of course, is the origin of the 'viewing' traditions. Only in situations where Aconite fear has been taught need this be a problem.

Petrea King, who runs a residential self-help training school for cancer sufferers south of Sydney, had developed acute myloid leukemia after the death of her brother, who was lost from a mountain trek in Katmandu. She attributes her cancer, which was diagnosed eighteen months after the death, to the unfinished nature of the event - there was no return of his body, no funeral, no possessions to disperse. He simply was there one day and gone the next, no goodbyes, only a massive shock and unfinished business. Finally, during a healing meditation, she realized there was no-one to blame, and no need to blame, and was able to move on out of the cancer. She had been given three months to live. 'Strange thing,' Petrea says, 'you are always given either three months or six months to live, never four or five; and really, they have taken away fifty years!'

Nat Mur lives an outward life at odds with the inner self. There is some of the Staphisagria hypocrisy in Nat Mur - never let your right hand know what the left is doing; and put a different face to the outside world from that which you know is the real face.

The reason Nat Mur people suppress grief is because they have a belief that no-one must ever be allowed to feel sad. Sadness is a massive guilt to the Nat Mur type, whether male or female. No-one must be sad, and if they find sadness, they do everything they can to brighten the sad person up. They all cultivate the art of coping without tears in public, keeping a stiff upper lip, controlling their emotions so that the only tears that fall, manage to escape in the privacy of the darkened bedroom. Never let anyone know you are an emotional wimp. (Arnica is a common precursor to Nat Mur, in my practice - 'I must be tough.') They never admit to feeling grief and sadness, and some manage to suppress it so successfully that they literally do not feel it at all, even under extremely sad circumstances.

The funny thing is, it is only the emotionally sensitive who feel the need to do this. Those who feel spiritually understanding and philosophical about death are not so emotional over it, but if they do feel like crying a bit, they do so, knowing it is normal under the circumstances. Their inner knowing is greater than the social indoctrination given to boys (and girls), that only babies cry, and we must grow up tough, not make fools of ourselves.

When sensitive people like Ignatia and Nat Mur types get slugged by grief, their emotional sensitivity is not able to be talked out of reaction, and if there must be reaction, let it be taken inwardly rather than publicly.

This is where the problems begin. The suppression of grief, sadness and disappointment in the Nat Mur manner affect the cranium and the posterior pituitary in the same way as Ignatia grief. The same systems of the body are affected, though the symptom pictures of the two remedies are not identical. The clamping down of heart energy that happens to Nat Mur types is an extension beyond Ignatia and causes deficiency in the thymus gland, with resultant immune system breakdown and possible lymph and leucocyte malignancies.

The major difference is that Ignatia problems are caused purely by shock and perpetuated by unresolved shock, whereas Nat Mur problems are a creation of the intellect trying to dominate the emotions.

Some of our greatest comedians have been classic Nat Mur types. Most great comics are comics because they have a great sense of guilt over the emotion of grief. They feel compelled to be continually trying to keep everyone laughing - sadness is not allowable. No matter how grief-stricken or depressed he is, the Nat Mur person will do anything to keep it from others. Do not confuse this with the Ignatia person at the funeral, who laughs and smiles at everyone because the grief makes Ignatia changeable, and liable to display the most inappropriate emotions, laughing when she should be crying and vice versa. Nat Mur simply copes well at the funeral, has handled all the organising, stands looking suitably serious, then lets his hair down at the wake, full of jokes and stories.

The effects of not letting the grief emotion out, making it remain locked up in the musculature, are not manifest until many months or even years down the track, when the person may suddenly discover she has a malignant lymphoma condition, or he has developed heart disease.

One of the cleverest funny men of all time, Peter Sellers, was in Rome in 1967 making the film, 'The Bobo,' when his mother had a heart attack. Peter refused to leave the film set, knowing he had survived a more serious group of heart attacks himself, trying to convince himself she'd be all right. A week later she died, and Peter was notified by phone. The grief-guilt shock was so great it could not be expressed at all, Sellers could not bring himself to say the words to those around him in case he lost control. He held it all rigidly in and no-one knew for three hours, when the producer heard from England, about the death.[78]

Spike Milligan, another great, madly great comedian, is another Nat Mur character. He recalled an evening when he was with Peter Sellers and they were discussing their early days, the hard times, the wild times, the giggles that echoed and grew louder down the years. 'I'm an old nostalgic, Pete,' said Milligan, wiping the tears from his eyes. The past is so sweet and sad and beautiful for me.' Sellers looked at him for a long, silent moment, then with all the fun gone from his voice, leaving it tired and almost threadbare, he said: 'What do you mean the past, Spike? *Yesterday*. I get upset thinking about yesterday...because it's gone and it's so bloody buried, so irredeemable, and nobody seems to care. I can cry for yesterday.'

Such is the sentimental grief of Nat Mur, which, like its sister, Ignatia, and its brother, Ledum, lives more in the past and finds it hard to turn the mind away from old times, into the great new adventure of the future.

Nat Mur has benefit in some cases of cancer. Sodium is one of the most prevalent minerals in the body, being present in all the body fluids. It lives in critical balance with potassium in the nervous system, where too much sodium changes the electrical charge on the cell membrane and also disturbs the transport of water into and within the cells; and with calcium in the blood,

246

where too much sodium causes calcium to be laid down in the blood vessel walls, thus creating hardened arteries and hypertension. Excess sodium after metabolism also creates sodium hydroxide, caustic soda, in the bloodstream, which is an irritant that stimulates the development of tumour cells.

A Sydney doctor, Dr Maud Tressillian, in her book '*Does Diet Cure Cancer?*' described her theory of how tumour cells are formed in the body. She claimed that when sodium compounds in the stomach, brought in by taking salt with meals and by consuming any of a multitude of sodium based drugs, break down, their components recombine with other chemicals in the food. Sodium chloride, for example, breaks down into sodium atoms and chlorine atoms, the chlorine atoms combine with water to form hydrochloric acid to aid digestion, and the sodium combines with other chemicals. However, once the available chemicals that can combine with sodium have been used up, there is nothing left for the excess sodium to combine with except water. This gives you caustic soda, and droplets of caustic then run through the bloodstream, irritating and burning the tissues where they may be susceptible.

Dr Tressillian then demonstrated how, in order to relieve the burning, the body calls upon lactic acid, the by-product of cell replication, to come and neutralize the caustic. This is a normal process and all would be well, if the body were not continually being assaulted by more sodium, so that it was constantly having to find more supplies of lactic acid. When the sodium level is too high, the smart body, with its infinite intelligence, then says, OK, let's turn these cells into the form they were in prior to birth, when cell replication was taking place at a much faster rate, and much more lactic acid was being produced. That way, we may get enough lactic acid to neutralize the sodium hydroxide. So cells become tumour cells, for that is what tumour cells are, cells that are multiplying at the rate of foetal cells. Dr Tressillian felt that common table salt was the most common, preventable, cause of cancer.

We now know that in addition to sodium in its many forms, other chemicals are giving the body cause for erratic multiplication of cells. This does not give us any reason to discount her theory, and the fact that Natrum Muriaticum is a primary remedy for some forms of cancers in the blood and lymphatics indicates to homeopaths that salt gets out of balance in the body in these people and this balance must be set right if healing is to take place. We also know, from our texts, that people with Nat Mur problems frequently have a desire to add salt to their food, though eating salt has not been postulated as a reason for needing the remedy by anyone in homeopathic literature, to my knowledge. Until me, that is.

Excess sodium in the body comes through the use of salt, bicarb soda, monosodium glutamate and various other food additives. It is also introduced in many common drugs, and in the water supply of many cities in Australia as sodium fluoride, not to mention in all tinned foods where fluoridated water is added, and juices from trees watered with town water.

Excess sodium is eliminated through sweat glands. When antiperspirants are used, the sweat elimination is suppressed, and sodium as well as toxic waste products are forced to stay in the body and be recycled, adding to the irritants already in circulation and putting further strain on the organs of elimination.

Excess sodium can also be neutralised by taking the remedy Natrum Muriaticum in 10M potency, the best antidoting strength for any substances. This way, there is no over-kill, the imbalance is restored to order rapidly and easily by providing the energy that alters the electromagnetic field of the sufferer, converting harmfully charged particles to a healthful resonance and in essence, correcting the body's galvanic fluids so that both chemistry and physics are normalised.

CHAPTER 13

Humanity is never so beautiful as when praying for forgiveness, or else forgiving another.
- Jean Paul Richter

LEDUM - 'I CAN'T LET GO'

Ledum (ledum palustre, *Marsh Tea, Greenland Tea,* N.O. Ericaceæ) is native to damp regions in the north of America, Asia, Europe, Ireland and Scandinavia. Mrs Grieve makes little mention of it, except to say that 'the leaves are reputed to be more powerful than those of L. latifolium (*St. James' Tea,* from Canada) and to have in addition, some narcotic properties, being used in Germany to make beer more intoxicating.' Hahnemann said that in his day, 'many intoxicating beers were adulterated to a hurtful extent and in a criminal manner with Ledum, to which the police authorities should pay more attention.'

According to Dorothy Shepherd, the great Swedish botanist, Linnaeus, in the *Flora Lapponica,* was the first scientist to introduce it as a medicinal remedy. Linnaeus suggested it for contagious septic throats with spasmodic cough and glandular swelling, and for pertussis (whooping cough). Swedish doctors had used it since the 13th century as an insecticide and for infectious skin complaints such as scabies. In Sweden, it was also used to make beer more intoxicating, and in tanning, and a decoction was used for freeing oxen and pigs from lice, according to Clarke. Linnaeus says that this same decoction, if taken internally, has cured 'violent headaches and a species of angina.'

Hahnemann mentioned 'Ledum has often been given to horses when they go lame and draw up their legs.'

British and North American doctors never took it up, and it is not used in modern herbal medicine anywhere in the world.

LEDUM IN HOMEOPATHY

Hahnemann took up Linnaeus' suggestion and gave it homeopathic provings to determine its specific actions. He said of it, 'The subjoined symptoms are enough to show that this very powerful medicine is suitable for the most part only for those chronic maladies in which there is a predominance of coldness and deficiency of animal heat.' Hahnemann recommended it for 'parts where cellular tissue is wanting, and where a dry, resisting texture is present, as in the fingers and toes', which corresponds with my own discovery that it is primarily a tendons remedy; also for a 'bluish or violet tuberosity, especially on the forehead, and an eczematous eruption, with tingling itching that spreads over the whole body, penetrating into the mouth, probably also into the air passages, and occasions a spasmodic cough, sometimes very violent, which might be mistaken for whooping cough. It is especially useful in bronchitis with emphysema of the aged; renders bronchial secretion less viscid, lessens dyspnœa, stimulates circulation and lessens cyanosis. Haemoptysis alternating with rheumatism.' He quotes symptoms of 'feet held to the earth as if by a magnet when attempting to move: when moving, felt as if pricked by needles; pain rising from feet to head.'[79]

Lameness and gouty soreness in the feet has long been a field for Ledum.

Its parasiticide aspect led the homeopath Teste to think of it as a remedy for puncture wounds such as rusty nails, thorns and insect bites, and it is now used for mosquito bites, stings of bees and wasps, rat-bites, snake bites, caterpillar burns, needle-pricks resulting in whitlows, and even burns and scalds. As it acts quickly, it prevents tetanus. It can be used to relieve the soreness after intramuscular injections, where the needle may have touched tendinous tissue, and must be remembered as a post-immunisation remedy.

While the patient is chilly generally, and his injury or sore joint may be cool even if inflamed, the pain is relieved by cold applications. To test whether Ledum would help, apply cold water and see if it feels better.

Pain in Ledum problems tends to shoot up the limb towards the body, in contrast to most other limb problems, where the pain travels down the nerves. With Ledum problems, the nerves are not the parts most damaged, but pain shoots up the damaged tendon and muscle to its point of origin further up the limb. A 1cm thorn that embedded itself in my foot at age 13 sometimes used to hit a tendon and send a pain shooting up the tendon to the extensor muscle body and its attachment point below and behind my knee, causing me to not be able to point the foot at all until it subsided. After 18 months, the thorn moved closer to the skin and was able to be extracted. Gouty pains behave the same way, and these often have an origin in a blow, such as from dropping a weight on the foot, or falling and jarring. The injuries are often Arnica blows or falls, but Ledum works on the tougher muscle connection tissues rather than the body of the muscle, where Arnica excels.

Although the sufferer may be chilly, the heat of the bed only aggravates his problem, and the limb must be put out into cooler air. Walking about will also aggravate if the problem is in the lower limb. Swelling, puffiness, purpleness, extreme pain, sensitivity to touch. Arthritic, chalky deposits in joints of the spine and extemities. Shoulder pains, hip pains, thighs, knees, ankles - all joints of all limbs and even the jaw and ribcage can be affected.

On the psychological level, there is discontent with others, even to the point of misanthropy.

Clarke lists the following conditions as helped by Ledum:

Clinical.- Ascites. Asthma. Bites. Black eye. Boils. Bruises. Deafness. Ear, inflammation of. Eczema. Erythema nodosum. *Face, pimples on. Feet, pains in;* tender. *Gout.* Haemoptysis. *Hands, pains in.* Intoxication. *Joints, affections of,* cracking in. Menière's disease. Pediculosis. Priapism. Prickly heat. Punctured wounds. *Rheumatism.* Skin, eruptions on. *Stings.* Tetanus. Tinnitus. Tuberculosis. Varicella. Whitlow. *Wounds.*

To this I can add: Chronic streptococcus infections settled in joints. Post-injection asthma, pneumonia, arthritis, fibromyalgia. Repetitive strain injury. Tendons, torn. Tremor, parkinsonism. Viruses.

LEDUM IN MEGAPOTENCIES

We noticed back in the early days of our research that Ledum's tendon tension had a lot to do with inability to let go. Many Ledum people were people who had a need to keep muscles very tense, holding a tool or a machine very firmly in order to prevent it from getting out of control and creating havoc. Doing this for continuing lengths of time resulted in inability of the muscles to relax fully, once the controlling tension was relieved. We were getting clients who had tendon injuries, for this reason. Those fibres that were retaining tension would tear, as if the fibres had dehydrated while the tension was imposed, inhibiting the flow of fluids to the tendons. Such people included power tool operators like builders, earthmoving machinery operators and tractor drivers, truck drivers, process workers and computer operators whose job required that only certain muscles be used, leading to tenosynovitis, carpal tunnel disorders and repetitive strain injury.

Tendons are the hanging-on parts of the muscles, the ends that attach to bones. When we use a muscle, the body of the muscle fills with blood and becomes tense and strong, and the muscle shortens, so that the two bones it is linking are drawn closer together, creating movement of the bone structure. While Arnica affects the muscle body, the part that fills with blood, Ledum works on the holding parts, the tendons at each end, particularly when these tendons have been held tight too long.

We then found that certain sports fitted the Ledum picture. Wherever the grip must not be relaxed for fear of calamity, this is the remedy. Water skiing, abseiling and mountaineering, motor racing, stunt driving, cycling and trail bike riding, rodeo work, gymnastics and high trapeze work are all situations conducive to Ledum injuries. The need to be in control is essential for life and safety. It also relates to precision instruments, surgery, shooting, archery, darts, signwriting, needlework, tennis and squash racquets, all situations where fine accuracy and a steady hand are required.

Control is a major issue for Ledum people. They fear loss of control, want their life to be under control every minute of the day, feel totally torn apart if their life or circumstances get beyond their control. It reflects into every aspect of their thoughts. They will hang on to the bitter end to an idea, an ideal, a relationship, a tool or piece of equipment, for fear that the consequences of letting go will tear them apart, or destroy the framework of their structured life. There is often a sense of having no alternative path to choose, no option. He must hang on for grim death until the time comes when he has mastered the situation.

Remember the union boss, Kite, in the Peter Sellers film, *'I'm All Right, Jack'*? He was a great example of how Ledum can always find a grudge of some kind, in pursuit of his ideal.

Loyalty is a big thing for Ledum people, and misguided loyalty often plays a part. Ledum helps people to let go of the past, of other people and situations that may not be in their interests, and helps those holding on to departed loved ones, alive or dead, to let them go and to move on into the next stage of life. It also helps dying people to let go and die peacefully.

Holding on to the past is a big handicap. Ledum types find it very hard to move on after circumstances change their lives; but most significantly, they find it difficult to forgive, so they may develop a set mouth and eventually, deep grouchy resentment lines running down from the sides of the mouth. These are often quite a lot more pronounced than the small downturn shown on the face of Ignatia sufferers, who simply look long-faced and sad. With long-term Ledum, there is a perpetual grievance look, and because a lot of the lack of forgiveness is suppressed, it can alternate with smiles and the person is often not conscious of the underlying grievance, which relates to something long ago. He or she may wonder why the face carries this aggrieved expression.

Where the acute Ledum condition may be accompanied by conscious bad temper over something someone has done or said, it becomes less conscious when the physical hurt heals up without resolving the mental injury. Because of lack of forgiveness, which locks into the facial muscles and sets the jaw tightly, and into the locomotive muscles, firming them taut as piano wires, chronic disease is enabled to develop. This sets up a process of reduction of blood and nerve supply to these muscles, which results in severe muscle weakness and, in many cases, pain - fibromyalgia . Dehydration can bring in a tendency to tear tendons off the bone, either partially or totally.

The interesting thing is, talking out their problems usually releases a lot of this tension, and they feel better able to survive the day. Those who discover this, and who can find someone to listen to them, off-load some of the stored energy and get some relief, albeit temporarily. Those who do not, may remain disagreeable, misanthropic, vocally dissatisfied or silently unforgiving.

Even the most optimistic and generally happy, loving people can have something niggling in the back of their consciousness, eating them away. Chronically Ledum people eventually become thin, anorexic, undernourished and begin to suffer malnutrition. Their strong, wiry muscles become shrunken. If it is a grief problem, that they cannot let go of a deceased partner, excessive loyalty is preventing them from enjoying life without the other. If the grievance is accompanied by indignation that is suppressed because even righteous anger is 'not nice,' Staphisagria may be needed first.

Being unable to let go of the past makes it hard to move on into a better future. The present is dominated by thoughts of the past, instead of looking at the present moment and welcoming the opportunities it brings to create a joyful tomorrow. Contrast this with Hypericum, who is racing into the future without regard for the past and unable to stay in the present.

The desire to control life equates to an inability to accept that life is a constantly flowing stream, ever-changing. When people come to a crossroads in life, when a phase of their life has ended, it is time to reassess and select a new direction. If you have not let go of the past, if you do not want to get out of your established comfort zone, even though it is no longer comfortable to remain in it, Ledum does wonders in enabling you to make the shift. Whatever age you are, whether it is a matter of leaving home to study or work elsewhere, or of taking up a new line of work when your job peters out, or of needing to face the impracticality of living in your own home alone at the age of 95, Ledum helps, giving you the ability to make the shift with enthusiasm rather than resistance.

Ledum people tend to be long-living. They expect to live long, unlike Hypericum, who find it hard to imagine themselves old. They hang on to life stoically, not to be found among those seeking euthanasia. However grim life seems, whatever the resentment or grievance he harbours, Ledum always hangs in there, determined that sooner or later, things will improve. Under stressful conditions of living, it is Ledum who outlasts all others through sheer, stubborn *nil bastardi carborundum* - 'never let the bastards grind you down.'

One of my old friends was a gentleman in his nineties who had had a nasty fall some years ago, tearing one of his biceps tendons off the shoulder. A clean break, that part of the muscle then slipped down and bunched up beside its other half, further down the humerus, and nothing could be done with it. We gave him Ledum 30 with Arnica 30 and Ruta 30, and the combination gave him considerable benefit over some months. Later, his wife died, after a grim illness.

At that time, his daughter had got into his bad books by going off on a holiday with a new mate. The combination of events was perfectly suited to Ledum. The poor fellow was so distraught with grief over losing his wife, and grievance towards the daughter's friend for taking her away at the time of

253

mother's decline, that he could not speak to him, was very irritable with both and spent his time, when not grumpy with them, in floods of tears, sitting looking all day at all his wife's photos, that he had arranged around his chair. Ledum M worked like a charm, he was sociable the very next day. When he looked like sinking into depression again, I gave him more Ledum M.

A few years later, he had another fall, hurting his wrist with the classic Ledum symptoms - black and blue, right up the arm, swollen purplish hand, could not use it for weeks. Ledum 30 again, in the same combination with Arnica and Ruta, slowly got it back to rights, but eventually M was given again. It worked so well on his mind that I never needed to give him megapotencies, and he finally died at 96.

Ledum works well on forgiveness of people, situations or circumstances, no matter whether they are creations of others or your own. We knew a woman who came to Australia with a new teaching that she found very hard to get established. She was a determined, courageous woman with a strong, jutting chin, and a lot of resentment over various little grievances. She had not allowed for our relatively small, and somewhat conservative population; her knowledge was a little too esoteric for the average materialistic Aussie, and she was ahead of her time, here. After some years of teaching in different parts of the country, she left Australia and went back to England, disillusioned and bitter at her lack of a great following. I wish I had known of Ledum in those days.

I took Ledum CM myself on 12th April, 2002, because of crippling needle-like pains in the tendons of the feet. This was no better next day, and as I had intended to take 10MM first, I took this the next night. There were no further pains in the feet, which I had had for a month. A return of old hay fever came on, as had also happened when I had taken Ignatia five years before. My eyes, which had been very dry and itchy for a few weeks, returned to normal moisture, and urination increased in power and volume. My energy seemed to slow down for a while - as can happen, the relaxation of undesirable muscle tension makes you feel very lethargic at first, until you get used to having relaxed tendon tension. I don't know what I was letting go of, mentally, but it felt good.

A mother of two boys came in September, 1994 about her sore joints, which had been a problem for 'years and years, and I'm always tired.' She was on the go all the time. Blood tests ruled out osteo and rheumatoid arthritis. She was allergic to several grains and to pork. She played competition tennis on summer evenings, this seemed to start off the pains in the legs, which would come and go. She had weakness in the lumbars and legs, so that to get up from the floor, she had to lift herself with her arms - a common indicator for Hydrastis. She had guilt over her marriage bust-up years ago, saying 'I do everything right, what am I doing wrong?' And grief over her brother's death - he had died while on drugs, at a time when she was refusing to have anything to do with him - 'I was judgemental,' she said. On these grounds I gave her Staphisagria MM, and four weeks later, Nat Mur CM. Her father died a day after she'd taken Nat Mur. I saw her once or twice over the next few years, and she appeared again about the joint soreness, which had been worse again for a year, in July 2000.

At this stage she was feeling tired, cranky and depressed, very tense and sore. She had given up the sports and the knee was no longer swelling, though still sore. She said she lacked ambition and initiative, just cruised along, but would like to have achieved something; pessimistic, never optimistic. She talked about how devastating it had been to find out her first husband was homosexual. She had blocked it out for two years, then left him, and had been unable to tell his family why, so they were not friendly. She was most stressed now about her state of underweight, said she would do anything to look better. I gave Hypericum 10MM, which made her generally better.

A month later, she was still sore from the neck down, but was dealing better with the aches, was not as conscious of the underweight, but found she was getting breathless, sighing, and tense and racy premenstrually. She still had grief over her father, disappointment over loss of expectations in her first marriage, and a severe tendon contracture of her left thumb. She had been a book-keeper, held the pen too tightly always (left-handed). This time, the penny dropped and I gave her Ignatia CM and Ledum MM.

Two months later, she felt she was no longer dwelling in the past. Still sore all over, still Ledum symptoms. Ignatia and Ledum were repeated in November 2001. If I had looked with different eyes at the story she had been telling me all along, I would have given Ledum from the start. But I did not know it well enough in the earlier days.

A much more straight-forward, totally Ledum woman of 46 came in 1998. She had painful feet, sore to touch, and had had gout as a child (familial problem). Her right elbow had lost strength and was getting shooting pain through it. Her joints had been swollen since having a mosquito-borne virus in 1990, which had also given her Menière's syndrome, with 10% loss of hearing in the right ear. She had had asthma since getting a smallpox vaccine and a BCG shot when she started nursing, and she had also had pneumonia the following year, in the right lung.

The gouty feet had a sensation as if the feet were full of crystals, she could hardly put her feet to the ground. She was still getting dizziness. Fevers were coming on every couple of weeks, with temperatures up to 40°C. To top it off, her feet were getting hot in bed, and she hated her feet being hot. She also hated the cold weather in recent years. We had started her on Ledum 30, which helped wonderfully, and I now gave her Ledum 10M. In five weeks, I gave Ledum 50M and in January 1999, this lapsed and I used Ledum 10MM. Nine months later, pain was coming back into feet and wrists, her ankles felt sprained, and her chest, she said, was 'filthy', requiring a puffer. In many ways, she was still improved. She had not noticed the winter as much that year. I gave her Ledum MM, the final clincher. (Notice how it can take a few years for different potencies to complete the healing. Ledum types have usually been so for a lifetime.)

Inability to let go of fixed attitudes creates rigidity that leads to hands or fingers that grasp like crabs' claws and will not let go or straighten (du Puytrene's contracture); or to leg and hip muscle tensions, that prevent you from stepping forward into whatever lies ahead. The extreme of this is spasticity and spastic paralysis. Think of Ledum also for muscular atrophies, motor neurone diseases and dystrophy and other forms of myopathy including tremors and parkinsonism, or even multiple sclerosis: significantly, I remember hearing many years ago, one of Australia's great women athletes proclaiming from her wheelchair, "This country does not appreciate how much I did for it!" - a typically Ledum grudge.

Think of Ledum in lower potencies for the bites of insects, ants and spiders that will not let go - ticks, bull-ants, funnel-web spiders - and remember, if the remedy is given while the tick is still embedded, it will get the benefit of the remedy and be more inclined to loosen its grip. Similarly, for dogs such as bulldogs and rottweilers who have a natural inclination to hang on and not let go. Ledum will help them with many of their health problems.

Using Ledum against the chronic effects of injections and inoculations is something of which I have not had enough experience, to describe more fully. It is hard to say whether babies have a sense of losing control, or of anger at experiencing offenses beyond their control, or annoyance at having insufficient control over their bodies. I have always used Hypericum or Staphisagria with benefit for the cases that might have needed Ledum, who, I suspect, are the ones who develop hive-like raised swellings from injections, and later, joint soreness and growing pains. Certainly, there are plenty of wiry, tense little children around who have rigid attitudes and often, bad tempers, who could probably do with some Ledum.

Self-forgiveness is often a stumbling block. Some people blame themselves for events that led to their poverty, loneliness or discomforts. Self-forgiveness is usually given by Hydrastis. Ledum is only applicable if they cannot let go of the past.

Universal love is the keynote of Ledum. It will help those still carrying the idea that this is a great world with all its emphases on war, power, vengeance and control. Ledum opens the eyes to the necessity for beginning to love one's neighbour as oneself, and to do unto others as one would be done by, and gets it all happening. Like Arnica, Ledum people tend to think you have to be hard on others, but their reason is that they fear loss of control.

Many nations of the world need Ledum. Inability to forgive goes hand in hand with the Bedouin/Arab ego/fear-driven obsession with honour. To these people it is better, more honourable to kill a wife or daughter than to forgive any breach of their social code. Standing, in these male-dominated communities depends, it seems, on men's having absolute control over the hearts, minds and bodies of their womenfolk. Any independence of female spirit reflects so badly on the male head of the household that he is obliged to eliminate the offender, however much he may love her. Ego and its attendant, fear, override any such love. What massive guilt such societies perpetuate for themselves, when murder is preferred to loss of face.

This is the major remedy for those who rigidly hold on to their declared position for fear of losing face if they become reasonable. The wonderful thing is, Ledum changes such inflexibility overnight. You see the same attitude in parents who impose rigid disciplines or punishments on their children and will not be talked out of it by any appeal to reason or kindness. Ledum people have greater capacity for cruelty, mental or physical, than any other remedy.

Where Hydrastis behave badly to others because of alcohol or drugs, Ledum is an extension and intensification of the Staphisagria righteousness. 'You will do what I say is right or I'll never forgive you - I'll punish you severely.'

Use Ledum to help you to forgive those who have contributed to your present situation, and those who put others into hardship, grief, poverty or whatever, through their ignorance, recklessness, cruelty and/or greed. It is helpful for those who feel unappreciated - 'after all I've done for you.'

Use Ledum to help you let go of outdated ideas or situations, to accept and welcome changes, to bring in much needed change. With Ledum there is a considerable fear of the future, because it is an unknown over which you may not have control. Fear of loss of control prevents a shift into the perceived unpredictability of the future. Ledum helps you to create your future as you want it to be, by freeing up the belief that you need to, but may not, be in control.

One year, I was approached by a woman for help to detach from the past and get on with new things. A seven-year relationship had ended last year, and after September 11, her travel agency job had ran out. It was a year of big changes from which she was still having trouble healing. She had kept her contacts and a few good clients were keeping her going, from home, via the Internet. It was the relationship that was really still getting at her. Her Hypericum mate had abandoned her in favour of greener pastures, and even now, less than a year later, this was falling through and he was seeking her company again. She was not willing to forgive the woman and not sure about him, and did not know which way to turn. She found it hard to rise above the grief and injustice of the events over the last year, felt there must be something new on the horizon but could not see what it might be, yet.

A comparison with Ignatia helped to determine which remedy was needed here. Ignatia is not afraid to move ahead, but feels stymied that plans for the future could not progress, through events beyond her control. There is

257

a sense of grief, but with Ledum, there is blame, aggressive grievance and a real desire to hang on to the past. This lady also had strong Staphisagria lines across her forehead, raised eyebrows, and definite pulling down of the upper lip muscles on each side, as of Ignatia. So I gave her Staphisagria MM and Ignatia 10MM for starters.

She felt a lot better, less emotional after these. Life was easier to handle, and she was letting go of 'what was not happening'. Benefits were lapsing after only a couple of weeks, so I cut in straight away with Ledum 10MM.

'On the way! Even sight has improved.' She now admitted to long term constipation, a common 'inability to let go.' After Ledum, she became very aware of the tension in her jaw and realized how much she had been holding it. 'Letting go' is really starting to kick in now,' she told me. I asked about fears. These were: of letting go of her job; of lack of options; of feeling unable to move on because of her aged mother nearby; of being alone, although she had previously lived alone for ten years without any trouble; and she feared for the safety of her oldest son, who had had three big accidents. I noticed she had an Aconite type of nose, and she said she had always had this kind of profile. She had been through a prolonged birthing and was small and blue when born. I gave her Aconite 10MM and more Staphisagria, 10MM. It was not long before she needed Ignatia again, her son's six-year relationship was breaking up. This time I gave Ignatia followed by Ledum CM. Her skin began to demonstrate the outward expression of her healing energies by getting very dry and itchy, and the next time I saw her, the grief issues were dissolving and life was looking much more positive.

Needing to be in control, of yourself, your life and that of another or all around you, has a relationship to Staphisagria who knows how things should be for everyone, but tut-tuts helplessly when they do not see the rightness of his ideas. Ledum is deeper, goes further into the rigidity of control and the resentment towards those you are not influencing. Many Staphisagria people also need Ledum to help them relax on this strictness. Whereas Staphisagria people want a fair and just reward for both good deeds and bad, Ledum can go overboard on punishment in order to set an example to others who may commit the same misdemeanours - even if they are but little children. Society must be taught early that rigid discipline and control keep the cogs running smoothly (for the controllers). Such Ledums love to rule by fear.

George W. Bush, former President of the USA, demonstrated his Ledumness in his grim and unforgiving goading of Saddam Hussein, on the one hand, and his declared determination to seek out and destroy terrorists threatening the US, on the other. The very idea that a situation could happen over which he had no control, threatening his country, to which he had absolute loyalty, was already showing effects on his health. Bush was determined that war was the only way by which he would retain control; and the Ledum mindset will fight to the death to hold on to his standpoint.

This is something I have taken a long time to realize, and as I look back over many cases, I find instances where Staphisagria did the majority of the work needed, but Ledum had been missed as a follow-up. In the Staphisagrian social culture, probably about 40% also need Ledum, and there is an overlap with Ignatia, who could need either or both of the other two.

On the other hand, it is rare for a Hypericum type to need Ledum. They are polar opposites in many ways. While Hypericum believes in rapid revenge, rapid-fire machine gun or swift knife-in-the-back killing, Ledum stores his grievances and plans for years to wreak vengeance, as did Osama bin Laden. Ledum believes in capturing alive, interrogating and putting to torture before death. Ledum the torturor loves to prolong the agony. 'Killing is too good for him - make him suffer.'

Even where there seem to be points of overlap, the reasons are usually coming from a different standpoint. For example, the current attitude amongst those in power is 'tell them only what we think they need to know.' Both Hypericum and Ledum people are ruling this way, fearing loss of their power seat if people become too knowledgeable. Staphisagria people always believe they know what is best for everyone else, and how much it is best for you to know. They all fear freedom of information once they get into power situations. They encourage education but prefer to restrict the availability of information by regulating what can be taught in our teaching institutions into a conformity that discourages opposing or alternative ideas in the controlled curriculi. In Australia, this attitude has created a stated plan, determinedly pursued, to reduce the number of small, independent colleges by two thirds and thus gain more government control over curriculum content. The cost of conformity is beyond the incomes of small colleges.

From government departments, information is released on a 'need to know' basis, which now means 'we do not need you to know'. At the same time, new, draconian gun-laws, tax laws, civil laws are being introduced at an alarming rate. The Hypericum top-dogs fear losing their top rung on the ladder; the Ledums fear a population getting out of control. They both know that over-control is tyranny against which a people may be incited to rebel; but instead of relaxing the trend, they expect to see more and more compliance and conformity. Staphisagria types in top positions go along with it, thinking they are doing the right thing and knowing they are helpless against the more forceful Hypericums and Ledums. Needle-shocked, the lot of them. Help them to greater, more loving leadership!

Of course, those who are in control and are enjoying having other people under their control, do not necessarily have the strong facial lines of grumpy resentment, though they will have been through times when they did not have the control they wished. They may still show a thin, set pair of lips and can just as easily develop muscle disorders from the stiffness of their control.

Think about Hitler, the worst Ledum we can remember. True to the nature of the most negative Ledums, he set up torture chambers in the form of concentration camps, for concentrated, cruel maltreatment of his fellow men and women. When he finally began to lose control of his own officers and his war machine, he developed such tension in his body that he could no longer control his limbs or his jaw, and began to splutter and tremble badly. There are plenty of 'little Hitlers' around still, in every country. If you get the chance to treat any such person, remember Ledum and help the world. And do not change the remedy until you have been through all the megapotencies. Ledum is very reluctant to let go of his 'controlling' belief, and the problems and attitudes keep recurring for a few years.

Contrast Hitler with a strong, positive Ledum. Ledum's great loyalty to his community is amply demonstrated in our former Prime Minister, Malcolm Fraser, who, though now at an age when others would have long ago retired, is still working determinedly to unify the black and white populations of Australia. He will not let this issue go, and will very likely pursue it to his dying day. His great love of humanity and Staphisagria training drive him on to ensuring that all Australians get an equally fair go in every way. His concern also goes to all who have chosen Australia as their home, even those who come illegally seeking asylum, of whom we have had a great number found recently, all placed in detention centres.

Mr Fraser called for a parliamentary enquiry into conditions in some of these centres, which are situated in isolated desert areas at great distances from towns and have very basic facilities. The refugees protest, are treated harshly and driven to rebellion and some then are placed in gaol, separating them off from their families. 'We wouldn't treat our worst enemies the way these people are being treated,' Mr Fraser said. 'Illegally here or not, they are human beings. We should treat people as we would wish to be treated.'

Whatever your religion or your politics, this is spiritual consciousness in action. I recently heard a journalist describe Malcolm Fraser as 'a great spiritual leader,' and I heartily concurred. He is going to great lengths to see reconciliation fulfilled in his lifetime.

CHAPTER 14

A house divided against itself cannot stand.
- Abraham Lincoln

RUTA - 'UNITED WE STAND'

Ruta (ruta graveolens, *Rue*, N.O. Ranunculaceae), is an evergreen, shrubby plant that the ancients knew well as a remedy for resisting contagions and poisons. The name Ruta is from the Greek *reuo*, to set free. It is mentioned in the Hippocratic writings; by Pliny, who recommended its use for the preservation of sight, especially after the overuse of the eyes in painters, and from too much reading; and by Dioscorides, who used it as a counter to the poisons of toadstools, aconite, serpent bites and the stings of bees, hornets and wasps.

Rue is a very old plant. It disappeared entirely from the earth during the glacial periods, and was lost from view again many thousands of years later, during the dark days of the early Middle Ages.

Rue was introduced to England by the Romans and naturalised in the gardens of the monks. It grows well in dry, neglected, barren soil. Culpeper recommended it to be applied externally for sciatica and pain in the joints, and internally for malaria-like shaking fits. Also, 'the juice warmed in a pomegranate shell and dropped in the ears, helps the pain of them.'

The plant was strewn in the later Middle Ages in the Law Courts and judges' chambers at the Assizes to protect against typhus, the common gaol fever of the times, caused by overcrowding and lack of sanitation. It was regarded by Piperino, an Italian physician in the Middle Ages, as a specific against epilepsy and vertigo, and was much used in religious ceremonies, called the Herb of Grace, presumably to protect against evil spirits (infection).

In modern herbal medicine, leading Australian herbalist, the late, great Dorothy Hall[80], recommended Rue for the portal circulation, as it strengthens the portal vein and bowel and supports the elimination of toxic materials discharged by the liver. She suggested it for high systolic and diastolic blood pressure resulting from the Rue person's belief in 'keeping the lid tightly on a pressure cooker of unspoken emotions.' Pelvic venous congestion, varicose veins, blood clotting and coagulability, haemorrhoids and pelvic congestion with periods can all be regulated and normalised with Rue, in the type of person who needs it. And you will get a clear picture of this person as we go along.

RUTA IN HOMEOPATHY

Homeopathically, many of the herbal uses of Rue are found to still apply. Ruta in low, medium and high potencies has wonderful, strengthening effects on sprained joints, particularly wrists and ankles, knees and the lower spine. It covers sensations of bruising of the periosteum of the bone, from overstrain of the ligaments and cartilage, or from major injuries such as falls from heights, motor vehicle accidents, football injuries; weakness in the thighs causing stumbling; shooting sciatic pain from strained lumbar ligaments allowing spinal subluxation, such as you may get from lifting heavy parcels and turning to place them somewhere else.

It also assists eyestrain with heat, smarting, itching, watering, aching and fatigue from too much close work, causing weak vision. Ruta acts on the ligaments behind the eye that are strained when prolonged close focusing creates tension in the neck, and the first cervical vertebra is pulled slightly out of position, restricting nerve energy to the front of the head. This can also be a reflex effect from a lower lumbar spine problem.

There may be spasms in the tongue causing speech difficulty; sensations in and around the ear as of a blunt instrument moving inside, or a bruised sensation of having had a blow or knock to the ear cartilages; or prolapse of the uterus, bladder, anus, rectum and/or bowel resulting from weakness in the pelvic ligaments (Ruta has been helpful to some bowel cancers); pain, heat and tenderness in the feet, causing difficulty walking on them; and at rest, legs restless and heavy, all parts lain on feel sore as if bruised - cannot get comfortable (Arnica also has this). He wakes frequently at night, even without body aches.

The Ruta patient's problems are worse for cold in any way - cold air temperature, cold applications. He feels coldness in the spine and legs, yet enjoys the bracing quality of winter as long as he is warmly dressed and in good health.

Ruta acts on the etheric body, the energy matrix of the physical tissues, and quickly acts on simple breaks and tears of ligaments and synovial membranes, removing inflammation and pain. According to Dr Dorothy Shepherd, 'it has a hammering effect on the etheric, altering the flow of blood through the ligaments and the periosteum covering the bones. Those who are sensitive to the vibrations will tell you they resemble the musical rhythm of three short beats and one long one; in Morse, it would be three dots and a dash.' Think of the first bars of Beethoven's mighty Fifth Symphony, and you might wonder if, perhaps, many lovers of this work are not of the Ruta type.

Clarke lists the following conditions as amenable to Ruta:

Clinical. - *Amblyopia*. Anus, prolapse of. *Bone, bruised; pains in. Bruises*. Bursitis. Cartilages, bruises of; pains in. *Chest, sternum, pains in.* Constipation. Dislocations. Dyspepsia. Enuresis. Epistaxis. Exostosis. *Eyes, sight weak;* pains in. Facial paralysis, from cold. Fevers. *Fractures. Ganglion.* Haemorrhages. *Hands, pains in.* Paralysis. *Perichondritis*. Periostitis. Rectum, affections of; prolapse of. Restlessness. *Rheumatism. Sciatica*. Spleen, affections of. *Sprain*. Stammering. Tongue, cramp in; swelling of. Urination, difficulty of. Varicocele. Veins, swollen; varicose. Warts.

To these I can add: Cancer, from lumbar spine damage. Eyes, macular degeneration. Spine, disc rupture.

RUTA IN MEGAPOTENCY

We found that Ruta people were always a bit mystified that their body had not been able to take the load. They did not do anything unusual, they often said, almost always it happened during the usual course of the job or sport. Something must be happening on a less physical level to undermine the strength of the connective tissues.

My first understanding of the mind of Ruta, from 1993, was that the people needing Ruta had no sense of limitation in respect to strength, and felt that they ought to be able to lift or carry any weight they needed to, and I began to call this my 'Hercules' remedy.

Strength matters. The Ruta strength is the glue that binds a body together, structurally. Ligaments and cartilage hold a skeletal structure together at the joints. They have no power to move limbs or spine, they simply hold the bones fast in balance with the pulling power of the muscles. If this holding-together ability is undermined, the bones shift apart, and joints subluxate. In the person needing Ruta, it is the fear of loss of might, loss of strength in numbers or of unity of purpose that causes the joints to be weaker than the muscles.

It is the binding quality of Ruta that causes a family or a community to pull together in times of adversity. Positive Ruta people can return a community that feels a loss of unity and strength to being close-knit, supportive and collectively powerful. In the body, Ruta problems develop when a person feels the family, spouse, employees or community are not standing together to achieve great things. These people know the value of strength in unity and combined effort.

There is a sense of need to be strong through all life's ups and downs. Standing firm against adversity, the Ruta person is a survivor, always takes the bit between his teeth and pushes on through the hardships and traumas life offers. Unlike Hypericum, who prefers to run for his life when the going gets tough, Ruta stands steadfast and true, is firm and reliable and always copes. He or she is the natural independant, admired by others for this great inner strength. Ruta does not try to fight against life but accepts whatever comes that cannot be changed and changes what he can, back to the status quo, or towards greater strength and stability.

Ruta does not panic easily, but he can act very swiftly in emergencies. He thinks, assesses and takes appropriate action, without appearing to be moving rapidly. He is a plodding, solid, salt of the earth type who gets there by perserverance and determination and patient acceptance of the natural order of things.

Ruta says, 'You just get on with it, don't you. It is what you do, that's life - make the best of it.' We find Ruta people with all levels of education, from the professor to the peasant farmer, always with a 'live and let live' expectation that all others are living from the same standpoint, in charge of their own lives. They do not try to take responsibility for others (Hydrastis) or shirk their own responsibilities (Hypericum); they avoid hypocrisy (unless they are also strongly Staphisagria), so that you know where you stand with them, which is beside them, squarely on two feet, taking your share of the burdens.

Many women have said to me, 'I have to do everything, he does nothing.' The feeling is not that of having too much to do, but of regret that so much more could be done, with greater satisfaction, faster, if others were pulling their weight. Ruta strengthens the person who is not succeeding in getting this unity of purpose from others. It also strengthens the person who has been mightily invincible beyond his body's capacity and broken under the strain of pulling his own weight without help from others. 'Many hands make light work.'

The young Ruta is invincible. He can lift anything, drink or eat anything, expecting his body to adjust and deal with everything he takes on. His conventional and conservative nature does not let him indulge in self-destructive activities unless they are those accepted as conventions by his community - in Australia this means, or used to mean, drinking beer, smoking tobacco, playing rugby football.(All these are Arnica conventions too.)

The pull-together consciousness of Ruta brings great team spirit. They will throw their whole weight into team effort, whether sport or work. The team is all-important, can't let the team down, must be strong for the team, the ones who are relying on everyone pulling their own weight.

There is also a great sense of the level playing field in Ruta. Unlike Hypericum, who likes to bring down the tall poppies to a low level so he can feel higher than all, the positive Ruta person likes to bring his whole community to greatness by a co-operative effort. He makes a good leader, inciting others to participate in creating his visions on a non-competitive level. He is not interested in winners and losers so much as in everyone being a winner, gaining benefits, profiting from co-operation and pulling together.

Unawareness of one's (human) limitations to strength and endurance is common to lots of Ruta people. It is different from the Hypericum rebellion against limitations, with recklessness and unawareness of risks. With Ruta there is a feeling of extending the boundaries, of expanding the power, that reminds me of the great British colonial song, 'Land of Hope and Glory': *'Wider still and wider Shall thy bounds be set. God, who made thee mighty, Make thee mightier yet.'* England knew no boundaries in the eighteenth and nineteenth centuries, and even up to the mid-twentieth century. It was inevitable that 'the colonies' would eventually rise up against her despotic takeovers and take action to gain self-rule, yet very Ruta in mentality that they remained a unified Commonwealth of Nations, each independently ruled but commercially inter-dependent for the common wealth.

We saw the mightiness of the British spirit of cohesion in adversity during World War I and even more so, in World War II - the War Effort, it is referred to - where the whole population willingly worked together in the most amazing community effort ever seen. Forty million people changed their lifestyle, eating habits, style of government (to an all-parties-in Parliament), agricultural and manufacturing priorities and products, and even occupations. Women, for the first time, were accepted in men's jobs, in farming and industry, and some formed a Women's Army and a Women's Air Force.

Never before, and never since, has a large nation been so totally aligned in this way, for the benefit of all. You could think it was a Staphisagria sense of duty and a Ledum loyalty that were operating here, and indeed they were, but it was the Ruta people like Winston Churchill who were the backbone of the whole organisation, the leaders who pulled on team spirit to hold the country focused on the good of the whole rather than the individual.

The Ruta spirit is indomitable, patient, undaunted, persevering. He and she alike stand firm against adversity, whether personal, local or general, and always make the best of things. In spite of such great perseverence, Britain was really brought to its knees by World War II. The long years of struggle took their toll and the war threatened to come to an impasse, the day being saved eventually by Hitler's increasing loss of control of his cohorts and his mind, and the injection of a little fresh energy from the US.

Like Britain, then, the Ruta person will struggle on, defying the odds until his back is broken and knees are on the ground, forcing him to lay off and allow time for rest. He will not let the side down if he can possibly help it.

I remember a man who came to me long ago, wanting help to keep on with the job he had started, alone. 'I'm digging the foundation trenches for my new house,' he said, 'I've been shovelling all day, and now my back is out and I can hardly walk, let alone dig. I want you to give me something that will enable me to keep going through the weekend, I must finish the job because the concreters are booked to come on Monday with the Ready-mix.' A pretty tall order, I thought, but I gave him a vial of Ruta M and said to keep taking it throughout the weekend, and hopefully it would keep him going. His part of the job was the digging, and he was not going to upset the schedule for the others, if he could help it, even though he had no-one to assist.

Ruta is like this because he or she believes this is the right and proper way to live, for all people. He gets upset when others fail to pull their weight, and he is even more guilty if anything prevents him from pulling his weight and doing his bit. Compare this with Hydrastis, who takes on responsibility for others. Ruta encourages self-responsibility. He is able to teach the young this value, even if it means giving them harsh lessons, where Hydrastis weakens and goes soft on others, doing their share for them, paying their way. Ruta gets disheartened when others are 'bludging' their way through life, living off the efforts of others.

Like Staphisagria, Ruta has a strong duty consciousness, but on a much broader scale. While Staphisagria's duty is towards obedience to the rules and regulations and towards the respect owing to parents and authority figures, Ruta places cohesion higher. The family, the team, the village, the town or country must be held together. Unity is strength. Without it, we collapse, like the skeleton, into a collection of individual units - divided, we fall.

Compare this with many Hypericum-style politicians. The nature of Hypericum is to have sympathy for the underdog, so long as he stays below you. Hypericum seems to love people, but it is conditional upon their remaining underdogs, youth or children. Therefore, he works tirelessly to get more and more government support for those at the lower socio-economic levels, thus keeping them totally dependent on support and preventing them from ever rising to his level. This way, he gets their love - that is, until someone wakes up and stabs him in the back. Hypericum also is the nature of the underdog himself, with his attitude of 'Let's all over-tax the rich and strong and let the government provide for us, the work-shy, the fun-loving, although it means bringing the capable down to our jobless state in the process.' The thinking is right out of balance, so he shoots himself in the foot by making a situation that it is impossible for either the bosses or the government to sustain.

The Ruta leader is quite different. He believes in personal integrity and inner discipline. He seeks to inspire others to greatness through their own efforts, thereby building a community of greatness. He is not interested in providing for others but in teaching others to provide for themselves. He will not take on responsibility for others who could be taught to handle their own responsibilities. He believes that strength builds unity, as well as the converse, and is always willing to teach and lead others to personal strength.

Compare the current medical/government attitude of a Hypericum nature to the emerging Ruta trend in naturopathic modalities, where we try to teach you about your mind and body and show you how to help yourself. Did you know that the word 'doctor' comes from the Latin *'docere'*, to teach?

Medical men in Roman times were simply teachers, helping people to help themselves by teaching them the principles of life and health. How far this is from current Western medicine! And how close to all the many forms of natural healing becoming more and more popular today. People want to know more and take reponsibility for themselves, nowadays.

Ruta personalities are very conventional and conformist. They like a solid foundation of community life with social mores that encompass sound guidelines for all to adhere to, and enjoy the secure sense of stability and coherence that this 'feet on the ground' pattern provides. They are hesitant to take up new ideas that might threaten this stability, hence can become resistant to change, new methods or more modern equipment. The old and familiar are fine, the simple methods tried and true - tried, in some cases, for tens of thousands of years and still good.

The first threat to the Ruta child's strength comes from within the family. A sense of grief over family disunity will affect the child subtly. It may be simply that another child in the family is continually in trouble with one parent. Or perhaps, parents argue or disagree. If there has been a family breakup, the guilt of this is great, and the Ruta child craves a unified, two-parent family. This child loves the sense of strength that family unity brings, he loves the extended family concept and all his relations even when more distant relations ignore his side of the family. He does not feel less worthy (as Hypericum does), simply mourns the loss of family strength and togetherness.

Ruta sporting injuries cause the sufferers to have great guilt over letting down the team by not being available to continue play, and they insist on getting back into the game before enough time has been allowed for healing. The injuries are usually severe - cartilage tears, ligament tears, joint dislocations, muscles torn from the bone - and require rest from play until the following season. Sometimes, Hydrastis or Arnica may be needed as well. (If he needs Arnica as well, he'll be trying to get back into the game immediately, even if concussed, mumbling hazily 'I'm OK, let me go on.')

The Olympic Games is a magnificent example of Ruta in its most positive aspects. Teams are sent from virtually every country in the world, representatives of large and small dominions. Each competitor has his own country's hopes and confidence to drive him, yet in the Olympic Village, all competitors, with few exceptions, become part of one mighty team, supporting each other with love, enthusiasm and sympathy. The public's contribution is also very much a part of this general support. Everyone knows and feels how much it has cost these competitors to reach the point of being accepted to compete. When the 2000 Olympics were held in Sydney, there were over eighty-five thousand unpaid volunteers teamed up to assist visitors, spectators and sportspeople, over and above all the paid workers. Love of being part of the team was their incentive.

On the other hand, at the same time, the International Olympic

Committee was being exposed as riddled with corruption, organised crime, extortion and bribery from the top down. Greed had dominated it since its beginning. Extraordinary, that such an inspiring concept should be used for such selfish reasons, with no concern for the individuals it purports to stand for, and still be able to excite millions. Thanks to investigators like Andrew Jennings[81], the days are numbered for these 'Lords', and the coming years will see much greater integrity entering the organisation.

Solidarity is important in life, for every Ruta person. He wants all his family to enjoy this solidarity, and feels grief if any member separates himself off from the family team. The benefits of family solidarity are manifold. The Ruta father always welcomes back the prodigal son, without question. (Not necessarily without some kind of punishment or conditions - but these would always be aimed at teaching the prodigal greater responsibility to family cohesion and beyond, to the wider community or the business, if this is still to be learned.)

The Ruta mother has a reluctance to see her children grow up and leave home, and makes sure they know they are still in a strong position in the family group, no matter how far distant they may roam. The grief of physical distance can be as great as the grief of emotional estrangement.

Within the Ruta family all members are expected to pull their weight, and this attitude is carried out into the groups, clubs and associations that Ruta joins and works within. When others fail to see the value of everyone working together for a common benefit, when they make excuses to be unavailable and leave the idealist Ruta unsupported, he watches, disheartened, as his society disintegrates, individuals pursuing their personal interests at the expense of the group.

Family breakdowns are a great grief to him, particularly when total separations occur. (Hypericum often thinks nothing of leaving his family to their fate, separating himself off from them, not wanting to take responsibility.) The Ruta, deeply concerned, feels that people would do best to support each other through changes of relationships, for the good of the whole and each member of the family. Ruta prefers to be and to live among people who believe in working through problems to find cohesive solutions. The strong Ruta encourages unity and strength in others. The weaker Ruta, at worst, maintains this attitude of unity at any price, though he may have failed to live up to it. Opposing forces are often great. He may suffer from silent expectations that are not being met, or guilt that he is not pulling his own weight in unity with another or others. His spine gives in.

We see Ruta in action in the defense forces, where success depends on team work, and smaller teams are employed as arms of a larger body, all pulling together for success. The encouragement of team consciousness, the need to pull your weight in defense of your country or to support your leaders, can often bring its own grief aspects, when it is brought home to the

Ruta person that the individual counts, as well. Theodore Roosevelt, a great Ruta who had encouraged his sons to enter the Army during World War I, was greatly guilty when his youngest son, Quentin, was killed: 'To know that one has inspired a boy to conduct which has resulted in his death, gives one to think long and hard about one's previously held beliefs about life.'

As it is in the military, so in business, and we see Ruta people at the top of large corporations and small family concerns. The belief in strength in numbers causes the Ruta-minded to buy up, take over and absorb, consolidate, amalgamate, combine forces and become corporate giants. They can feel quite cold and calculating about business, because they expect others to be strong or pay the price of weakness by losing their market unless they unite. It is the old concept of the survival of the fittest, the law of the jungle. They are not driven by the Hypericum desire to prove themselves or to win at any price, but simply by the pursuit of strength and consolidation.

Great corporations have been built by Ruta people. Consider, particularly, the great iron and steel company, BHP, losing its power in Australia because world consciousness is shifting away from needing the might and weight of pure steel. Size is no longer an indicator of strength since light-weight materials have been discovered that have greater strength combined with flexibility. Steel still has its place, but it is no longer the backbone of Australia's trading strength. Our steel industry has gone, we now sell the iron ore to China who is the world's biggest user now of steel.And this is indicative of Western world changes that have appeared to make the Ruta beliefs less and less useful as we have moved out of the industrial age and into the age of technology.

In all these situations, Ruta-type injuries and disease conditions can occur. We noticed early in our research work with chiropractic patients that the Ruta injuries often came from lifting very heavy objects which required a strong spine, usually with a twisting or turning action - shovelling, loading and unloading of trucks, shifting of heavy loads from one bench to another or from shelves to benchtop.

The injury occurs when the integrity of the ligaments is not equal to the power of the muscles. Extreme demand on the muscles causes the strong action of muscles-pulling-on-bones to override the opposite holding-bones-together action of the ligaments, with resultant strain causing tearing, to a greater or lesser degree, of the discs, ligamentous tissue, cartilage and periosteum. Compare this with Ledum, the remedy of choice when, in apparently similar accidents to Ruta, it is the tendons of the muscles that give way. Ruta has strong muscles and the connective tissues of the joints give way.

Anywhere in the body structure, joint integrity can be impaired by the repeated instruction that 'I must be strong', an instruction to the muscles. Too much muscular (pulling) strength leaves the ligaments without the corresponding strength to hold the body together. Muscles are strengthened up at the expense of the ligaments, cartilages and discs. The use of strength causes bones to be pulled out of their natural alignment, ligaments not being powerful enough to maintain joint integrity against undue muscle force. It amazes Ruta, who expects absolute strength.

The grief-guilt of loss of group unity and cohesion, combined with the belief that there is no strength without cohesion, leads to a great feeling of weakness that allows the most severe spinal injuries to occur. The 4th and 5th lumbar vertebrae are particularly at risk, and the discs here can be damaged severely during lifting and turning actions, which rotate the vertebrae beyond the point from which they can regain their natural position by the usual controlling tension in the ligaments, once the pull is released. The resultant 'slipped disc' is instantly felt as sciatic pain shooting from the spine into the leg, on whichever side the body is strongest in muscle. Similar problems can result from oblique or side-on landings from falling from a height.

In time, additional to the pain and inconvenience of spinal vertebral displacement, functional disturbances set in as a result of diminished nerve supply from the spine to the organs. These can be severe, leading to bowel cancer, for without adequate nerve energy cells cannot replicate properly.

My first use of Ruta MM for a bowel cancer patient occurred back in 1991. She was a woman in her sixties, always strong and healthy through life, and could hardly believe she had a cancer problem. She had been operated on and simply wanted me to ensure that her body was cleared of any risk of a relapse. I gave the Ruta in megapotencies several times, and the colon problem never returned, and she died in her eighties. (She used to tell others, 'You go and see Jill Turland, she won't let you die of bowel cancer.' Some came, including the woman described in Hydrastis.)

The reduced nerve supply from the spine also affects all the internal connective tissues. Pelvic ligaments weaken, causing bowel or anal prolapse. Ruta is renowned as a remedy for anal prolapse after the muscular effort and strain of childbirth, but it can occur from lifting, crouching or bending as you do when gardening.

Problems of the lower spine begin to reflex into the neck, causing poor nerve supply to the eyes, which are undermined by strain and overuse, causing myopia and slow accommodation to set in. In the Ruta type of personality, such eye problems may need to be treated with lumbar spine adjustments, as this may be the primary area, the source of the problem. The use of Ruta in high or megapotencies will often do the adjusting of both upper and lower spine.

Ruta's benefit to vision has always been noteworthy, and I found some great results personally, as well as for patients, in some kinds of visual problems. Eyestrain from doing too much close work - computer work or fine sewing, extensive reading, or work that requires microscopic detail and accuracy - is always benefited in the Ruta person.

I had been treating one woman for macular degeneration, a retina problem that was causing distortion of straight lines, giving a wavy effect to the printed word. She had hurt her back in 1991, four years before it came on, but had also fallen down some stairs as a child, running late for school. She had had eye troubles since childhood, frowned a lot, and her vision was worse for study and concentration or sewing, and for shifting the view from one page to another and back, or from the sewing to the TV, changing the focal length. She had benefits from several remedies and from a short period of laser treatment. In 1996, problems began to develop with a few workers at their factory, resenting her part in running *her* firm, with a lot of one-upmanship going on. She was losing enthusiasm for the business, with all the dissention.

I began with Ruta 200 in December '96 and progressed later up to M and 10M, and the eyes and back began to improve. At the end of '97 she hurt her back again, and the eyes were lapsing in benefit, so I used 50M. The eyes improved and did not give her as much trouble until prolonged bookwork at the end of the financial year in 1999 caused severe eyestrain again, and glare sensitivity. I gave Nat Mur 50M at this point.

In 2001, the diagnosis of the visual problem had changed to 'retinosa pigmentosa,' the symptoms being the same rippling effect distorting the vision owing to 'tiny holes in the retina', she was told. At this point, she could not drive the car and eye work was causing severe headaches. This 'new' problem had come on two months before coming back to me - that bookwork time of year again. She commented again that she was disheartened by failure of workers to pull their weight, and even her husband gave her no support (he also being affected by the workers). This time, I gave Ruta MM.

After this, she was able to use the computer without getting a headache, and her eyes were less strained and clarity better. She felt vastly better in herself, was no longer tired and grumpy and could work all day without exhaustion.

Ruta 10MM a month later, saw her back driving the car, and she had developed a temporary return of the old back symptoms, the old injury. Great sign! No treatment since.

Researchers recently discovered that bovine tracheal cartilage could be used to shrink the blood vessels supplying cancer cells with their nutrients. Cartilage is precisely the realm of Ruta. Ruta strengthens and tones ligament and cartilage tissue and all the connective tissues including blood vessel walls. It seems to cause tumour cells and giant platelets to resume normal growth rates. This is worth considering for people suffering from cancers and some blood disorders.

I believe there is still much to be discovered about the clinical range of Ruta complaints. Prescribing along the lines already known will lead to extended realizations that other practitioners will be able to contribute.

Where Ruta thinking can be cut-throat and materialistic, there is a positive side that is going to come to the fore more and more as time goes on. Give Ruta to those who need it and not only do their physical problems resolve, but they begin to bring out their skills in working and drawing others together for a common good. Their natural leadership, lapsed through disheartenment in the face of separatist attitudes, comes to the fore again. This is a profound remedy for leading us forward into the new millennium, to pull together for planetary, socio-economic and personal healing.

Ruta in megapotencies gives strength to Ruta personalities to encourage and use group power in ways that contribute to the healing and restoration of the ecology and the environment, the purifying of water and air and the fairer distribution of resources for the benefit of all. Megapotency Ruta changes the focus from the practical materialist to the practical idealist, so that mighty community energy is deployed without expectation of monetary reward.

Already, for example, in many parts of Australia, volunteer LandCare groups are putting their backs into regular community working bees to collect rubbish and tidy up wastelands, replant the eroded banks of waterways, plant desalinising shrubs and trees that restore salt-saturated lands to usefulness, eliminate introduced plants that have become a threat to the native flora and a wide range of related activities. Positive Ruta people do not wait for the elusive 'they' to do what needs to be done, they get stuck into it and show others how great the satisfaction is from a job well done by all pulling together. It is a matter of survival, and Ruta knows it.

CHAPTER 15

To thine own Self be true, and it must follow, as the night the day, thou canst
not then be false to any man.
- William Shakespeare, 'Hamlet.' (Polonius' advice to his son, Laertes)

STAPHISAGRIA - 'I KNOW HOW THINGS SHOULD BE'

Staphisagria (delphinium staphisagria, *Stavesacre*, N.O. Ranunculaceae), according to Mrs Grieve, is indigenous to Asia Minor and Southern Europe, and was well-known to the Greeks and the Romans. Dioscorides mentions it, and Pliny describes its use as a parasiticide. It was extensively employed throughout the Middle Ages, the dried, ripe seeds being used. They are extremely poisonous and were only used externally to kill lice and nits and to remove itch. The powdered seeds are violently emetic and cathartic and paralyse the motor nerves like curare. The alkaloid delphinine resembles aconite and conium in causing slowness of pulse and respiration, paralysis of the spinal cord and death from asphyxia. By depressing the action of the spinal cord it arrests the convulsions caused by strychnine (a component of Ignatia).

The name of this genus, delphinium, was given because the buds were said to resemble a dolphin. It strikes me as interesting that this remedy is arguably the most widely needed world-wide at a time when dolphin consciousness is at its height. Dolphin lovers, pay attention to this remedy!

Staphisagria is not used by modern herbalists. However, after they saw homeopathic doctors using it with success, it found some favour with American doctors in the nineteenth century. They prescribed the toxic tincture in doses from five to fifteen drops, for many of the same conditions the homeopaths were treating, using potencies to eliminate the toxicity. Finley Ellingwood describes it as a remedy for hysteria, mental depression and hypochondriasis, melancholia, despondency and accompanying outbursts of passion. He lists in its physical sphere of influence, conditions of prostatic disease, prostatorrhea, spermatorrhea, gleet; irritation of the prostate gland, testicles and vesiculae seminales, overcoming impotence and increasing sexual power. It arrests excessive prostatic discharge and mucopurulent discharges from the urethra, and dysuria with feeble expulsion of urine. It soothes the nervous excitement accompanying these genito-urinary disorders 'especially (impotence) occurring in men who have been excessive and dissipated in their habits, appearing usually about the age of forty five.' Bladder prolapse in men and women, uterine disorders, facial and cervical neuralgia, eye conditions of amaurosis, ophthalmia, floating black spots were also treated with this tincture, as well as night sweats.

STAPHISAGRIA IN HOMEOPATHY

In homeopathy the use of Staphisagria has been found to have even greater scope. In addition to the eclectic uses, homeopathic provings revealed that in potency, this remedy could be safely used for a very wide range of conditions, but particularly those resulting from fits of anger, 'justifiable ill-humour over what has happened or has been done by oneself; weeping and dejected over the supposed ill consequences of it. Hypochondria and hysteria after unmerited insults (or sexual excesses), with complaints of flatulence' (Clarke). Also, 'Staphisagria is a remedy for anger and the effects of anger, especially if the indignation cannot have its natural expression. "Was insulted; being too dignified to fight, swallowed his wrath, and went home sick, trembling and exhausted."'

Clarke lists the following conditions as being suitable for the consideration of this remedy:

Clinical.- Adenoids. *Anger, fits of.* Anus, itching of. Backache. Bashfulness. Blepharitis. Bones, diseases of. Cauliflower excrescences. Chalazion (a pea-sized tumour in the eyelid). Condylomata (warts). Cough. Cysts. Dentition. Dysentery. Dysparunia (difficulty or pain in coitus); in newly married women. Eczema. *Eyes, tumours on.* Fistula dentalis. Gastralgia. Glands, affections of. Hip-joint disease. Hypochondriasis. Impotency. Iritis; syphilitic. Jaw-joint, easy dislocation of. Lumbar abscess. Mania. Masturbation, effects of. *Neuralgia.* Night-sweats. Nymphomania. Ovaries, affections of. *Pediculosis (lice). Perspiration, offensive.* Pregnancy, nausea of. *Prostate, affections of.* Psoas abscess. Ranula (a cystic tumour on the underside of the tongue or the floor of the mouth). Rheumatism. Sciatica. Scurvy. Sea-sickness. Seborrhoea. *Self-abuse.* Spermatic cords, affections of. *Spermatorrhoea.* Steatoma (fatty tumour or sebacious cyst). Stiff neck. *Styes.* Swallowing, constant while talking. *Teeth, caries of.* Testicles, affections of. Tibiae, pains in. Tobacco, effect of. Toenail, ingrowing. Tonsillitis. *Toothache.* Tumours; tarsal (glands in eyelids). Voice, nasal; hoarse. Warts.

To this I can add, in the light of experience, many common complaints of our times, particularly PAIN arising from bodily indignation after things done to it in the way of procedures, drugs, surgery, dental and orthodontic work, manual therapies, some accidents; social or job-related offenses of injustice; assaults, rape and many more: ADD-ADHD. Allergies. Arthritis. Chronic Fatigue syndrome. Endocrine gland hypofunctions, all glands. Homosexuality. Hypertension. Osteoporosis. Rapism.

Snoring. Systemic yeast infections. Tumours, of any endocrine gland. Uterus, complaints of.

However, Clarke stresses in the preface of this work[53], 'Homœopathy is from first to last an art of individualising. We have to individualise patients, and individualise remedies. However convenient it is to think of remedies in connection with the diseases in the treatment of which they are most frequently called for, it must never be forgotten that this is a convenience and nothing more. To allow our conception of our remedies to be limited by any list of nosological terms is to accept again the mental fetters of old-school therapeutics. To understand and utilise our remedies to the fullest extent, we must know them as powers ready to serve us in any case, no matter what the name of the disease may be, when the indications for them come to the front.' In order to recognise the essential indications for Staphisagria it is necessary to know the personality picture of the person who needs it.

STAPHISAGRIA IN MEGAPOTENCY

The one characteristic of the Staphisagria person that has done most to change the world, for better and for worse, is the belief in Justice as an essential factor of community stability. Associated with this idea, throughout time, has been a Christian belief in Divine Retribution and Judgement Day based on the ancient Jewish Scales of Justice belief (Mene mene tekel upharsin - 'you have been weighed in the balance and found wanting'). Jesus tried to get people to ease up on this belief because of its rigidity and lack of tolerance or forgiveness ('Let he who is without guilt throw the first stone', 'Judge not, lest you be judged') but the pattern is just as widespread now as ever it was.

It is an erroneous belief that any person has enough knowledge of another to be able to make an accurate assessment, a judgement of that person in terms of what he has done, said or thought. Judgement also implies a right and a wrong way of being and doing. Right for whom? Wrong by whose standard?

Mine? What is right for me may not necessarily be right for my brother or for you. Yours? How can you know what is right for me, in my best interests? Do you know my past, my intentions, my dreams, the amount of my learnings from my experiences? You are just as limited in your perspective of me as I am of you, and you would not have me sit in judgment over your life, would you?

God's? No way. We are all blinkered, as humans, and have little knowledge of the broader workings of the universe in these terms. That is, until we look within and begin to listen to the voice of the inner god, which tells us that all is one, all people are united in a balanced, harmonious oneness that we have forgotten, and judgment is yet another manifestation of the alienation resulting from that forgetting.

275

Alongside the belief in judgement came the development of the judiciary, and a system of laws became necessary to enforce a code of living that was believed to be Right, by punishing those who were seen to be Wrong. Judgement and Law somehow became the tools for creating true justice, which, as I have shown, does not even exist in human capability. In reality, they are only the tools for gaining and keeping power over other humans.

Ho, hum. What a mess we have made of this world, because of this Man-trying-to-be-God scenario.

From the perspective of the Staphisagria person, there is certainly a Right way to be and a Right way to live, and he/she knows exactly what it is, lives by it and expects everyone else to do the same. Anyone who wants to march to a different drummer is automatically Wrong. Righteousness and self-righteous justification is the way of their life.

For this reason, when the Staphisagrian British first came to Australia, as they had done earlier in America and Ireland, the natives, who had a completely different, intuitive, way of running their lives and their societies, were immediately branded Wrong, lesser, inferior, ignorant of the Right way to be. Many lives were destroyed and tribes made extinct as a result of this belief.

Britain brought its class system with it to Australia. The native population could only be placed at the bottom of the ladder, and were relegated to a level even below the Irish, who, because of their Hypericum impulsiveness and lack of Staphisagria/Ledum discipline, could only be seen as worthless trouble, all the more so because most of them were convicts.

Later in Australia's 'civilisation', over a period of many decades in the twentieth century, that century that was the blackest in all history, aboriginal children were taken from their families and put into homes and institutions where they would be taught the Right things, and have all those Wrong ideas knocked out of them. Most of them never saw their parents again. As a result of genocide and the segregation and ill-treatment of the black population, we now, still, have a major 'them against us' problem both in the country and in the cities, which, as I have described in the Hydrastis chapter, needs a vast amount of healing. Use plenty of Ignatia, Ledum, Hypericum, Hydrastis, Staphisagria, Nat Mur and nowadays, even Conium, for these people.

Which brings me to the opposite side of Staphisagria, the helpless victim of injustice. There are just as many victims as there are people who perpetrate injustices against others. They are at opposing poles of the same belief. As long as we have a lack of allowing, a lack of tolerance and respect for the differences of each other, we will have the Staphisagria scenario replayed over and over again, as it has for thousands of years. It stands as a specific thought frequency, and those whose thoughts and beliefs are set to that frequency will continue to create their lives according to the Staphisagria patterns. Giving the remedy in megapotency is the fastest and surest way to lift people out of such a treadmill.

You can tell when people are locked into this Right versus Wrong belief by the way they speak. They get very hot under the collar over any sign of injustice, telling you how there should be a law against it, 'they' should not do such a thing, it is not right, it is not fair. The word 'should' comes into every sentence - I should, I shouldn't have, you should ... always according to how it would have been 'best'. There is, for most of them, a great desire to do the best thing, the right thing, whether it is for themselves, for the community, for the environment, for the poor, the suffering, the underprivileged, the ignorant, the nation or the world in general.

I am not saying that this is inherently Wrong; it simply is, as a manifestation of Staphisagria's inability to allow people to be who they are and where they are, do what they want or feel they must, think the way they think, and have the opportunity to learn from their own situations in life, which are, after all, their own creations.

Staphisagria leads a well-controlled, disciplined life, on the straight and narrow path, down the midline of life. He is not usually an extremist or a rebel, unless driven through extreme circumstances to take a firm stand, usually for justice. Many of the world's most highly evolved, reliable, trustworthy, admirable people are Staphisagria types, including the Dalai Lama. They all have high standards of ethics and morality, and often hold prominent positions of authority which they handle very creditably, probably creating more beneficial change in society than any other type, once they rise out of the crippling conformity imposed upon them in youth. They make fine parents and have dutiful children.

The person needing Staphisagria is often a sweet-natured, gentle person who wants a fair go for everyone and frequently puts himself last in order not to inconvenience anyone. He never seeks the frontline place or centre stage unless he knows he has earned it and is the best person for that position. On occasion, life becomes just too unfair, and she may become a little teary, crying out of frustration and the injustice of it all (for self or for others). (Do not confuse this with the person who cries tears of self-pity, from missing out on attention, not given enough importance - this person needs Pulsatilla.)

In times of bereavement, there may be a sense of remorse over love left unexpressed, of injustice over the suffering and the death or over the distribution of the estate, and this person may need Staphisagria as well as Ignatia, particularly when he is unable to articulate the feelings. 'The bitterest tears shed over graves are for words left unsaid and deeds left undone,' said Harriet Beecher Stowe.

Many Staphisagrians will have an English, Scottish or European background, or be of aristocratic lineage, where the social emphasis has been on withholding emotions and keeping a calm, clear, sound mind in a healthy body. These countries are areas of the highest historical distribution of gonorrhoea, and also of widespread smallpox vaccination - both of which cause genetic patterns of the Staphisagria or suppressive type, setting up a framework of rigidity in mind and body.

A simple illustration of this rigidity comes with the attitudes of many educated Staphisagrian types, who get very indignant at the new trends in spelling and language. They want these to remain 'as they should be' (i.e., as they were taught in their formative years), and desire that children today should be taught and forced to learn the rules of English expression.

While I am also a great lover of the English language with which I grew up, I have to remember that my form of English is one that has only existed for the last century or so, and that the language, particularly the written language, has been very fluid and flexible throughout time. When we look at documents written five or six hundred years ago, we can hardly understand them, so many words have gone out of usage now, and spelling has changed so much. This degree of change is not acceptable to many Staphisagria people, who believe they know the correct rules for written language and everyone should apply them.

They are disciplined with money, sometimes to the Ledum point of being parsimonious, not generous in parting with their hard-earned wealth - 'mine by right,' they think, and they make every cent count, and expect others to do so, too.

There is not the big sympathy for the less well off that Hypericum has, but a desire to see all brought to an elevated position of well-being through justice and fairness, equal opportunity and equal rights, but tempered with deserving, earning those rights. In this way, a great many Staphisagrian people are amongst the world's best campaigners for better conditions, or for peace; a great many also will put themselves behind military might or police departments in order to enforce their ideals upon others, 'for the betterment of all'.

You will also find Staphisagrian people amongst terrorists, political agitators, guerrillas, spy rings and organised crime, but not as many as need Hypericum, Ledum and Hydrastis, as Staphisagria usually prefers to get his results from within the 'peaceful law and order' framework of his society. He is not a backstabber, and does not seek vengeance, more justice and fairness.

On the other hand, many Staphisagria people feel helpless to do anything about an unjust situation. They may suffer indignities or injustices, or they may be upset on behalf of others - either way, they feel they are just a lone voice in the wilderness, no-one will take any notice of them, there's nothing can be done. So they remain silent, helpless, while often, the offending event is perpetuated.

This kind of helplessness is felt by those who are harshly treated by parents, punished for being 'naughty' (i.e. not conforming to the rules, which often make no sense to an inquisitive, experiential child), unjustly treated in a marriage, victims of rape or incest, of bullying, teasing or unfair accusations.

Inner rage builds up but the anger and indignation must not be expressed for fear of further blame or punishment, of creating another opportunity for unjustified anger or harsh words. This reinforces the helplessness feeling. From not acting in a way that might upset, they shift to not doing anything at all. All this achieves is to become despised for their weakness, their gutless inability to put up a fight. If they are spineless enough, Silica may also be needed.

The fear of making others angry towards them creates a desire for peace at any price. A great number of Staphisagria people are peaceful, peace-loving, gentle, kind, sweet, generous, helpful, fair and even tolerant. These are the ones we all know and think of as the nicest people you could ever wish to know. They really hate dissention and argument. They never tell you what they really think, it would not be 'nice', it never does to offend anyone (as if speaking your truth is necessarily offensive!), and nothing is gained (their training tells them) from creating a disharmony. Such people seem to be very well balanced and in good command of themselves and their lives, but I can tell you they suffer Staphisagria problems as surely as do the noisy ones. They much prefer to tell you what they think you want to hear (and they are always sure they know what you want to hear), so you will get white lies and hypocrisy rather than honesty, and the suppression of feelings required to live like this creates just as much muscle tension and resultant internal disorders as the more aggressive and militant ones get.

And who was it said, 'All it needs for evil to triumph is for good men to do nothing'? The inability to stand up for what you believe in is the reason that those who have no such helplessness, and also no good community conscience, gain control over how the land is being run.

A respect for law and order and the establishment brings a respect for orthodoxy and a determination to obey the law and live by the customs, rules and regulations set up by society and government. For this reason, many Staphisagria people find it very hard to come to terms with the fact that the doctors they have worshipped for centuries are not helping them. They have been led to believe that all that was worth knowing has been taught the doctors in the halls of learning, and if it was not taught it cannot be worth knowing. Doctors are taught this, too.

Nothing could be further from the truth, as we have already seen. These are people who blindly follow the medical system despite much suffering and pain, fearful of offending the god in case he refuses to bestow his favour upon them in some future hour of need. They would rather die at the doctor's hands than stand up for themselves against the one in the authority seat.

You can see that this state of affairs can only arise out of the unfortunate fact that these people have suppressed their self-preservation instincts along with their intuition and their love of truth. If you have a 'rest-of-your-life' belief, told that you will never be free of the condition you have developed, take Staphisagria 10MM at intervals of two or three months, and you will find yourself rising free of the helplessness and hopelessness that medical drug-pushers like you to have, and you will disprove their propaganda.

Sexual innuendo is prevalent in the Staphisagria brand of humour, and those who would be offended by the 'not-nice'-ness still titter and smirk over it. Staphisagria people have, because of their distorted pituitary functions, a high degree of sexuality about which they feel embarrassed and guilty, a common feature of 'suppressive' types. In conjunction with this is the 'not-nice'-ness guilt over eliminatory organs and their functions - unmentionable except in jokes, cartoons and situation comedies. It is only embarrassment, an unnecessary guilt/fear if ever there was one, that makes such things funny. Much of the world's humour for several centuries has reflected sexuality guilt.

I find it a sure indicator for Staphisagria when I hear people complaining indignantly that they are really 'pissed off' with someone or something. It comes from the Staphisagria tendency to bladder weakness!

Lavatory jokes are also the precinct of Hydrastis, the great bowel remedy. 'Dirty' minds are guilty minds, and Hydrastis cleans up the guilt filth. Hydrastis jokes, like a lot of Hydrastis language, are full of references to 'bums', 'arses' and especially to 'shit.'

The sexuality of Staphisagria is specifically characteristic of the whole remedy. The mind dwells on sex a lot, but because of the training, this is believed to be unacceptable, so all too often, it is suppressed, not a hint gets out to others; suppression of sexual expression becomes physical - all too many Staphisagrian people, not wishing to offend, or to be embarrassed themselves, or to break the taboos of society regarding availability, avoid getting into close relationships, instead, developing a high degree of frustration. Sooner or later, an explosion occurs. All that pent-up energy has to get out, eventually.

Staphisagria is the primary remedy for promiscuity, for sexual harassment, for prostitution, for rape, even pack rape, for incest, for paedophilia (which means 'love of children' - where do they get the idea that sexual obsession and abuse can be termed 'love'?), and for needing all the extraordinary paraphernalia and practices people get up to in sexual expression. Staphisagria lifts the mind and body out of the imprisonment of sex and into a greater heart feeling, so that love can be the main driving energy towards a far more spiritually rewarding sexual experience, and there is no need for violence or offense to anyone. Many homosexuals need Staphisagria for their hormonal imbalance, too, relating to their suppression of emotions, living according to society rather than to their truth, and also, I believe, because of an inherent pituitary suppression from the start of life, which may have resulted from a forceps birth distorting the cranium, or some other offense at birth, or from a Staphisagria condition in the mother being passed on to the foetus.

Frustration and impatience over imperfection dissolve, once you get Staphisagria, into an allowing that the inner tutor is always in charge, and all is moving in accord. Staphisagria brings trust and knowingness that any frustrating hindrance is purposeful, allowing you time to learn, do or experience something important that could not otherwise have happened if the stall in proceedings had not occurred.

Clenching the jaw to hold words in causes tension in the facial muscles involved, which often has the effect of retracting the jaw to a point of under-shot (the 'chinless wonders' of the 19th century British kings and aristocracy) or if unilateral, of pulling the jaw laterally so that the horizontal alignment is still parallel between upper and lower jaws but the central point of the mandible has shifted noticeably to one side. The upper and lower central incisors do not align perfectly.

Often the eyebrows are perpetually raised in an expression of 'Where's the justice in this? or 'I don't understand how this can be happening', 'What have I done to deserve this?' - or, judgementally, 'How could you behave this way?' Even newborn babies can exhibit this expression - 'What have I come to, how could you treat me like this? What have I done, to deserve this?'

Often the forehead has horizontal creases or parallel lines, usually four or more - related to raising his eyebrows so often. The muscles involved in raising eyebrows become permanently in tension as time goes on.

Often the upper lip has vertical creases, lots of them, from continually pursing it in judgement over one thing or another - the 'tut-tut' expression.

The sternocleidomastoid muscles of the front of the neck often stand out in tension, the result of clenching the jaw. There will be pain and tenderness on palpation of any of the attachments of these muscles, at the mastoid, sternal or clavicular ends.

Staphisagria helps after all kinds of dental work by releasing the bodily indignation that sets in over having procedures done while in a position of powerlessness, and over having to hold the mouth open for long periods, straining the jaw joints. But if your face is not indicating a Staphisagria mind-set, you will not need it.

To be technical, suppression of anger, frustration and indignation has a twofold effect on the head - firstly, by generating heat in the cerebral cortex which restricts the release of pituitary hormones, thus disturbing the function of glands throughout the endocrine system; secondly, repeated and prolonged clenching of the jaw causes undue tension in the muscles of the neck and head, which will perpetuate the pituitary imbalance already begun: the sphenoid bone becomes fixed, locked by tension in the tendons attached to it, so that it is unable to perform its normal microscopic movements; tension flows on to the diaphragm sellae which in turn cramps the flow of nerve and blood to the pituitary, with sometimes disastrous results flowing on to the rest of the endocrine functions.

Muscles involved in this process include all the muscles of the face, the sternocleidomastoids, epicranius frontalis and occipitalis, the medial and lateral pterygoids, the splenius capitis, levator scapulae and the upper trapezius. All of these muscles store the powerful, unreleased energy of pent-up rage, anger and indignation and the seething simmering of frustration, arising not only from offensive words but also from bodily indignation felt at things done to it, such as painful, violent adjustments or massage, dental and orthodontic work, surgery, injections and other procedures, and drug effects; such indignation sometimes being expressed as allergy reactions.

The belief that anger and offenses must be swallowed or ignored in order to keep the peace, avoid offense, avoid unpopularity or simply because 'nice people do not get angry' causes the angry one to bite back his words, containing the energy of the emotion in the jaw and facial muscles.

When all these muscles begin to become chronically tense, they exert pull on the cranial bones, including the sphenoid bone, altering the shape of your skull, restricting action and movement at the cranial sutures, and locking up the various processes that take place in normal health within the head structure. (Refer to Chapter 2.)

By releasing these emotional tensions out of the facial and cranial muscles, the skull's bones are enabled to return to their normal positions and microscopic movement. Staphisagria benefits the posterior pituitary's nerve connection with the hypothalamus, and the anterior pituitary's blood vessel connection with the hypothalamus. Hormones such as anti-diuretic hormone sourced from the hypothalamus are assisted by Staphisagria. The hypothalamus is responsible for regulating body temperature, appetite, metabolic rate, water balance within the body, sleep patterns and your response to stress, and all of these are influenced for the better by Staphisagria (and Ignatia).

Diabetes insipidus could also be helped. Dwarfism and acromegaly have benefited. Endorphin production is enhanced, hence Staphisagria's great reputation for pain relief.

Its particular action is on the pituitary hormones: growth hormone or somatotropin (GH), prolactin (PRL), thyroid stimulating hormone (TSH), follicle stimulating hormone (FSH), luteinising hormone (LH), adreno-corticotropic hormone (ACTH) and melanocyte stimulating hormone (MSH). Through enhancing these hormones a vast number of conditions can be dealt with.

One twelve-year-old girl, stunted in growth by congenital ACTH irregularity for which she was, all her life, on cortisone, gained five centimetres in height within two months of taking Staphisagria MM, and her general health improved immeasurably. She continued to grow normally into adulthood, against the expectations of her paediatrician, whose textbooks tell him such children are lucky to live to adulthood. She is now a mother and in very good health. Thanks to the use of Staphisagria, her adrenal cortex function is close to normal, despite her former genetic chromosome fault in the pituitary.

By using Staphisagria to reduce the patient's anger and sense of injustice, messages sent by the hypothalamus to the pituitary to initiate action that never eventuates (aggression) are reduced. Conditions caused by storing unused action hormones in the body include hypertension, coronary artery disease and stroke.

All endocrines are affected by pituitary compromise, and Staphisagria assists every endocrine gland. One of the big issues receiving publicity in recent years is that of osteoporosis. Much misinformation is being promoted in the media regarding the need to drink more milk and take calcium supplements to keep up one's calcium levels - in addition, of course, to taking your HRT estrogen supplement. The truth is, however, that for most people, low calcium intake is not the issue, so much as what is happening to the calcium within the body.

Osteoporosis arises from failure of the parathyroids to regulate the activity of calcium in the bloodstream. Under the leadership of the pituitary gland, the parathyroids send instructions, via the hormone parathormone, to move the calcium from bone to muscle and back to bone all day and night, depending on messages sent from the sympathetic nervous system. Muscle activity draws calcium out of the bones to be used by the muscles, and in rest, this calcium is then freed up to move back into the bones.

When something happens to diminish the supply of energy to the parathyroids from the pituitary, the messages to the calcium molecules become enfeebled. Calcium heading back into bone fails to reach its destination, sometimes remaining in muscle tissue, causing polymyalgia, sometimes being deposited in other parts of the body, such as arterial walls, causing atherosclerosis and arteriosclerosis, as the blood seeks to off-load its excess. Meanwhile, the bones remain depleted and osteoporosis sets in. In some cases, the calcium will reach the bone but somehow, be unable to penetrate the periosteum, so that spurs of calcium are built up in the tendon attachments.

Another aspect of calcium transport failure is the Chronic Fatigue problem, where any attempt to exercise is met with increasing levels of pain and weakness. Normally, exercise builds strength in muscles. When you have a pituitary under-function, the parathyroids fail to draw enough calcium out of the bones for muscle usage. Almost every sufferer of Chronic Fatigue who has come to my office has benefited from Staphisagria, usually dramatically.

There has been much promotion of exercise as a preventive of osteoporosis. I cannot endorse this, particularly for elderly people, as exercise pulls calcium out of the bones, and if the pituitary and parathyroids are not functioning well, as is frequently the case, it fails to go back into the bones at night.

You can forget the menopause/oestrogen tie-up with osteoporosis - men get osteoporosis too, and the only real link is that oestrogen and calcium movement depend on good pituitary function keeping the parathyroids going well and oestrogen manufacture in order. Taking extra calcium is not going to get it going to the right places; taking HRT is not always successful, particularly if you are male. Staphisagria enables the body to adjust to reduced ovarian oestrogen smoothly, regulates oestrogen in males and females, regulates calcium activity in males and females and thereby eliminates spurs, strengthens bones and heals some forms of arthritis.

A very tiny elderly lady consulted me in 1994 because of frequent fracturing of bones. She had loss of disc height at the L5-S1 disc, with end-plate compression fractures at L4 and possibly L3 and L2 vertebrae, and a 5mm posterior slip of L1 on L2. X-rays also showed calcification of the aorta and iliac vessels, the right carotid artery and the carotid bulb. There was degeneration of the lower cervical facets; signs of fractures at T10-12, with some scoliosis in the upper lumbars and mid thoracics, all to the right.

Her symptoms were: eyebrows permanently raised; cannot walk far, the legs get painful and go to jelly; even standing for ten minutes leads to pain across the lower ribcage spine, both sides, better sitting again or leaning on a walking stick. She had had a fractured hip ten years before, when a big man collided with her in the city and lifted her off her feet, so that she landed heavily.

Staphisagria CM gave her a short period of relief from pain, but it returned. Next visit, I gave her Staphisagria MM and Symphytum MM (history of breaks), and kept her on Staphisagria 12C twice a day. At the next visit, her comment was, 'feeling a lot better altogether. Energy is better, back is not too bad.' She did well, but failed to keep in touch with me. A year later, after a trip to Sydney by coach, she carried her light suitcase up her stairs, holding the bannister with the other hand, when she felt her back go suddenly, in the kidney area. She had forgotten she had still some Staphisagria 12 left, and the pain eased off when she started to take them again. I gave Staphisagria 10M and advised to continue with some more 12C, giving her Symphytum 30 three times a day for the fracture. Two weeks later, she rang to say, 'Very much better, thank you!'

While Symphytum knits the bone-breaks, Staphisagria, by kicking-in the parathyroids, draws the calcium back from the blood vessel walls, into circulation and back into the bones.

Spurs on the heels are a common problem in our clinic, and while I have had success with a few remedies, Staphisagria is the one of choice usually. Bryan has his own way of treating them. One woman we both visited once in 1994 had spurs to both heels, the left being particularly painful on getting out of bed in the morning, it was hard to put her weight on that foot. It also played up in the evenings, with a pulling, drawing sensation, with cramping in the calf. Six months, she'd had the problem. Three cortisone injections two months earlier had been no help. An operation to bad varicose veins had been badly performed on the right leg, some years ago. Bryan found the medial aspect of the calcaneal tendon too tight, and advised her to roll her foot over a glass Coke bottle to massage the heel. To get the calcium out of the tendon and back into circulation, I gave her Staphisagria MM. We heard no more until she met us in a shopping mall 18 months later. 'You don't remember me, do you, but I remember you. You fixed my foot! I did the exercise and took the pills and the spurs went away rapidly. I was very impressed, and have had no further trouble.'

Osteophytes on the spinal bones fall into the same category as spurs. A man of 45 came in December 1998 for some help with his neck, which had been giving him some trouble for five weeks, and chiropractic was not getting it fixed. Bryan had suggested X-rays and a CT scan and when he did so and Bryan saw the situation, he realized it was not just a manual problem. He had osteophytes at C5, C6 and C7, causing narrowing of the intervertebral foramina and C5-6 disc. This compressed disc was bulging towards the left C6-7 foramen and into the thecal sac, contacting the spinal cord and causing severe pain down the left arm.

He had been to his insurance company doctor that day and was angry with him for being told nothing. (Yet how could the guy tell him what he did not know?) He was very tense in the neck, and his jaws were clenched and immobile as he spoke to me. Neck movement was restricted, naturally. I gave Staphisagria MM. He rang Bryan the next morning, to ask, 'Bryan, is this possible? Could those two little pills I took last night have fixed this neck pain I've had for five weeks?' Bryan just said, 'Well, I suggested you see Jill a while ago. Of course, it is possible.' I saw him ten days later. He was still amazed at the immediate benefit, had had a little pain in the left knee (old injury) and was going back to work the next day. 'I feel like having a game of golf,' he said. He has used the remedy a couple of times since, with continuing benefit.

Thyroid tumours and thyroxine output are greatly benefited. In cases of thyroid tumours, I have seen Staphisagria MM reduce one tumour of two years standing to nothing within ten days; others have taken a matter of months.

In the rapid case, symptoms had begun three or more years prior, as tiredness, with aching all over on waking (very common Staphisagria symptoms). A multi-nodular tumour had been found, and her pituitary was taking on the load of thyroid hormone functions. She had developed heavy periods, and had been on thyroxine for three years when I saw her. This lady was a nurse and had had enough contact with medical methods not to want orthodox treatment for the growth. Lately, she had been getting pressure feelings in the throat, felt claustrophobic and was conscious of pressure from her car's safety belt. She had also begun putting on weight.

Where had all this begun? She had never been on The Pill, had never smoked or taken other drugs, since childhood, when she had had 'lots and lots of antibiotics for chest problems, including pneumonia.' As a result, she had developed glandular fever at age 18.

She had also had operations to her knees - from age 5, they would dislocate easily, and operations were done to change the muscle insertions to different areas in order to keep the kneecaps in place. Her feet were now turning in.

She had felt better and saw the weight coming off when she stopped eating bread. This is a common sign that the body has been given more carbohydrate than it needs, which gets converted into fat for energy storage. Eating less bread, pasta and rice is the fastest way to get your body using up the stored fat without adding more in replacement.

She had a retracted lower jaw that belied her inner anger, which could only be expressed by hyperventilating when anxious. She was emotional, sometimes teary, suppressed emotions and suffered inner rage over her husband's moodiness and sulking. She also suffered bloating and rumbling of wind in the abdomen. All signs for Staphisagria. I gave Staphisagria MM. When we met ten days later, she exclaimed joyfully, 'The lump has gone!'

I saw her a year later, as the pituitary was still not functioning well. She still had low thyroxine output and low ferrotine levels, needing iron injections once or twice a week. I gave more Staphisagria MM as well as Hypericum MM. Nine months later, she called again, the thyroxine dose was high again and the iron injections were down to monthly, picking her up for a bit but not long enough. Her energy was good, she was achieving a lot, doing everything that had to be done. Sugar levels were normal. She admitted to having hurt her coccyx three years before, falling on an iron bar frame of a trampoline, and it was now sitting horizontally in her pelvis. I gave more Hypericum, 10MM, and followed it with Nat Mur MM for the iron levels. Everything came back into balance.

In cases of thyroidectomy the thyroxine levels improve greatly (the improved pituitary gland makes up the deficiency in supply) and medication can be reduced, while general health and energy are greatly improved.

A forty-year-old mother of four came in September 1995 with symptoms of dizziness, spaciness, low blood sugar, and within half an hour of being given Staphisagria CM, these symptoms had settled. She had had thyroid imbalance and overweight all her life, with a history of tonsillectomy at age 2, hepatitis age 9, chicken pox, measles, mumps and rubella in childhood, as well as immunisations. After leaving school, a doctor had given her injections of gonadotrophin to help her lose weight, which worked and she lost a couple of stone and 'looked good'. After her first child was born she had an appendectomy; during the second pregnancy she put on five stone (70lb/34kg) and was put on to the same injections, losing the five stone again.

Before long, her eyes became bulgy and her grandmother said she had a goitre. She then had had four miscarriages, and more thyroid symptoms developed, mental and physical. An endocrinologist gave her the chemical propylthyurisyl (which eats up red blood cells) and she had a miscarriage followed by a thyroidectomy. 5% of the thyroid gland was left. After this she felt like 'a new person' for some time.

At the time of seeing me she had had erratic periods for a year which had ceased two months before, and her weight had built up again. Her eyes were bulging again and her legs were filling with fluid for the last two weeks, something which had happened a year ago and her local doctor had increased her thyroxine for it. After the Staphisagria CM, the periods began again.

Her stomach was her biggest worry - she was suffering bloating, with pressure upwards under her breasts. She feared cancer, sometimes. She also had sleep apnoea, dyspnoea and felt excitable. She is a loving and generous, appreciative and very kind-hearted person.

All in all, she was Staphisagria through and through. She had a retracted jaw, almost to the point of losing her chin in the folds of her neck. Her life had been one long series of offenses to the body, beginning with immunisations and the tonsillectomy, and nothing had ever been done to correct the under-functioning of the pituitary gland.

Nothing ever is done in Staphisagria cases - the medical world seems to have no concept that there may be a problem with the pituitary, and even if they did, they would not recognise that structure governs function, that cranial musculature tension was the cause of the pituitary compromise, and that this tension resulted from indignation lodging in those muscles after their own treatments were perceived to be so offensive by the child and her body. The guilt of ignorance over the effects of emotions and of structure on bodily functions prevents most doctors from ever looking into osteopathic and chiropractic knowledge of body mechanics, much less homeopathy.

I gave her Staphisagria 10MM on 1st October, 1995 and MM on 6th December 1995, repeating 10MM on 26th January 1996. When I saw her again in April 1996, she claimed to have been 'the best ever in my life, this last three months!' and was only just now starting to lapse. Repeated Staphisagria 10MM.

This time she began to get Thyroxine overdose symptoms and went to the doctor, who put her on Premarin (which caused intensely painful, profuse period), then Primolut to reduce the bleeding (which it had not). So her Thyroxine was reduced to half. Staphisagria MM was repeated in July 96, and she did well on this again. In April 97, I gave her Staphisagria 10M, which kept her improving until March 98, when I gave Staphisagria M. She had developed persistent erratic menstrual bleeding, so I introduced Phosphorus 10M with Staphisagria 10M in June 98, which corrected that. I left her with a vial of Staphisagria 10M to take whenever needed and have not seen her since. In view of the thyroidectomy I believe that a total cure would be a lot to expect, and she was very happy to have had the corrections she had from this amazing remedy.

The thymus gland responds particularly well. Immune compromise conditions ranging from Glandular Fever to AIDS - this is by far the best remedy. Many cases of Chronic Fatigue in all its varieties have vanished rapidly under Staphisagria in megapotencies, as the remedy counteracts the adverse effects of eating sugar and therefore of candida and other yeast infections that undermine vitality, thriving because the immune system is not keeping them under control. Most of the Chronic Fatigue patients I put on Staphisagria are greatly energised in only a few days. One man rang after a week to say, 'I told you I'd had this for two years, but I'm feeling better now than I've felt for seven years.'

A young woman I had treated years previously returned in November '98 with depression and fatigue, and suffering teariness, moodiness, dizziness or fainting, pre-menstrually. She had also endometriosis, thrush, sugar cravings, pain on coition, rashes on her knee and neck, frontal headaches behind the eyes and to the scalpline. She was 'too tired to get angry,' no energy for it, and needed a sleep just after lunch every day (This whole picture including 2pm sleepiness is indicative of Staphisagria). I gave her Staphisagria CM. 'I couldn't believe the improvement,' she said in December, 'just starting to lapse now.' Staphisagria MM fixed the lot.

The prevalence of sugar cravings definitely puts history into great guilt. Aa I mentioned in Chapter 3, the awful slave trade opened the world up to sugar. I say awful because slavery was seen as OK by England and the rest of Europe. This was a most enormous (Staphisagria-type) suppression of love in the name of power over the 'stupid, ignorant savages only fit to be servants and slaves.' The class system predominated over common respect. Fear of loss of respect kept the political scene in blinkers for two hundred years. The great thing is, the people used as slaves still kept their love in spite of their stress situations, and it was this that finally won them respect, shaming their former controllers.

Staphisagria people today are adversely affected by sugar because they still carry this guilt of inhumanity to man, via the patterning of social consciousness passed down the generations and held in cellular memory. Every contact with sugar sparks the guilt memory in the cells. By removing the guilts of our forebears from our cells, Staphisagria frees us to move forward, freed of the same attitudes. (Hydrastis guilt applies here, too.)

The Staphisagrian English originally employed indentured labourers in the canefields, but allowed themselves to get hooked into the more predominant use of slaves through their sense of Staphisagrian helplessness to stand against the trend, despite the unfairness, just as they perpetuated their own class system. They were happy to accept that that was just how things were, and true to conservative form, could see no need for change for a long, long time. Being in a position of power in the trading world, glowing good followed all around the world, once the English saw the light.

The filthy guilt of two hundred years of slavery in the cotton fields is still affecting the cotton itself. Cotton holds dirt and oil, unwilling to get free of it - unlike the synthetics, which were created with a sense of wonder and excitement, and are very easy to clean. Once we get ourselves free of our guilts, we also get free of dirt and grime in our homes and environment - our thoughts are not of the guilty polarity that attracts and holds dirt, instead, dust particles are actually repelled from our airspace. The more we clean up our own act, the cleaner we live.

The adverse effects of sugar take the form of yeast colonies growing within the body, thriving on the sugars eaten and creating, in their turn, alcohol, which enters the brain and creates the same kind of disorientation as inebriation gives you. Symptoms range from mental blanks, spaciness, lack of concentration, poor memory and vagueness, panic attacks, anxiety and loss of confidence to poor eye focus, incordination, sleepiness, heart palpitations, breathing irregularities, bloating in the abdomen, indigestion, diarrhoea, frequent bowel motions and constipation, weak, frequent and ineffectual urination and many other symptoms mentioned through this chapter. Stress situations intensify the effects.

Staphisagria has a profound effect on the health of the thymus gland and it is this that makes it so excellent for all the sufferers of chronic fatigue, fibromyalgia, myalgic encephalitis, call it what you will. Many of these people developed their problems as a result of having antibiotics repeatedly.

The pattern is always the same. The antibiotics are given, initially, for congestion in the ears, tonsils (which are lymph glands) or bronchi, which may seem to clear up the effect of the problem (the 'infection') but never get to the source. People are still unwilling to believe in the inherent power of the human body to cleanse itself of toxins, bacteria, viruses, wastes and parasites. In childhood, especially before the immune system is developed to the sophistication of later years, the method used by the body to achieve this purification is through heat. A fever is engendered for the express purpose of cleansing, just as you might throw your rubbish into an incinerator. This fever is all that is needed, in most circumstances. Any bacteria that have formed revert to virus form and then back to normal cells as the matter that has been causing the distortion of cell reproduction (bacteria) is burned away.

Nature Cure methods through many thousands of years, revived in the nineteenth and twentieth centuries, have always sought to support the fever process rather than suppress it. When it is suppressed with cold baths, antipyretics and antibiotics, the cleansing process is halted, put on the backburner until the suppression factor is discontinued.

There is an apparent recovery from the inflammation of the ears, tonsils or the general fever - for a time. Sooner or later, once strength has been regained, the body, in its infinite wisdom, decides to have another try, and the same set of symptoms comes on again. *If, time after time, this self-healing process is thwarted, the vitality of the immune system is reduced and the problem becomes driven deeper and deeper into more vital organs or tissues.*

It may sit, latent, for some years. Allergies are almost inevitable by this stage. Finally, a stress period, such as high school or university study or a stressful job or relationship, brings about an increase of toxins that overloads the lymphatic system and creates swollen glands with fever, now called glandular fever, or mononucleosis, a term that simply means that the blood now contains large white blood cells with a single nucleus, that act as macrophages or pac-man gobblers to devour the undesirable material and bacteria and cleanse the blood. These white blood cells are part of your immune functions, developed out of necessity when your normal lymphocytes are insufficient for the job. Again, *the body is using fever and has introduced reinforcements.*

This condition is self-limiting but once again, if the process is not given supportive, energy boosting herbs and homeopathic remedies to push through to a speedier resolution but instead, attempts are made to halt the fever cleansing, it can become recurrent.

By this time, the patient is already suffering from the adverse effects of things done to the body and the mind, by drugs and by stresses, and the immune system is often further compromised by overlay conditions developing from the destructive antibiotics, which have killed out large volumes of friendly bowel flora, thus allowing unfriendly yeasts to gain mass and strength. This adds to the immune depletion, as it struggles to deal with these extra invaders. Energy becomes depleted. Sugars that in other people might have provided energy, to these people become simply food for yeasts, which thrive on the sugars and multiply, while leaving the person deprived. These yeast invaders also thrive on hormones like progesterone which many women take as their birth control Pill.

The poor sufferer is now left with a more complicated pattern of disorder. DNA is altered by the damaging effects of the yeast invaders, and many body processes become unable to function efficiently. Anaerobic fungi develop and send filaments throughout the body, penetrating even the brain, causing short term memory loss (Alzheimer's), and the muscles causing weakness and easy exhaustion; penetrating into the bowel wall causing Irritable Bowel Syndrome, or through the bowel wall, into the pelvis and through the walls of the uterus, causing endometriosis (endometrium, the inner lining of the uterus, leaks out into the pelvic cavity). Because of the deterioration of the thymus gland and the immune system, allergies become a real problem, sometimes a big one. Untreated holistically, this whole scenario has developed into cancer problems, or even acquired immune deficiency disease, which, incidently, is not a new disease of the late twentieth century but is known to have been around for the majority of that century, not necessarily related to human immune virus.

The pattern goes on. Uterine problems may develop. If you did not have it to start with, the Pill is given now and only makes things worse, leading to hysterectomy - if you cannot fix it, cut it out, who cares about women anyway? Energy depletion and feeling constantly weak and ill creates emotional releases, teariness - ha! can't contain that suppression any longer! - and this is where I usually get to pick up the pieces with Staphisagria. If you are lucky enough not to have gone too far down this track, or taken your kids there, take heed and get back on track before it gets risky.

I use Staphisagria also in every case of auto-immune disease. It will benefit most cases of rheumatoid arthritis and most malignancies, in conjunction with other remedies, and is the major remedy for systemic lupus erythematosis.

One of my first cases of systemic lupus (SLE) was Jenny, a very sweet, gentle woman of thirty four who came in December '94, having been diagnosed the previous year in July. Soon after that time, she had had a severe allergy attack of swollen, painful joints, crippling her so much that her mother had to sit beside her in the hospital, feeding her sips of water through the day. She also had thrush in the mouth, and a perpetual rash on her face and body. These symptoms were still with her on this first visit, although she had been given cortisone initially. She wanted to discontinue the cortisone because of side effects and wanted me to provide an alternative.

Jenny had been highly allergic all her life. She had had immunisations as a baby, for diphtheria, tetanus, whooping cough, oral polio serum, rubella, tetanus boosters later, and malaria and yellow fever prior to going overseas, on each of two occasions. At age four, Jenny's allergic sensitivity (Staphisagria-type effects of so many needles) had shown up in a reaction to a wool wash detergent, which caused a violent reaction - she became swollen all over, went black and blue, a real blood toxicity such as some snake poisons give. In later years, she had been given a series of allergy injections, and had had lots of dental anaesthetics.

Her life put her into contact with toxic chemicals, though she was unaware that it was her job that was undermining her health, and I was not given any details of this until much later - she had, her mother always said, a kind of disconnection with her body, was not aware of herself and was not forthcoming with information, and most of the knowledge I needed did not come until too late: prior to coming to my district, and at the time of her lupus diagnosis, she had worked for fifteen years bagging fertilizers and other powdery chemicals and packeting seeds for a large horticultural seed company, and was also constantly exposed to dust containing mould and insect deterrants.

I found her allergic to petrochemicals, grass pollens, antibiotics, dairy products, yeasts, moulds and fungi, paints and herbicides. Her symptoms were: weakness, recurrent swollen joints, a blotchy rash always on her face and sometimes other parts or prickly feelings in the skin, constantly dry mouth, raised eyebrows, eyes angled upwards at the outer corners, suppressed angers, money worry, fingers sensitive to cold and going blue and red if cold. She had poor memory of her earlier life, a common Staphisagria feature. She had come to live with her parents after her brief marriage failed, because she was so ill.

I gave her Staphisagria MM followed by Conium MM, and a great number of benefits set in. At the second visit, she was feeling sufficiently better to start looking for a job. Benefits lasted for about four weeks every time I repeated the remedies, and each time, some old symptoms returned from the past, briefly. By May 1995, she was off the medications and blood tests were discontinued. Symptoms developed for Arsenicum, which helped in 30C, but it was not until much later that I learned she had visited a mine, eighteen years earlier, whose walls were lined with precipitated white arsenic from the smoke and fumes of the mining process. She continued to get benefits from the remedies through the first year, did a training course and started a job in February, 1996.

Jenny was still very ill, though she was unaware of most of her disabilities and kept active and busily involved outside the home, enjoying her job and working late. She took up going to Toastmasters meetings to get more confidence in facing people and talking to the public, which she had never had to do before - she was very shy and lacked confidence, and her main mental, from her parents' point of view, was that she still had a dependency belief. Although she took on 'more than she can cope with, she does not take on her own responsibility for herself or her health.'

1996 began with quite a few new symptoms I found hard to clear, and I left the original remedies sometimes in favour of others, with some gains. In mid year, Jenny took it into her head to do a course in lead-lighting. I had explained to her that this kind of lupus was always caused by chemical poisoning, but she forgot this in her excitement over the new interest. The course lasted for six weeks, one night a week, and this worried me somewhat, but I expected to be able to pick her up if any downhill symptoms developed again. I had treated all her allergies individually, and by June 1996, she was feeling a lot better and stronger, so I could not blame her for, as we all do, forgetting how sick she had been from chemicals.

Unfortunately, this was the beginning of the end for Jenny, for all her problems came back with a vengeance. For the rest of the year, nothing I gave her helped much at all. It was quite a mystery to me, she had been doing so well. She continued to work and go to Toastmasters, and developed a craving for starches, which I realize now was her body's way of creating more fat in which to store the toxic chemicals it could not eliminate. Inflammation and swelling began again in her joints, and she developed a lump in her neck, another sign that her body was trying to isolate and contain toxins. I could not understand why this was happening. Remedies gave temporary benefit only. I had not yet discovered Symphytum's extraordinary powers against chemical destruction in cells, and liver toxicity damage.

Finally, at the end of the year, she became very ill and weak, but refused to be taken to hospital, her previous experience there had been so terrible. Her chest felt caved in, she was weak and trembly and had pain in the left chest. (It was at this point that I was told about the arsenic-lined mine, and that Jenny had still been going to lead-lighting group, throughout the last six months! as well as continuing doing it at home.) Within two weeks she died, and the autopsy reported pneumonia, septicaemia, multiple organ damage from lupus - heart, liver and spleen greatly enlarged. One lung was full of fluid, and the lining of the other was decaying.

Enquiries revealed that lead-lighting involves the use of many chemicals - zinc chloride flux, tin and lead solder, turpentine, kerosene, methylated spirits, whiting powder, and in the patina, copper sulphate, nitric acid, fluoboric acid and selenous acid. We did not win this battle, but we all believed we were winning, prior to this dive into the old chemical exposure.

In another case of chemical toxicity, a woman whose hot flushes and jumpy legs had been sent packing with Hypericum 10MM, came a couple of years later about her migraines, which had not let up. They had originated at age 12 or 13, felt like a steel band around the right eye; began at the base of her skull, followed with spots in her vision, sudden pain on the right side of her face to the temple, giving a feeling as if the top of the head would blow off; and if not caught early enough, would put her in hospital. Her blood pressure had never been a problem, usually low. Her legs were jumpy again, as well. She had inhaled too much insect spray, and was using a Pulmacort puffer. I tried Hypericum again, as it usually matches vertex headaches and hypersensitivity reactions, but it did no good to either the jumpy legs or the migraines. Finally, I used Staphisagria MM. Gone, both, in no time. Two months later, a headache began to come on, but went away. 'You are a bloody marvel!' she pronounced emphatically.

I could not count the number of Chronic Fatigue, 'allergy to the 20th century' and post-viral syndrome cases who have recovered quickly with Staphisagria in megapotencies.

Pancreatic imbalance is often corrected under Staphisagria, particularly where immune impairment involves hypoglycemia and associated low blood pressure. These people usually have Chronic Fatigue or, at least, a yeast infection, following some kind of virus or overwork.

A man of forty came about his chronic fatigue that had begun three years previously after a virus, and about a new crisis in his life - his wife was leaving him for another man. He still loved her, and they had come to an amicable arrangement over their farm and sons, and he was to move out. His main feelings were shocked, mystified, lonely, and needing to take charge of his life and get into gear again - somewhat indignant, yet accepting the situation, trying to keep happy and peaceful. Having CFS had force-taught him to give more time to the boys and less to work. Staphisagria MM, followed four weeks later by 10MM, fixed all the issues, and his energy picked up wonderfully.

Ovarian and uterine problems are particularly exciting. Hormone imbalances caused by, or in spite of the use of The Pill can be regulated through the pituitary benefits of Staphisagria. Many hysterectomies have been avoided when Staphisagria has been used (sometimes in conjunction with low potencies of Phosphorus) for endometriosis, irregular periods, flooding, pain, tumours, fibroids and other conditions, particularly when these patients have had a history of sexual abuse, rape, or ignorance and fear of the reproductive processes. Premenstrual syndrome becomes a thing of the past, headaches go, life becomes enjoyable. Check out Hypericum as well, for endometriosis, this may also be needed.

A mother aged 40 came about her endometriosis, which, she said, she had had 'forever'. She had had one or two days off school per month with serious pain, ever since periods had started, particularly in the right ovary area, which had had three drainings of cysts over the years. More recently, the pattern had become pain for two weeks and bleeding for two weeks, so a hysterectomy was done at age 37. The symptoms returned a year after the op, and she was now getting constant pain. A doctor had put her on a male hormone tablet, which helped for a few weeks, then led to pregnancy symptoms of weight gain and nausea and the threat of lowered voice and beard growth. She was in her second marriage, and had been addicted to sleeping tablets for 12 years, a result of stress in the first marriage.

Although I generally begin endometriosis cases with Staphisagria, there were quite a few Hypericum characteristics to this lady. Her father had left the home on her eighth birthday; mosquito bites came up in hives; meningitis as a baby; and a Hypericum line on her face - vertically, midway between the eyebrows. I gave her Hypericum 10MM at the first visit. Two months later, she returned. 'Incredible benefit - no pain, just an occasional twinge on the right side (ovary), otherwise delighted.' She felt a lot better in herself, thought the Hypericum was wonderful, was sleeping better now, not needing the drug so much, and felt good on rising.

At this visit, I learned something new, which had come to mind and could not be put out of her mind this day (a sure sign for the next remedy - people always tell me what I need to know). At the age of 16, she had had an abortion performed on her by her mother, with a plastic spoon. She felt she would probably not have needed the hysterectomy if this abortion had not taken place. Needless to say, such a gross offense warranted Staphisagria, and I gave 10MM, with Phosphorus 6 daily for a while. No further trouble.

The post-operative effects of hysterectomies can also be ironed out well without the use of HRT or any hormone treatment. Indeed, for many people, HRT can be totally avoided or replaced when Staphisagria is put to use, it solves all the problems that HRT purports to solve.

Commonly occurring menopausal symptoms also respond well. The mental characteristics are critical, this is not the only remedy and you must be one who suits the remedy 'picture' if it is to work for you. I have had great results also, from Aconite, Conium, Hypericum and Ignatia in mega-potencies, for heat flushes and sweats, and there are other good remedies in common use. Some people need more than one guilt-release remedy.

Sexually transmissible diseases such as gonorrhoea, genital warts, gardnerella infection, pubic lice, rashes and skin disorders, vaginal discharges and gleet can need a good hit of Staphisagria to get rid of them. Here is a letter I received from a young mother who had been cured of gardnerella. She had been hooked for a long time to a man who was on drugs and unreliable. She had finally taken a stand and extricated the child from his father's society; he had retaliated by kidnapping the kid and making off, and eventually she tracked them down and took the little chap to live in a different state. I had given her heaps of Staphisagria and Ignatia previously, and now sent her Staphisagria and Ledum so she could forgive and leave the past behind.

'One week on the remedies and I feel a whole lot better. My gardnerella is gone! It's absolutely wonderful. I think I must have had it for seven or eight years. I feel lighter in my mood and body, clearer and more relaxed in my thoughts and in my head and skull. And I've had no heart palpitations, which I was having a bit lately. Lots of good things are happening with other people, improved relationships. I think it is the remedies that have allowed things to happen. The changes in me somehow affect the change in circumstances. I wonder why I was attracted to, and spent so much time with someone who treated me so poorly and was addicted to drugs. I cried with the Ledum, got itchy on my chest with the Staphisagria, feel so full of energy now and I'm getting small bursts of a love and ease of life, a feeling I had in abundance when I was 15 or so. It's not that long ago that I can't remember the smells, the joy, the eagerness, the ease of my body, and it's something I want more of. I appreciate your skill and insight in finding the right remedies for me, Jill, I really appreciate it.'

Testicular and prostate hardening and growths will respond well if caught early enough. At later stages the body has more work to do to reverse the process and longer time is needed, and this can be discouraging. Even if you need surgery, you still need Staphisagria to deal with the offense to the body of the cutting, to reduce the likelihood of further problems and boost your immune system against malignancy. Conium may also be needed.

A classic Staphisagria man (horizontally furrowed forehead, raised eyebrows, judgemental, impatient) developed prostate enlargement in his seventies and dutifully went to hospital to have the urinary tract reamed out, a bizarre procedure which is thought to help, when pressure from the enlarging prostate gland narrows the urinary tract and slows down the urination. The surgeons go up the urethra with a razor-sharp blade and cut a larger tunnel, actually cutting away the wall of the urethra, which opens the prostate to contact with the irritants in the urine until a new wall forms from scar tissue. (They wonder then, why the benign growth becomes cancerous.)

When this happened, our man was of the belief he had had his whole prostate removed. A couple of years down the track, problems developed again, of frequent urination especially in the night, and many little symptoms that he tried to ignore. Eventually, after nine years had gone by, he began to suffer falls, losing his sense of balance suddenly. These were infrequent at first, but became more regular and frightening after a couple of years. Eventually, he became weak and ill, and was hospitalised, where he died. The diagnosis had been 'prostate cancer metastases in the brain,' which really confounded this man, as he had thought he had no prostate left; his mystified eyebrows went up even higher.

Prostate cancer metastasises to the brain and/or to the bone. Even if the prostate had been removed, this does not remove the cancer, which is not a localised thing but a problem of the immune system, influencing every cell of the body. Cutting out tumours does not cut out cancer; all it does is give you a bit of breathing space to make the changes necessary in your life that will get your immune system functioning again, to reverse the processes that are heading towards destruction.

As we have seen in the earlier chapters, this means a big change in attitudes and beliefs, resolving shocks, throwing off guilts and griefs, angers and resentments, fears and lack of loving. With a cancer problem, Staphisagria is only one of several remedies that could all be needed, together with a willingness to change.

Many teenagers need Staphisagria for excessive sexual hormone activity. It helps them cope much better with maturing by removing the extremes of sexuality that otherwise lead them into promiscuity, excessive masturbation, or rape. The typical Staphisagrian attitude to sexuality is that seen in many English films - all under-the-covers secrecy, guilt and embarrassment, unmentionable except with much snickering and giggling. And I find also, that excessive sexual needs in the elderly will also be mitigated and life becomes more comfortable.

This is the greatest remedy for fear of the opposite sex, in male and female, and by releasing the anger tensions out of the muscles, it really helps you to put the past behind you and get on with living to your best potential. Coping and relationships improve.

Many sexuality problems can be ironed out, including homosexuality, in cases where the mentals fit, the guilt and indignation effects of rape and incest or simply of sexual harrassment, many other forms of sexual offense, pain with intercourse, bladder irritability, extreme sexual desire, impotence, loss of libido, gonorrhoea, suppression of sexuality or excessive masturbation guilt through social 'niceness' conditioning and fear of offending or fear of being knocked back on advances.

Homosexuality is a condition that I am convinced is caused by pituitary imbalance, and most of the gay men I have known have needed Staphisagria for many reasons, which makes me think they have always needed it.

A school principal came to me in November, 1998 about his back problems, which had given him trouble all his life, particularly the lumbar area. At this time, he also had had a painful left arm for nine months. He had seen Bryan in February, with no benefit. Doctor, physiotherapist and orthopedic specialist were all confounded by it, and he had come back to Bryan again in November, twice, to no avail, before consulting me. Exercises had helped the lower back, but the arm pain remained, causing him to lose sleep, as he could not lie on it without pain worsening. Sitting and lying both aggravated, and heat improved it. Despite the pain, movement was unimpaired, he could move the arm in any direction.

He could relate it to no injury or illness, but recalled he had had to take time off school two years earlier because a very upsetting person was causing trouble for him and for a lot of parents at the school. He had had a tetanus needle three years ago, as well as an operation for kidney stones, and a broken arm sustained slipping on wet ground while doing someone a good turn. Not a good year, 1995.

He was also waking with a headache at the top of the head, the tension making it hard for him to straighten up after rising. He felt very lonely, as no-one had been able to understand the problem. He was also lonely and suffered guilt relating to having been gay all his life, unable to let it be known. He said he had a violent temper inside, but let it out in a very controlled manner. 'I can't stand injustice,' he proclaimed firmly. He had had a nervous breakdown some years previously, after being let down by some people he had trusted. He said he was a perfectionist, and impatient to get everything done that needed doing, could not tolerate time-wasting. He had been waking up the last few days with intense aching in the jaw.

Naturally, I gave him Staphisagria MM. Six weeks later he reported in, saying 'It's a miracle. The shoulder benefited in two days and was fixed within the week.' He could not believe he had been to all the best of medical experts with no benefits, yet these tiny pills had fixed in no time. Prior to taking Staphisagria, he said, he had been debilitated by the pain, and facing threats of fusion, all treatments being unable to help. He had been taking morphine-based tablets, and he had been about to retire early from his job. 'I sing your praises everywhere I go,' he enthused.

A young woman came to me in 1998, suffering severe stress and hay fever, with a lot of gynaecological problems dating back fifteen years. She was one of eleven children and had been sent from the family home at age 15. Beginning in 1985, she had had five miscarriages and three ectopic pregnancies, interspersed with three children after taking fertility drugs, and finally a son without the need for drugs. The final ectopic pregnancy had resulted in the removal of one fallopian tube. She had been raped by two men at age 18 and it took her nine years to be able to tell her husband. To add to this, she had endometriosis and scarring and was about to have a hysterectomy.

Just to complicate things further, in 1987 she had had a car accident where her husband, in one car, ran up the back of hers, giving her whiplash and a broken jaw. She had jaw trouble for ages afterwards, and many thousands of dollars of orthodontic realignment, paid for by an insurance claim. She now, also, had hay fever. All this was classic Staphisagria, and I gave her MM, followed six months later by 10MM, thanks to which her life changed for the better, stress reduced, hay fever went. At the first visit, I also gave Staphisagria MM to her five-year-old son. This poor child had been placed on dexamphetamines for ADHD, hyperactivity that had come on after immunisation. At her second visit, she sought help for her two-year-old's skin, the elder boy being now well again.

Skin rashes such as from mosquito bites are common - indignation at being bitten, but also after being 'stung' by hypodermic syringes and other surgical procedures. The rashes have the appearance of flea bites, mosquito bites or chicken pox and are often misinterpreted as chicken pox. Always look at 'chicken pox' in relation to recent offenses to the body such as blood tests, immunisations and such, and also psychological offenses or frustration.

I remember a seven-month baby brought to me once who had had **'eczema'** since 10 weeks old, that had come on after being treated for seven weeks with antibiotics for a chest infection that began at age three weeks. (How can they do this to such young babies?) His mother had also begun a Mini-Pill when he was eight weeks, and he was immunised that week (while still on antibiotics!) and at four months and six months. A lot to feel indignant about. Mum had taken him to another homeopath, resulting in an aggravation of his symptoms, and someone had suggested me.

On this day in 1993, his skin was fiercely irritated by an outbreak of violent spots and pus-filled blisters aggravated by the remedies given by the other practitioner - not a harmful sign, indeed, generally regarded as a sign of progress taking place, the undesirable material making its way to the outside of the body - but the condition was not relieved yet and the mother was impatient, a strong indicator for Staphisagria - they want things put right fast! I gave him Staphisagria 10M for several days.

In two days, Mother rang to say he was much better, very happy and the inflammation was going down. Next week the rash had moved and the worst areas had calmed and crusted off. Still very irritated by the skin but happy. Staphisagria MM was given now, and also to both impatient parents. Three weeks later I saw him again. This time his skin had changed to a spotty rash like chicken pox, developing blistery tops and then merging together like measles. Very itchy, waking hourly in the night. He was still very happy. I recommended epsom salts baths and carrot juice, green vegetables and some fruits in his diet. Five years later, I was consulted about his sister and I asked about his skin. 'No eczema since the remedy, since the spots cleared up.'

Indignation and frustration at things done to you take many forms. A father brought his ten-year-old son to me, suffering from slow intellectual learning and poor retention of schoolwork. He had had immunisation shots in infancy. He had been a very strong baby, lifting his head at birth, crawled at four months, walked at nine months, then suddenly things changed.

It was noticed that he was walking oddly. Experts at the Children's Hospital had his parents tie his legs together every night, to prevent him from pulling them back under his tail. Father said 'He used to look at me so reproachfully, he could not understand why we were doing this to him. I still do not know, but I've learned so much since those days, I'd never do such a thing again.' Speech problems began after this. He did not speak until two and a half. By four he was stuttering badly. Even today, he was averse to reading aloud, feeling unable to put sounds together to make recognisable the words he was trying to read. He felt very frustrated and depressed, and had started to dislike himself and life generally. His teachers had given up on him, and he now had a tutor and was improving slowly with the reading. He is the second of three children, none of whom were ever much wanted by their mother, who no longer lives with them, though they see her frequently.

He had had chicken pox, Christmas 99, 'the worst Christmas ever!'

He is very intelligent in all ways except the reading; has a great memory for items in a spoken list, but could hardly recognise his own printed name. It seemed like a disconnection or block in that part of the brain.

I gave Staphisagria MM, to him, his father and both sisters. A month later, '100% better.' Even his teachers and friends were noticing the difference. He was now coming home from school and getting into his homework without being reminded, and doing other household jobs without being asked. Father said he was no longer hanging around him but getting out into the fresh air, down to the creek. His depression had gone and his self-esteem was well up. He seemed to be losing weight as well. Father and the two girls had all received benefits to their sense of wellbeing from their doses.

Researchers have identified the ethyl mercury-based preservative thimerosal used in the DPT (diphtheria, pertussis, tetanus) and HiB serums as being the culprit responsible for 'the increasing prevalence of neurological disorders among boys world-wide'. This is claimed to have been phased out of these vaccines but is still being added to Hepatitis B vaccine Engerix.[82]

According to Margaret Burgess, the head of immunisation at Sydney's Westmead Hospital, Australian infants under four months could have received six doses of thimerosal vaccines, which was the equivalent of 3.2 micrograms of mercury per kilogram of body weight per week for the average baby. In the same article, mention is made of 'a landmark report', Autism: A Unique Type of Mercury Poisoning, by American Sallie Bernard, who claims that 'children exposed to thimerosal presenting with neurological delays and disorders had excessive mercury in samples of their blood, urine and hair, and their development problems improved once treated for mercury.'

Corporate knowledge (demonstrated in drug company documents) of potential health hazards from injecting mercury has been around since the 1930s, according to the same article.

In homeopathy, we have understood and been counteracting the toxic effects of mercury since the earliest days, that is, for two hundred years, with Staphisagria and other remedies. (Mercury compounds were standard practice in the treatment of a wide range of complaints, from skin conditions to syphilis and epilepsy, and many people today suffer the chromosomal damage such treatments caused in their forebears' genes.) How long must we go on patching up after this deliberately perpetuated ignorance?

Many hyperactive children need Staphisagria. It may begin when they have been shocked out of their normally good behaviour by an occurrence of some sort, usually a treatment or an immunisation at which the child and/or his body have taken offense. Many ADD/ADHD children have benefited from Staphisagria and from Hypericum and even Ledum, while I have found the historically favoured remedies, Tarentula Hispanica and Stramonium to name but a couple, to be almost invariably useless when I have used them. Many children feel helpless indignation at being given painful medical assaults 'for their own good' - difficult to convince a baby of that, and the pituitary and hypothalamus constraints begin immediately.

A thirteen-year-old boy was brought to me for his 'behavioural problems.' All his life, he had been easily angered. A pædiatrician had been consulted for sleep problems, a year before, and he had prescribed anti-depressants. At first they had seemed to help, but no longer. The boy was frustrated to boiling point. He had no patience with his father or his younger brother, yet was OK with his mother and little sister. Very strong-willed, tired and touchy after poor sleep, he was a real 'couch-potato,' hard to motivate. (Typical teenager, you say?) He had been hyperactive since crawling age, and always wanted his mother's attention while rejecting his father. He had had croup a lot as a younger child, and antibiotics in plenty for ear infections and urinary tract infections.

My first remedy was Staphisagria MM. He did very well for three weeks, then began to get into bad moods, especially angry and resentful towards his father, who was also moody and angry, and was trying to separate from the marriage. The boy had always a lot of inside anger - black, gloomy. This time I gave him Sepia MM. Ten weeks later, I heard that he was vastly better and has remained so.

Sepia is a magnificent remedy for black moods, oestrogen imbalance and lazy apathy, and invariably, I find the major mental issue with Sepia is a great disappointment over father, a grief relating to father in some way - father is not the kind of father you would have preferred to have, he has died or left home, he mistreats you or your mother - always this great sense of grief over who he is or is not, whether you are male or female, of any age. It is like Ignatia and Nat Mur, but specifically father-related. Sepia is just as deep-acting and powerful as any remedy could be, and rarely needs repetition.

If you see yourself as a pure Hypericum type rather than Staphisagria, yet you have hormonal problems, another good remedy to consider is Pulsatilla. Pulsatilla is the 'expressive' person's hormone corrector, whereas Staphisagria is greatly 'suppressive' in character. Pulsatilla is invaluable for correcting the adverse effects of antibiotics - glue ear, tonsillitis, diarrhoea - and has the mental 'fear of abandonment' or of being left out of what others are doing, that leads this person into the Hypericum abandonment. Pulsatilla is the endocrine sister-remedy to the nerve remedy Hypericum.

It is not only children who suffer immunisation traumae. Contrary to popular medical belief, people are not stupid, and they recognise the origins of their problems, and stick to their knowledge even when doctors ridicule them. A man came to our centre for the second time in four days, with very severe pain in his left hip area, felt mainly on coughing. I began to massage and found his muscle tensions mainly in the mid-thoracic spinal muscles and above, while the lower back muscles were quite free of tension, having been freed up four days ago. I began to ask about the cough.

'I cough day and night, since I got pneumonia a few months ago. I put it down to the flu needle, myself. I was pushed into having it, I'd never had one before and I never get the flu. I said to the doctor, 'I hear a lot of people say they got the flu after the needle.' He said, 'No, you won't, you'll only get a cold.' Well, I got pneumonia. Now he wants me to have a pneumonia needle. I said, 'What do you get after that? No, thanks!'

On these grounds, I gave him Staphisagria MM:

(i) he had allowed himself to be talked into the needle against his better judgement,

(ii) he was still, months later, suffering the effects of the introduced rubbish, trying to cough it out,

(iii) he was still indignant about the doctor, who had not done anything that helped his cough or his hip pain, and

(iv) he had heavy (Staphisagria) creases of mystified indignation across his forehead, with raised eyebrows.

Knowledge of a similar event came to me the same week. Because of a chronic renal problem, an elderly man was advised by his well-meaning doctor to have a pneumonia inoculation. Within two days of the shot, he was in intensive care, unable to breathe without extreme pain. At first assumed to have had a heart attack, he had undergone tests which disproved this, and he was diagnosed as having pleurisy. The hospital refused to acknowledge any link with the serum. He was left with a 'spot' on one lung and was having monthly X-rays to monitor this. He had been enjoying a good period of wellness before the needle; now he has a problem at risk of being made cancerous by repeated X-rays.

Is it not common knowledge that children are not given inoculations if they have a cold or other illness, as they are too vulnerable then? Yet doctors are happy to inject the older, more frail population regardless of their inherent vulnerability. One could understandably conclude that forces are at work to reduce our growing population of elderly as fast as can be done, to reduce their drain on social security and other welfare services.

Any time a treatment is given that is inappropriate for the job, the body is likely to develop Staphisagria symptoms of indignation. Sometimes, these symptoms take the form of allergic responses; sometimes as drug toxicity reactions. Sometimes, the reactions can kill rapidly, unless Staphisagria is given (or Hypericum in the Hypericum type of person). Chemotherapy is one such cause of indignant over-reaction that can affect not only the person getting the treatment but all the family.

A woman came to me in 1994 suffering period problems for which the doctor wanted to give the customary hysterectomy. Her symptoms were pre-menstrual craving for chocolates and sweets, really tired, lacking energy to keep up with her daily jobs, apathy, aggro temperament, held-in griefs and biting her nails badly. I gave Nat Mur MM which corrected. Five years later she returned, having been unwell since a bad virus seven months earlier. She had been given anti-inflammatories, and an antibiotic had given a severe skin reaction on her chest with the first dose, so she took no more. Her residual symptoms were recurrent dull headache, ringing in the ears, very frequent periods, heat flushes, putting on weight, poor energy still, abdominal bloating, stress from her mother's frequent phone calls - and she and mother had a store of indignation over the appalling medical treatment of her sister, two years previously.

She told me the whole story of how her sister had been killed by chemotherapy, how she had even accused the doctor of killing her - and not without good cause. The sister had had a flu needle every year, and every year the resultant flu kept her in bed for weeks. The doctor would prescribe antibiotics, one after another, the residual cough hanging on for months. (Staphisagria people keep on doing the things that are harmful to them, if the doctor advises - he must know best!) Finally, blood tests revealed inactivity in the white blood cells, which were down in numbers. 'Leukemia' was diagnosed and immediate chemotherapy was initiated. The woman, who was well, apart from the mild cough, was put into hospital and given five days of continuous IV chemotherapy. The family sat by her bedside watching as she deteriorated, her mouth so burned out by the drugs that the skin was coming off. What was happening further in? Within two weeks she was dead.

Staphisagria set my patient to rights, first in 10MM and later in MM, and three months later, she brought her mother in.

Mother was a spare, tiny lady with arthritic knees, 'windswept knees', she called them, for which her doctor recommended knee replacement surgery. (See how they are always helpless to offer you any remedy that would cure?) Mother said 'No way, I'm not going to hospital, they kill you there.' Her grief and indignation had not receded over the previous two and a half years. Because her eyebrows were perpetually raised and her forehead full of horizontal lines, I gave her Staphisagria 10MM, as well as a low strength twice a day for the pain. She also needed Nat Mur for her grief, and to help strengthen her knee ligaments, which were too slack, but as she did not return, she never received this benefit. (She lived some distance from town and travel was difficult for her.) I now have a policy of following the plant remedy immediately with the needed mineral remedy wherever this is clearly seen, as it does no harm and allows the benefits to set in much more deeply.

On this occasion I had allowed myself to be diverted by the medical diagnosis of 'osteoarthritis', instead of focusing on the real problem which was the slack ligaments. The term arthritis, and even osteoarthritis, we find in our practice, is frequently a misnomer, a convenient term that covers, in the medical mind, a multitude of problems often not remotely related to arthritis in the true sense of the word, but used because it carries that aura of hopelessness that doctors have and want you to have, about its curability. This lady did not have much chance of benefiting from knee replacement, as it was not the real problem.

Notice how the daughter's problem of 'leukemia' was totally the result of medical treatments, the flu needles introducing toxicity that the body tried valiantly to eliminate via fever and expectoration, which was suppressed and driven inward, impairing her immunity (white blood cells) even further with indiscriminate use of antibiotics. Staphisagria was all she needed to get back on track, but unfortunately she did not know this. (We heard, not long afterwards, of a doctor in another nearby town who died rapidly on the same treatment, the same mis?-diagnosis.)

I had had the same condition many years earlier. A situation of leucopenia [shortage of leucocytes (white blood cells), often called leukemia these days, though leukemia was always an excess of white blood cells] developed, which was, again, a case of vaccinosis. Flu inoculations began my downhill trend. My father had had us all immunised against flu when he was getting his factory workers done, when I was 13, 14 and 15 years old. A good Staphisagria type, knowing what was best for everyone else, Dad had no compunction in insisting that we all line up for our jabs. I had previously had a polio needle at age 11, with no apparent adverse effect, but after the first flu shot, I found it increasingly hard to remember my schoolwork. This had never been a problem, I had always had no need to study, having a photographic memory.

After the second shot was given, my ability to learn maths and physics formulae, chemistry, history dates and events and language vocabulary went out the window. Exams suffered, I was put down into lower standard classes, out of the top, and even failed a few subjects. My high school and another twenty five years were blighted by this foggy memory. (In hindsight, it was protective, because if I had continued as I had begun, I would have gone into pharmacy and probably, would have been brainwashed out of the chance of seeing the greatness of homeopathy.)

By the time I was eighteen I had become allergic to lots of environmental things, including cats, which I love, and suffered a lot of hay fever. In my twenty-fifth year, a doctor friend who feared smallpox coming to Australia persuaded me to have a smallpox vaccination. Being a compliant Staphisagria, I let him give it.

Within six weeks, I was hawking up lots of yellow mucus from the back of my throat. Overnight, it would build up and take me ten minutes of hawking over the bathroom basin every morning to clear the build-up. The local doctor gave me penicillin, no help, and for six months, one antibiotic after another, with no benefits. In fact, I became sicker and sicker, and hawked all day. After six months, the learned doctor sent me to an ENT specialist, a doddery old fellow who told me to get my tonsils out and all would be well. (Tonsils are lymph glands that filter toxins and pollutants out of the bloodstream and dispose of them through the lymphatics, via the bowel. Mine were clogged to the point of not being able to shift the rubbish along.)

I had my tonsils out and was no better, in fact, only got worse, which is only logical, as nothing had been done to clear the lymphatic congestion. Logic escaped the doctor. After another three months, he sent me to an allergy specialist, and the antibiotics and vaccines having reduced my immunity still further, I reacted to everything tested for in the RAST test. I was then given three months of weekly injections (further Staphisagrian insults and more pollutants) of antigens, intended to stimulate the immune system to get itself back into gear, but its energy was not up to the job. By the end of the series of needles, I was so bad that the mucus accumulating in my throat was choking. I could not lie down at night, and had to sleep sitting back in an armchair.

Eventually, light dawned. 'Strike me lucky, this is the pits', I said to myself. 'These guys haven't a clue what is causing this, I am just one long experiment, a year of trial and error and I'm worse than ever. If they don't know, I had better find out for myself what is going on and how to fix it.'

Having made the decision to take responsibility for myself, new doors opened and information came to me about how to fix the problem. Within three weeks of making changes to my diet, the whole mucus problem disappeared and remained away for ten years, until I relaxed my dietary programme. Since I had not fully eliminated the cause, the vaccine toxins, I still had to face these at a later date, as described in Chapter 12.

Once I learned about homeopathy, I also learned about recognising and treating vaccinosis with Thuja, in medium and high potencies. I had some benefits from this remedy, but it did not stop the vaccine virus that had settled in my spleen and mesenterics, which was the direct cause of the toxic lymphatic problem, until I took it in megapotencies in 1999. It also did not improve the chronic effects of all that had been done to me, and I did not discover these until my white blood cells went on strike and I began to look into how to fix this new aspect. By this time (1988) I was forty six and had been suffering many, I now know, symptoms of Staphisagria for many years - allergies, short term memory loss (Alzheimer's-type), chronic fatigue, candida problems, poor eye concentration, muscle pain, sleepiness after lunch. I remember thinking, when I turned forty, 'If I feel like this now, what am I going to be like at eighty?'

Finding that Staphisagria was the remedy for the lymphocyte deficiency was purely done by standard repertorisation as taught to all homeopaths. Once I realized the fuller implications of this - that offenses done to the body were as destructive to it as were offenses of a psychological nature - I was able to apply this knowledge to many patients, each of whom confirmed my realisation. This magnificent remedy, given in megapotency, is a primary one needed throughout the world by all who suffer from vaccine toxicity in all its manifestations. Medicos, for the love of humanity, please take note and take action.

The use of Staphisagria in megapotency would have solved the problem of the poor woman who was killed by chemotherapy, by overkill of offenses done to her by her doctors. I say this quite unequivocally, having seen it work powerfully for all the people who have come to me with such problems over the decades. Unfortunately for most Staphisagria sufferers, they are very conventional and believe their indoctrination that the doctor is the first line of defense, as I used to, and do not seek alternative help until they have continued to go downhill too long - if they seek it at all.

Immune deficiency and offenses done to the body can result in tumours. Even offenses from environmental pollutants, not medical drugs, respond to Staphisagria. A man came to me back in 1993 for help with his lung problem, 'Polensky's pleuritis tumour', otherwise called asbestosis, for which he had been given a poor prognosis. He had worked with asbestos, lagging pipes in a factory in 1955. Nearly thirty years later, he had had two attacks of pleurisy and antibiotics, and X-rays taken at that time showed the presence of foreign material in the lungs. He became ill again in 1991, with pain in the lower lobe left lung, developing into fluid and infection in the bottom of the lung, and he was on antibiotics again for three months. Antibiotics always caused diarrhoea and upset stomach. He was tested for brucellosis and TB, negative.

Over the next year he had developed severe temporal headaches and chest pains running up to the sternocleidomastoids and down to the groin; and a sharp lowering of blood pressure over the last five weeks had caused dizziness and blurred vision. He had had twelve months of aching in his Achilles tendons. He had been a fitness freak and had had three torn hamstrings, the last of which had been severe, and the chest pains began after that. He was now low in energy and breathless on exertion.

He had had a smallpox vaccination, tetanus, BCG and five other inoculations in the Army, and had had regular chest X-rays when younger. He was still at the same factory, now manager and looking forward to retirement. Staphisagria, to clear the effects of vaccines, injections, X-rays, four minor operations and antibiotics; Silica, to drive out irritating matter from the lungs; Hydrastis for his lower spine, and various strengths of Arsenicum for his lung symptoms were the remedies that brought him back to health, at a cost of less than five hundred dollars over three years. He still takes Arsenicum 200C once in a while for weakness and breathlessness, which always go quickly with the remedy. Despite the effective and inexpensive cure, his Staphisagrian sense of needing justice to be seen to be done caused him jump on the compensation bandwagon and sue the asbestos supply company for damages, which he was awarded. I had a phone call of thanks in 2011, to say that he had passed his twenty-year check-up and had been told he was the only one to have survived twenty years after the diagnosis (with none of the orthodox treatment) and what's more, the only one to have lived beyond ten years. No wonder I enjoy this kind of work!

Urinary tract infections are often the result of 'things done to you' - the body starts to get a bit 'pissed off'. A 22-year-old girl came after twelve months of UTIs and antibiotics, and she was sick of them. She had a permanent cough, some asthma (cortisone puffer) and eczema and had been quite allergic in childhood: her first immunisation had given a bad reaction and she had only had homeopathic immunisation since then. She also had skin outbreaks - pimples and boils that took ages to get rid of. She had sinus congestion, tightly spaced teeth that had had braces when younger, and her jaw was pulled half a tooth to the right. A PAP smear two years ago had indicated 'irregular cell growth', and her periods were heavy and only two to three weeks apart. A recent PAP smear was 'normal'. She is a person who likes to be liked, tries to please others, is determinedly perfectionist, feels society says she should have achieved more by now. She is a real doer, having three jobs going at once.

My first remedy was Staphisagria MM, which did well until, three weeks later, she developed nausea and vomiting for two days, which went after Aconite. Since Staphisagria, she had been discharging a lot of mucus from the sinuses and chest. There were no more urinary tract infections.

Offenses done to the body in the form of operations usually need Staphisagria. It has always been known as a primary remedy for pain after surgery, or any blade wounds, where the flesh has been carved into by any sharp-bladed instrument or tool, such as an axe, meat cleaver, carving knife, vegetable parer or fine scalpel. Staphisagria speeds healing of such wounds, without infection, and is as good as Calendula here. But once I learned about the chronic effects people suffer after surgery, I began to apply Staphisagria in megapotencies with remarkable results. Here is one case that comes to mind:

A man of 54 had a heart by-pass operation in 1992, from which he had recovered very quickly. He had been an officer in the British Army, and rules and regulations were always a feature in his life, as was knowing how other people should be, and the necessity of keeping emotions in check. In 2000, I was consulted for his 'intermittent claudication' in his legs. He had had a by-pass operation in the right leg which had failed, the right foot was slowly dying from lack of supply, and an angioplasty and vein graft was done. Life was slowly coming back into the foot, which was still swollen and numb and the skin was peeling off. He had lost five or six kilos and suffered night sweats every night after midnight, since coming out of hospital three weeks ago. An angiogram and Doppler had indicated 'calcification' in the arteries in the legs, and his earliest symptoms had been very bad pain in the legs on walking short distances.

My diagnosis was that he had iatrogenic cardiovascular damage caused by irritants in the blood, from the anti-malarial drugs he had had to take for years while in the tropics, and from the numerous vaccines.

I gave him Staphisagria 10M followed two weeks later by 10MM, for the adverse effects of things done to him with the surgery, to speed up the correct healing of the leg, and to get the calcium out of the blood vessel walls and back moving between the muscles and the bones; and Cinchona (China) 200 daily until the sweats ceased, to counteract the anti-malarial drugs. I suspected he still needed China in megapotencies, and probably needed Ledum as well. Problems that have been so long developing need longer treatment than he was prepared to allow, but he was happy.

The effects of high potency Staphisagria on teeth is a continuing source of excitement to me. Dental work is an affront to most people, even with modern pain-control methods, and Staphisagria should always be considered for post-dental or orthodontic care, as well as tooth and jaw pain and gum sensitivity. The use of orthodontic appliances, braces and plates usually indicates a need for Staphisagria, particularly when the teeth are crowded rather than too spaced apart. Orthodontists need to consider whether Staphisagria ought to be given, in MM, before beginning to re-align jaws, as the release of muscle tensions often does a lot of the realigning for you. It needs about three weeks to give its full benefits, and can be followed by 10MM after four or five weeks if considered beneficial. And it helps to give kids with bands on their teeth a vial of Staphisagria 200, so they can have a dose every time they go for adjustments. It clears pain and tension in the jaw afterwards and allows the teeth to settle more quickly into the desired positions.

The dental indications for Staphisagria are:

- grey teeth
- crowded, poorly aligned teeth, or teeth evenly, tightly spaced
- upper teeth are not centrally aligned over the lowers which are pulled, often as much as half a tooth, horizontally, to left or right, by tension in the jaw muscles and/or temporo-mandibular joint subluxation; and/or -
- a noticeably pulled back jaw, overshot by the upper teeth, causing the chin to look small and even merging into the neck
- tension in the sternocleidomastoid muscles up the front of the neck

I had orthodontic work for about six years when I was young, from age 13 to 18, with a variety of methods from bands on the upper teeth, bands on all teeth, rubber bands connecting upper and lower jaws, and finally a series of plates with wires. Prior to starting, I had had two molars removed from my lower jaw, which was made all the more offensive when the dentist confiscated the gold fillings he had only recently put in, which had cost my mother a lot of hard work. While the upper teeth were helped to spread a little and make space for the canines to align themselves, the lower jaw was forced out of joint. Yes, the perpetual pulling of the rubber bands, thought to be pulling my teeth back, actually pulled the entire jaw backward, subluxating the temporomandibular joint. And was it also the muscles of indignation that became too tense and pulled the jaw back into an abnormal position? When I took Staphisagria MM in 1992, these muscles released and the jaw went back to its original set, along with the improvements to my blood cells.

You may be interested to hear that curing snoring is one of the unexpected benefits of taking Staphisagria MM. Numerous times, wives have reported that their husbands, after getting their Staphisagria, no longer snore! It would seem that realigning the jaw removes constriction from the airway space. Tension in the pterygoid muscles between the jaw and the skull at the back of the mouth, each side of the palate, is reduced by Staphisagria, thus enlarging the naso-pharynx.

One of my former students, who had had great gains herself from Staphisagria, went off to do a full Naturopathy Diploma. She wrote a long letter telling of her studies and how the classes were going, and said: 'I gave a lady Staphisagria on Thursday. This lady had come off The Pill six months ago and hasn't had a period since. She said she does anything to keep the peace in her house, and whenever she gets frustrated, she cuts herself. I asked her to hold her mouth open and then force it shut and her jaw went click. So I thought all those things tied up nicely with Staphis. And if the pituitary is not sitting right, maybe it's not secreting her hormones right either. Worth a go. This lady is a second-year Homeopathy student so the lecturer is going to hear about it. She asked if she would feel any side effects from it and I told her she may tell someone to piss off but not to worry as they probably deserved it.'

Good reasoning, good advice. Staphisagria people rarely say what they would really like to say, and the remedy can initially free you up verbally. You soon notice yourself finding the right words to get your message across without rudeness, white lies or need to suppress anger - the anger ceases to be felt, the injustices cease to be injustices.

Another warning we often give is to refrain from alcoholic drinks while taking the Staphisagria. The release of anger tensions, combined with the release of inhibitions that alcohol gives, can bring on a real explosion of anger that is a lifetime's accumulated frustrations and indignations.

It can be very embarrassing afterwards, to realize that you have behaved so uncharacteristically as to belt up your boyfriend at a party, when he had done nothing and it was only ancient emotions finally being released.

Staphisagria is a greatly under-used remedy in England and all the British Commonwealth countries. Time and again, I read of cases where Staphisagria would have solved a complaint in no time, yet practitioners miss the remedy and apply second-best, plodding slowly towards benefit. I believe that this is because more than half the population of these countries have the Staphisagria beliefs, and when whole societies are based on common beliefs, attitudes and reactions to life, they regard themselves as normal and therefore discount these characteristics as part of a total symptom picture.

This is just another result of Staphisagrian hypocrisy. It amazes me constantly, to observe how the Staphisagria mind deceives itself while trying to deceive others, even with the best intentions. White lies, created out of the fear of dissention, disharmony or of upsetting someone, are practised so smoothly and so often that they come to be believed by the ones who speak them. Our repertories list Staphisagria as a primary remedy for liars, yet most Staphisagria people would be highly indignant at being thought of as liars or hypocrites. The British do not realize that this is the main reason that other countries do not love them.

When you confront them with their manipulation of the truth, they are self-righteous in their defense of it. 'Oh, yes, but I couldn't say that (truth), though, could I, it might upset them, and they would not think well of me.' Can they not see that it is far more upsetting, and makes people think far worse of them, when they realize how they have been lied to and conned into believing a falsehood, or 'protected' from knowledge of the truth? They can be acting in the nicest possible way, from the best intentions, but the harm is just as great in the long run, as if they had been malevolent. Often, too, the intent is purely selfish, and you can find yourself being manipulated in the nicest possible way, and not know how stand firm against it.

Always think of Staphisagria for liars, manipulators and confidence tricksters. Gonjesil says, 'Fill fraudsters with Staphisagria, too. It is a great remedy for people who think up ideas for conning people out of their money.'

For some, only taking Staphisagria in the megapotencies will give them the enlightenment to see themselves as others see them. Many a patient of mine has said, after a few months on the remedy, 'I used to think I knew what was best for everyone, and how things should be for the best. I used to think it was best not to tell people the cold, hard truth, in case it upset them. I don't think that way any more. I can see how wrong I was.' Remove the restrictions, and see what happens! Ignore the rules, turn the rules around, and see how much it broadens your scope. Hypericum people have found this out, and are changing the world (yes, for worse, and also for the better). We are never limited to the beliefs governed by 'should' and 'right way', or by the helplessness of being slaves to the rules of others. Staphisagria brings great courage, the genuine courage of your convictions. As Goethe is famous for saying, 'Whatever you think to do, begin it. Boldness has courage, power and genius in it.'

Many British political and religious reformers have been inspired by the high principles of the Staphisagria mind and beliefs, to initiate great changes to the world created by judgmentalism and self-righteousness, helplessness and subservience. Reform has also come through the writings of great novelists and playwrights, particularly William Shakespeare, Charles Dickens and A. J. Cronin, whose novels of the hard times of industrialisation struck at the heart of many. Here are a few quotes that illustrate Staphisagria beautifully.

'The fault, dear Brutus, lies not in our stars but in ourselves, that we are underlings.'[83]

'She shivered and tried to hasten her pace. But she could not go faster. The child within her, still without life, lay heavy as lead, pulling, dragging, bending her down. To be like this; at such a time! Three grown sons; David, the youngest, nearly fifteen; and then to be caught. She clenched her hands. Indignation boiled within her. Him, again, coming home in liquor, silently, doggedly, in liquor, to have his will of her.'[84]

'David jerked his head affirmatively. He could not speak now, his whole being was so tense with indignation. He boiled at the injustice of Jake's action. Wicks was almost a man, he smoked, swore and drank like a man, he was a foot taller and two stones heavier than David. But David didn't care. Nothing mattered, nothing, except that Wicks should be stopped from victimising Softley.'[85]

'He wanted with all his soul to win (an election), to prove the good in humanity rather than the bad. They had accused him of preaching Revolution. But the only Revolution he demanded was in the heart of man, an escape from meanness, cruelty and self-interest towards that devotion and nobility of which the human heart was capable. Without that, all other change was futile.'[86]

'Crime is the product of a country's social order. Those who make that order are often more guilty than the so-called criminals.'[87]

'Even if you believe there is a war between good and evil, be sure you do not enjoy the battle too much.'[88]

And finally, an Australian speaks: 'Where judgement is not, accusation is absent. Where accusation is not, guilt is absent. Where guilt is not, forgiveness has no purpose and a state without a need for forgiveness must, of necessity, be a state of pure Being, of innocence - a state of enlightenment.'[89]

There is always a choice. Quantum mechanics has shown that there is always an infinity of options open to us.

For Staphisagria people, the underlying belief that anger is bad and must be suppressed comes from the fear of war and aggression that a person has who feels helpless. He naturally craves peace and harmony because they are no threat to his helplessness. Suppression of fear and anger are not the answer. They melt away into nothingness, once we realize our own power to create what we want by generating positive (love) energy, rather than burying and harbouring destructive energies within our bodies. The magic of Staphisagria is that it empowers us, individually, to find peace within and courage to stand for our beliefs.

I'd like a dollar for every time a patient has said to me, after taking their Staphisagria, 'Why isn't this in the water supply? Everyone needs this!'

CHAPTER 16

A man is a worker. If he is not that, he is nothing.
- Joseph Conrad

SYMPHYTUM - 'WORK IS ALL THAT COUNTS'

Symphytum (symphytum officinale, *Comfrey*, N.O. Boraginaceae) is a
native of Europe and temperate Asia with a long reputation as a vulnerary
(wound-healing herb). In the Middle Ages it was a famous remedy for broken
bones. The name comfrey is a corruption of the Latin *con firma*, alluding to the
uniting of bones it was known to effect, and the botanical name symphytum
is derived from the Greek *symphyo*, to unite.

The comfrey plant contains a wide range of trace minerals, its finer roots
ranging deep down into the soil. It is loaded with catalysts and enzymes;
choline for liver regulation and cholesterol distribution; asparagin, a mild
diuretic; tannin, mucilage, iron and calcium in the same balance as in the
human body; and phosphates of calcium, sodium and potassium to nourish
the bones, brain and nerves.

In addition to bone healing, the roots' high mucilage content made them
ideal for stomach and intestinal complaints, ulcers, dysentery and diarrhoea;
comfrey root tincture is demulcent in lung complaints, quinsy and whooping
cough; and it is also helpful to internal haemorrhage anywhere - lungs,
stomach, bowels, bleeding piles.

The leaves are applied in poultices to severe cuts, boils and abscesses and
gangrenous ulcers, and the whole plant, crushed and warmed, has always
been deemed excellent for soothing pain in any tender, inflamed or
suppurating part. However, it is not antiseptic per se, and can heal damaged
skin so quickly that on occasion, bacteria in the underlying flesh remain
unaffected. It is usually used with Calendula, an aseptic herb for flesh
wounds, to prevent this.

Max Wichtl gives the following indications: externally, in the form of
poultices and pastes, for inflammation of joints, arthritic swellings, damage to
the periosteum and for promoting callous formation in fractures,
inflammation of the tendinous sheaths, arthritis, dislocations, contusions,

haematomas, in thrombophlebitis, phlebitis (varicose veins), mastitis, parotitis (inflammation of the salivary glands) and glandular swellings, as well as for poorly healing wounds and furuncles.

Decoctions are given as a mouth rinse and gargle in peridontitis, pharyngitis and angina (utilising, among other things, the emollient action of mucilage and the astringent action of the tannins).

Internally, the drug is given for gastritis and stomach and intestinal ulcers.

Finley Ellingwood says, 'Some writers have been very enthusiastic concerning its specific influence in all forms of bronchial irritation, with cough or difficult breathing, especially if there was hemoptisis. One physician who has used it for over thirty years, claims to obtain the best results from a strong decoction, made from one ounce of the root in a pint of water. He gives this almost ad libitum as a drink. In pneumonia, this decoction relieves the difficult and painful breathing. It aids expectoration, and tends to lower the temperature. In all serious cases, he depends upon this remedy. Its properties he believes to be not only soothing but demulcent, balsamic and especially pectoral.' He goes on to say,

'One writer, in his zeal and confidence, says, "It acts upon an inflamed surface like a charm, subduing inflammation as water subdues and extinguishes fire." Another writer says: "This agent has marvelous healing and cicatrizing properties. If the tincture be applied to swollen and painful parts, it quickly reduces the pain and swelling. It stimulates granulation in slow healing ulcers, and rapidly promotes healing in bruises of the muscles, ecchymosis, injuries to the tendons, and cartilaginous tissues. It is indeed efficacious."'

Allantoin is one of the active principles of the drug. It promotes granulation and tissue regeneration, and was isolated by pharmacy for use in chronic suppurating wounds and ulcers, where it promotes the rapid replacement of white blood cells, the scavengers of carrion within the body.

Comfrey has a long history of success in removing malignant large, round-cell sarcomas of the bone, skin malignancies and liver cancer, both in herbal form and in low potency homeopathy. Its action on tumours stems from the relationship between the fact that allantoin is present in the allantoic fluid of the allantois, an extra-embryonic membrane whose vascular mesoderm is the basis of the umbilical cord, and the foetal nature of tumour cell growth.

Comfrey has worked quickly and comfortably to reduce such tumours and normalise tissue cell reproduction, so much so that when doctors and surgeons have seen the results, they frequently denied the possibility, preferring, illogically, to believe in spontaneous remission or some other still unknown magical force. There is much to be learned about the mechanisms involved here, science is still light years behind empirical knowledge, which is happy to accept observation as a good basis for believing and accepting results. Seeing is believing, after all. Let science now find out how it works.

313

Comfrey has the ability to dredge up from the soil all its trace and major elements, and any other chemicals that may contaminate it. It has, on occasion, been found to contain higher levels of the pyrrolizidine alkaloids. In a long term (two year) study by Hirono et al, on animals, these alkaloids were found to be hepatotoxic, carcinogenic and mutagenic.[90] In 1978, Dr C C J Culvenor of the CSIRO in Melbourne published a paper, the majority of which had originally been published in 1912 (and still extant, I believe, in the possession of a friend of mine), to this effect, after which headlines in the press[91] sensationalised the 'killer' claims made in the article, with the result that our government was influenced to ban the use of medicinal comfrey. Culvenor's test plots had been grown on soil where other plants had previously been grown and *sprayed*. No attempt was made by the press to report on the benefits historically derived from comfrey.

Much research has been done on comfrey through the 20th and 21st centuries. The Henry Doubleday Research Association, which had researched comfrey and other biodynamically powerful herbs for many years, published a report on the alkaloids in comfrey which was challenged by Culvenor, without any evidence to refute the correctness of the conclusions in that report.

In 2006, a German study was published on the benefits of comfrey ointment in the treatment of patients with painful osteoarthritis of the knee. The randomised, double-blind, bicenter, placebo-controlled clinical trial investigated the effect of a daily application of the ointment over a three week period, on 153 women and 67 men, average age 57.9 years. On average, the knee pains had persisted for 6.5 years. At the end of the trial, a reduction of 58% was recorded for the treated group and a reduction of 14.1% recorded for the placebo group. The difference between the treatment groups increased systematically and significantly, in parallel with the duration of the treatment. 'The results suggest that the comfrey root extract ointment is well suited for the treatment of osteoarthritis of the knee. Pain is reduced, mobility of the knee improved and quality of life increased.'[90b]

Dr MacAlister at Liverpool University (UK) studied comfrey after reading in *The Lancet* of the leaf's being used as a cure for cancer, and wrote a report on his work, which dealt specifically with the allantoic acid in comfrey, leaf and root, as a very special therapeutic agent. Others have written of the protein content of comfrey - more pure, very high quality complete protein can be produced by one acre of comfrey than from any other known plant.[92] Yet of further interest is the very high Vitamin B12 content in comfrey grown with animal based fertiliser such as blood and bone, that accounts for its action in the production of red blood cells, and in sharpening the brain and memory.

All species of comfrey are efficacious, and offer no proven risk to man. The healing benefits can be seen to be truly homeopathic, for what a medicine can cure, it must be able to cause, in overdose amounts. If it can, fed in great excess to seven rats, and with the exclusion of all other foods over a long period of time (three months), cause liver cancer (in two of the rats), as in the animal experiment mentioned above, this is only further proof that Symphytum as a herbal medicine and as a homeopathic remedy, can cure liver cancer in the specifically individualised, appropriate case, and likewise genetic mutation disorders. Indeed, comfrey was used from 1960 in Japan for just this purpose, to heal those damaged by the atomic bombing of Hiroshima.

Fortunately, unlike Aconite and Staphisagria, the toxicity of comfrey is only to be found by isolating any alkaloids and giving them in concentrated amounts. In conjunction with the other ingredients in the plant, a balancing occurs that neutralises any potential harm when comfrey is used as a vegetable, a stock food or in dried, tablet form.

Being known to be so harmless (and therefore assumed ineffectual), comfrey did not attract much attention from modern medicine until its allantoin was discovered and isolated for use in patentable medications. The experiments on animals were done, in my opinion, with spurious intent, to discredit one of nature's most powerfully magnificent herbs, as the results were used to convince governments and medical scientists of the 'great danger' of using this herb as a medicine. The result was that it has been banned from use internally in Australia. We cannot have herbalists curing cancers, or anything at all, so inexpensively, with unpatentable, harmless plant medicine!

Michael Castleman[93] quotes cancer authority Bruce Ames, PhD, chairman of the Biochemistry Department of the University of California at Berkeley, who attempted to estimate the average person's lifetime cancer risk from exposure to hundreds of man-made and naturally occurring carcinogens. He estimated one cup of comfrey tea posed:

- about the same cancer risk as one peanut butter sandwich, which contains traces of the natural carcinogen aflatoxin,
- about one third the risk of eating one raw mushroom, which contains traces of the natural carcinogen hydrazine,
- about half the risk of one diet soda containing saccharin,
- and about one hundredth the risk of a standard beer or glass of wine, which contains the natural carcinogen ethyl alcohol.

SYMPHYTUM IN HOMEOPATHY

To the detriment of homeopathy, Symphytum is virtually unused in homeopathy except in the lower potencies, for its common herbal use as 'knitbone'. It is used most often in first-aid situations, in low and medium potencies, to speed the healing of bone injuries, particularly fractures, where it cuts the healing time by half and knits the bones together without excessive development of callous at the union. The first dose removes pain in the broken bone. Fragments of bone are broken down and re-absorbed into the blood, while new bone cells are being created to fill the gaps. Symphytum stimulates the brain to send the osteoblasts and osteoclasts in plenty to the site for rapid clean-up and rebuilding. I call it the 'White Brotherhood', this mighty team of workers. Our textbooks also refer to its use for psoas abscess, and there are recorded cases of tumour reduction.

In addition, it is renowned as a remedy for blows to the eyeball, where it reduces swelling and pain quickly.

I include Symphytum in my BandAid Cream with great results. Only this month my brother congratulated me on it, saying he had applied it to his skin cancers (?) twice a day for three weeks, and there was no sign left, not even a scar. I explained that two of the remedies in the cream were anti-cancer (Hydrastis and Symphytum) and a third was a scar minimiser (Calendula). Here's how I make it:

50g Aqueous cream, into which stir 2ml of each of Calendula, St. John's Wort, Golden Seal and Comfrey tinctures, until well mixed. Spoon into an ointment jar and potentise the mix to the combination of Calendula 10C, Hypericum 10C, Hydrastis 10C and Symphytum 10C.

The potentising makes the already excellent cream into a remarkably rapid healer of many quite serious skin damages.

Clarke lists the following conditions as applicable to the use of Symphytum:

Clinical.- Abscess. Backache, from sexual excess. Bone, cancer of; injuries of. Breasts, sore. Eyes, pains in; injuries of. *Fractures*; non-union of; nervous. Glands, enlarged. Gunshot wounds. Hernia. Menses, arrested. Periosteum, sensitive, painful. Psoas abscess. Sexual excess, effects of. Sprains. Stump, irritable. Wounds.

To this short list, I can add: Arthritis. Cornea, affections of. Dementia. Effects of toxic chemicals and radiation - genetic or acquired cell defects. Hernia, inguinal. Radiation, effects of. Skin, rough, sensitive. Ulcers, malignant, tubercular.

There are no mental symptoms recorded for Symphytum in homeopathy, to my knowledge. Proving groups, please look into doing this, in all levels of potency.

SYMPHYTUM IN MEGAPOTENCY

I had noticed years ago that patients needing Symphytum to resolve old bone damage problems were frequently very work-oriented. The word 'work' came into their vocabulary all the time, whatever they were discussing. A joint was not working, the memory was not working well, a plan was not working out, they could not work because of the old injury, they felt guilty if they took time off work to come for treatment, so they would expect us to work out of hours to accommodate their guilt; they were workaholics sometimes, who had had, subconsciously, to break a leg to give themselves an acceptable break from work. If retired, they were people who had to go back into a part-time job, the guilt of not working would not let them relax. They were not earning their keep and therefore did not deserve to be alive, without some work.

Putting several clues together, I began to extend this observation to people who had never worked - school leavers, fearful of not being able to get a job; older women who had left the workforce on marriage and had not worked for money for decades, but regretted this and did a lot of work, nevertheless, and felt guilty if not getting the jobs done - as well as to pensioners, to retirees and numbers of men and women made redundant by business closures or scale-downs. As there are several remedies in this book for the guilts of such people, you need to assess carefully to get the specific beliefs or attitudes behind them. With Symphytum, I found, there is a definite belief that *your existence is not justified if you are not working - whether or not you get paid for it.*

Looking back on history, I find that while people have always worked in some way for their livelihood, there has never been a time such as now when all the population were expected to work, to earn their keep somehow, for a specific number of hours per day and days per week. Centuries ago, most people earned their living doing what they did best, or in a skill passed down from father to son or mother to daughter, each fulfilling a respected role in a community, and those who were not fit to contribute to the communal strength were still fed and accommodated without question. Nobody watched the clock, and the main urgency for getting things done came when the harvest and seasons dictated. It did not matter whether your art or skill was simply singing, juggling, or telling stories, no-one denied you the right to food and shelter. The workers supported the others to that extent, happy to share. There are still places in the world where people live this way, but not in the industrialised countries. Here, it is every man for himself, and all too often, 'what I have, I've worked for, I've earned and you go earn your own.'

Nowadays, since the industrial revolution, we have lost sight totally of the realities of life as it should be lived. Most people, these days, think they must be in a paid job in order to justify their existence. They also think others, everyone, must be earning their living. We have been brainwashed into believing that the world will not function if we are not working. But the word 'work' is now extended in use in describing parts of the body that are not functioning properly. We say, if we need Symphytum, 'The old brain doesn't work as well as it did,' or 'My liver is not working as well as it should,' when we mean that function is not excellent.

Symphytum is a remedy whose great guilt-releasing powers were much less needed before two hundred years ago. Once the 'work'-guilt is lifted, it will become possible for the massive guilts of industrialisation to be lifted from the planet, and the damage caused by industrial pollution to be healed.

I had begun to notice that Symphytum was helpful for a number of cases in which the brain or head was not 'working' well. Dyslexia, cataracts and other visual failings, hearing loss, thinking processes all benefited. Sometimes, the problem had begun with a fractured skull. In many instances, the problem had been associated with chemical toxicity of some kind. People whose genetic predisposition had been of a syphilitic, destructive tendency seemed to suit Symphytum well. These people develop conditions of breakdown, degeneration or loss of tissue rather than malfunctions from blockages, from accumulation of matter. They are more prone, through genetic factors, to the destructive elements of industrial pollution and toxic chemical ingestion, drugs and serums.

Symphytum in megapotency has the ability to reverse such damage. We can, to a degree as yet unknown, reverse genetic mutation from these causes. Remember, the genetic pattern creates your structural form and gives you health predispositions of certain definable types, but your cells operate independently of their genes, unless or until your reactions to your life experiences - your shocks, guilts, griefs, frights - activate patterns genetically programmed. Only then can genetic predispositions become a disease reality.

However, toxic chemicals and radiation create such profound damage to cells, and particularly to reproductive cells, that deformities of shape and form are becoming prevalent. Functional disorders are no longer the only common problems we encounter. All too often, children are being born who have abnormal shape and structure of organs, bone deformities, large or small structural abnormalities in any part of the body.

But the greatest thing is, many children with brain and nervous system damage from, say, petrol sniffing or glue sniffing, or from radiation damage, or exposure to crop-dusting sprays, sheep dips or common household insecticides and weedkillers, may be improved greatly. In addition, the effects that these chemicals have had on the quality and health of their existing, previously healthy chromosomes within their eggs and sperm cells may be neutralized and order restored, before these young people grow into producing children of their own.

People who have had brain damage from injury to the head have been studied by neurologists trying to piece together the knowledge of what parts of the brain govern specific functions, by finding out what functions are lost when certain brain cells are damaged.

Recognition is one of the factors often upset by head injury. Sometimes this recognition is visual, e.g. a woman could not choose matching clothes to wear, yet she could know later that they did not match. Others could not recognize their familiar whereabouts. Some could not recognize familiar people, e.g. a man who did not recognize his wife, although he knew she was his wife - her face never was familiar. Some people associated the wrong name with an object, e.g. a man would call a cow a box, or some such totally unlikely word. Sometimes these effects can come without brain damage from injury.

Senile dementia is one of the deterioration diseases typical of Symphytum. We must be careful to differentiate this from Alzheimer's syndrome, which is not genetic but a medically created disease of the 20th Century, acquired through a specific sequence of immune breakdown factors (see Staphisagria). Dementia is less common, has been around for as long as syphilis, and is caused by a mutation in chromosome patterns resulting from syphilis in an ancestor who passed the gene change down to all succeeding generations. This syphilitic miasm is one of the easier genetic factors to clear away, and Symphytum is one of the remedies with which to begin the process. Or it may be resulting from cell mutation in this lifetime from exposure to destructive factors.

I had a patient who declined into total dementia while I treated him, unaware that Symphytum would have restored order to his brain. All this man could think about during this time was his old work situation. He had worked at a sawmill twenty years before, and for the majority of his working life. In his dementia years he lived and talked all day as though he was still there, chatting with the other workers and telling of interesting things that happened, or how the work must be done. He would get very confused when his mind was brought to the realisation that this was not the present-day case, that time had passed on. Without his work, he was quite lost. His earliest dementia signs were, indeed, of getting lost while driving. He would go to his local shops and not be able to find his way home. His wife took on all the responsibilities and suffered a lot of guilt and grief for him, finally dying before he did, from heart failure. From the onset of dementia to his death, the time period was less than four years, a lot less than the average Alzheimer's sufferer. Guilt of retiring triggered his breakdown, activating his genetic predetermination.

In homeopathic potencies, the greatest quality of Symphytum is its ability to get the message to the brain that something is wrong, somewhere in the body, and the brain and nervous system can then get on and do something about it. Arnica does something similar in that the Arnica mind does not perceive a problem. With Symphytum, the problem is perceived by the mind, but not by those aspects of the nervous system that deliver the warning alert to the brain. It is a problem of communication, the lines are down, the call for reinforcements is not heard.

The reason for this is a crucial fact of body chemistry that has remained unseen by physiologists to this day, which explains why it took me ten years to work Symphytum out. This is the knowledge that calcium, which is the second most prolific mineral in the body and present in every cell, plays an important part in the body's electrical workings. It is the primary cation, the principal activator of chemical functions.

Calcium forms the matrix upon which every cell is built. The electrically active calcium in every cell is that part that detects malfunctions and transmits the knowledge of them to the hippocampus for corrective action to be initiated; it also receives instruction via the silicon - the electronic 'chip' - in the myelin membrane of the hippocampus to begin restoring the malfunctions back to normal according to the DNA.

Lots of information is carried to the brain by calcium, inside cells. Most brain function is dependent on calcium in this way. It is when this electrical calcium function ceases in any group of cells, that a problem is enabled to develop outside the brain's knowledge, and therefore beyond its corrective mechanisms. Scientists, please look into this.

The hippocampus is that part of the brain that is used for storage and retrieval of semantic memory, our material world recognition that allows us to differentiate the things around us. Dementia is an information transport problem - calcium is not getting to the hippocampus to register the information conveyed by damaged cells. Recognition fails; and the lack of message leads to the physical death of cells, the very reverse of the child's developing brain.

In May 2002, I sent to a long-time patient of 69 years of age, three doses of Symphytum 10MM, and she kept daily records of its effects. They ranged from minor disturbances of function to some interesting mental effects:

'*Dose: Symphytum 10MM, going to bed, for 3 nights.*

'*Day 2:* Slight earache. More aware of things I should do - housework, paper work; hip sore - then improving; hands and feet worse.

'Slight breathlessness, ear twinges, sneezing, burping. Looking at the housework.

'Slow-witted; acting and moving slowly; time does not register.

'*Day 5:* After two years of thinking about it, I finally had a cleanout of the wardrobe.

'Irritable. Time passes, nothing done.

'Looking at the housework but nothing done; improving in other ways.

'Improving but lethargic.

'More assertive, for two days.

'*Day 10:* After sewing all day, went to night class for sewing and everything went wrong. I don't swear - but that night I wanted to use every vile word in the book; then when I came home, I walked up and down the enclosed verandah for three hours, couldn't settle and still wanted to swear. No more of those, please, Jill!' (This lady is by nature a good Staphisagria person and swearing is just not nice, not acceptable.)

'Irritable. Normally, I stand back and wait my turn, or let people push in - but this day I pushed in and asked for what I wanted, it was very rude - also, money does not mean anything. I spend. I have always been cautious.'

As the days went on, she settled down and became more and more aware of a need to plan for the future, book into a retirement village, although still wanting to remain in their own home.

'*Day 15:* Actually did some paperwork - I generally put off filling in forms for as long as I can - still looking at housework, the spirit is willing but the flesh is weak.

'Some days the swearing wants to come out - Jill, that just isn't me!

'Still pushing myself to prepare for the future, re retirement village.'

Finally, on the 19th day, 'not absorbing what I am told; rather casual attitude; feeling better.'

This short proving record was the most recent and the most insightful to date, for Symphytum. It demonstrated what I had long suspected, that Symphytum should be a major remedy for senile dementia, a syphilitic miasm disease. By giving the remedy to an aging Staphisagrian, previously sycotic miasm person, I unintentionally created a situation where I could observe what Symphytum could cause in the aging, and therefore what it could cure. I settled the whole episode down by giving her Staphisagria.

As our bodies age and lose the ability to regenerate our cells as well as previously, we tend to become of the expressive, degenerative miasm types rather than the suppressive. Symphytum, I realized, is a major remedy for breakdown of the body tissues, whether from chemical destruction, mineral loss or malnutrition, or radiation.

The apathy to work was unexpected, until I realized that it was actually a desire to be working and a guilt of not doing so, of not feeling motivated. Previously, I had only seen hard working people needing Symphytum. Every remedy has its opposite polarities. In this instance, the apparent opposite was still based on the same 'guilt if not working' feeling. (The remedy Phosphorus covers 'apathy' also, and Comfrey is very high in phosphates.)

The desire to swear was the most unexpected of all, and one I am still thinking about.

It is shock in one form or another that causes energy standstills in the body, and shock that activates pre-determined genetic dispositions. Symphytum can reprogram DNA so that not only is the shock redressed, but genetic patterns are corrected.

It is in the sphere of DNA that Symphytum does what few remedies can. It corrects faulty genes from diseases like syphilis, but its new benefits will come from its correcting gene damage from radiation and chemical poisoning. All who have had damage from pesticides and herbicides need this remedy. It is likely that this will be its major use. So much of the world is affected now by DDT and organophosphates, dieldrin and dioxin, fluorocarbons and many other chemicals that are indiscriminatory as to who they kill. Chronic 'allergy' fatigue from such exposures, creating great guilts over not being able to work, is one such man-made disease. Had I known of this aspect of Symphytum I would have given it to Jenny who died of systemic lupus erythematosis (refer to Chapter 15).

Symphytum's main claim to fame, its bone repairing ability, as well as the majority of its other healing benefits, stems from its very energetic calcium phosphate content. By adding the strong vitality of potentised Symphytum to the body, de-activated calcium is enabled to get itself back into working mode again. The brain starts to receive the distress calls that were not forthcoming previously, and begins to send the materials necessary to carry out the repairs.

Another aspect of Symphytum is its great ability to uplift people with seemingly hopeless diseases. Its glowing green energy transports people out of the fears of the solar plexus by energising the heart chakra and the thymus gland, the 'life-force' gland. It is great for those thinking they are never going to get better physically, and can be all you need when you seem to be at an absolute standstill. It is a princely remedy that allows great motivation to be instigated towards improvement, and even greater, it inspires hope and gives confidence to continue treatment.

The range of conditions treatable with megapotency Symphytum is quite vast (see Chapter 6), and some patients were found to have several problems at once. One such person was a dear friend, who was given Symphytum 10MM in May 2002, mainly because I recognised that she had a syphilitic miasm influence from her mother's line, and I wanted to find out how Symphytum could help her.

To my surprise, she reported two days later, that two patches of skin on her face - one at the top of her forehead and one above the top lip - which had been tender for years, had now cleared. Her right eye had had a white skin over the cornea at the inner canthus, and this was now clearing. The eye was watering sometimes. An old lump in her right breast had begun to hurt, some time before, aggravated by vacuuming or digging. This was now much better than it had been. Her ribcage had been damaged years ago in a car accident, the lower part of the sternum and a couple of areas on her back had still suffered bone soreness that was now better.

Briefly, two knuckles on her right hand began to hurt after gardening, writing and drawing - then this cleared. Haemorrhoids that appeared after gardening were gone. Her left ankle, that had been stiff and painful for months, was now better. She found that she was no longer expecting pain with everything she did. Her flexibility was improving a lot. Where she usually found it difficult to get into and out of her car, this was better now. A persistent infection in the bone of the maxilla, high above the teeth on the left, was finally going away. To cap it all off, she was no longer worrying about many little things, including things she could do nothing about, that were not her responsibility.

Ulceration of a chronic nature may need Symphytum in megapotency to break the apathy of the condition. At the end of '98, I had an elderly patient present with a twelve-year problem of *mycobacterium ulcerans*, or Bairnsdale ulcer, a tubercular ulceration of the skin of the left foot. She had lived for some time in the tropics. The disease is characterised by ulceration of an initial papule, sometimes followed by, as in her case, necrosis through deep fascia with involvement of muscle and even bone, with possible metastatic infection. She had been treated by the best experts including, she told me, Dr Hayman[94], had had BCG (TB immunising) injections (a homeopathic usage of BCG attempting to antidote the TB condition), spent 18 months on anti-leprosy antibiotics which nearly destroyed her bowel, she said, and the foot had not settled down in the two years since that time. She had been operated on three times in two months to cut away the infected tissue (including the base of her heel bone) and replace with skin grafts, which had been ineffectual, had had seven weeks of 40°C heat treatment 24 hours a day, and had simply got worse and worse. Three times, in more recent years, she had been nearly fixed by homeopathy, but the problem kept returning with a vengeance.

At the time I first saw her, the ulceration covered almost all the sole of her foot, most of the upper foot and all the skin above the ankle into the shin. Her heel op had not been successful and there was now a huge cavity where the calcaneus had necrosed, that was surrounded by raw, ulcerating, swollen flesh, and she could see the raw bone at the top of the cavity. I took photos. The foot weeped a burning, clear or yellowish fluid, which she said smelled of wet cement, sometimes with blood or pus, and there was a characteristic tendency to oedema of the foot. She was hypothyroid, overweight and dependent on crutches and her husband, who did everything in the home and garden.

I used several remedies over the next two years. After nine months, she fell and fractured her shoulder and was kept in hospital for three weeks. This should have told me to use Symphytum for the ulceration, but I missed the cue. I had given her Mercurius at the time, and it was helpful to the foot. Nights were always very painful, and the bandages seeped constantly. We used a lot of Mycobacterium ulcerans 10M with standard remedies, and by the end of two years, new papules stopped arising and the ulcerated areas were reduced. By two and a half years, there were only three small, healing spots left on the upper foot, the *mycobacterium ulcerans* was inactive. Still no cure in Western Medicine for *mycobacterium ulcerans*, according to a TV report.[95] The heel was still necrosed, though no worse. I gave Arsenicum MM and later 10MM, and it showed signs of filling in after a few months.

Around this time she developed a circular patch of red, raised, fleshy skin lesion medially to the heel, which burned greatly and gave her more trouble than the ulceration was now. This was never biopsied, so we do not know what was happening there. It gave some response to Staphylococcus Aureus 10M early in 2002. The necrosed heel was slow to show improvement. Finally, I realized that Symphytum should have been given long ago, and gave it to her on 7th May. 'Will it ever get fully right?' she used to ask. 'I am still hopeful', I would say, 'All you have to do is live long enough!' Alas, on her eightieth birthday in July 2002, she held a big party in the town, became over-excited and ill and collapsed that night with a fatal heart attack.

A young man of 32, father of three, consulted me in January 1994 about his back problem situated in the lower thoracic joints. He was all right during the day but the pain came on in bed, four to six hours after lying down, causing him to have to sit up, to get firstly twitching, then relief. It had come on after lifting a refrigerator on to a table, three years before. He had had chiropractic for two months at the time, with no real benefit. He also complained of sore wrists, quite painful, which his father and brother also had.

The fifth lumbar vertebra was anterior to the lumbar curve. He had had a bike accident at age 21, when, blind drunk, he had run into a brick wall, suffering a compression fracture of the tibia, which left him with a scoliosis from a short left leg, needing a raised innersole in his shoes. Because of these injuries, I gave him Hydrastis MM followed by Hypericum 10MM, which stirred up the old injuries for a few weeks, corrected the L5 but did nothing for the thoracic pain at night. I then gave him Symphytum MM. 'Symphytum worked like magic.'

He was not seen for nearly two years. At his next visit in December '95, the complaint was of heat flushes in the face for several months, very red face and sometimes with headache, coming on after lunch every day, straight after eating, sometimes even before lunch. He had had 'Texas flu' in July - sore throat, bad headache, pain in ears, violent eye pain, coughing up of yellow phlegm tasting of strong egg yolk, 'never-ending'. His eyes had been so sensitive, he had sought darkness. He also had pain in the joints and more recently had had an attack of RSI, his hand swelled up with the old wrist pain. His doctor had suggested he might have a malignant tumour of the liver, and wanted to do a biopsy, did a 24-hour urine sample and blood tests for Q Fever, leptospirosis and Epstein-Barr virus.

His job required a lot of clock-watching and hurrying to meet schedules and fit in with other workers, so I gave him Argentum Nitricum, another work-guilt remedy, though I think it was still a Symphytum guilt problem. Arg. Nit. did well for four months, then the problem worsened again, his face going 'so red it's purple,' his wife said. 'Definitely work-stress related.' He was lethargic, had double vision and now also a sore throat and chest infection, and I gave him Gelsemium.

Thirteen months later, he was back, this time with pain around the appendix area. His doctor suggested a tumour on or around the appendix or an infection in the appendix. He said the little tumour would also spread to the liver, if this was the problem, and gave antibiotics in case it was infection. He came to me 'for a better treatment'. My diagnosis was that a breakdown in the bowel wall was leaking toxins out through the wall, causing inflammation. Again, possibly a Symphytum problem, looking back. I put him on Aloe Vera juice, big drinks of it for three weeks, which fixed the damage and he had no further problem.

Four months later, December 97, a return of the back trouble came on after taking Hypericum for a tick bite. The pain was worse at night, all night, sometimes stabbing, below the ribcage and extending to the front of the ribs; hard to find a comfortable position to lie, and could also be painful and stabbing while sitting. He was having a lot of unfinished dreams, about the day's jobs and business.

Finally, his second dose of Symphytum! This time, 10MM. 'Magnificent results! OK in two days.' He would have been saved some of these other problems if I had used it a lot sooner. It has been a hard remedy to get clear on.

In another case of back pain, a young giant of a man had been helped in 1997 by Ruta MM, when he was hospitalised with severe back trouble that put him off his feet. He had let himself out of hospital the next day after the Ruta. This time, in February 2001, his symptoms were of right sacro-iliac pain and cramping pains in the right calf that woke him in the night. The pain was not always relieved by lying down. He had been coming to Bryan more and more frequently without results, so Bryan suggested he had better see me.

He had been on sleeping tablets for three years, until he could no longer cope with the side effects: they affected his vision, and gave him a very dry mouth. He had also had nervous tension affecting his stomach, for which he had had many different drugs that had caused bleeding and other side effects. He had given up hope of getting fixed.

He kept going to work, regardless of the pain, which he had suffered for twenty years, in one way and another. His specialist had told him to give up work, which, he said, had absolutely shattered him. He dreaded not working, and had been given work within the firm, doing light duties. He had always been very proud of his work. On these grounds, and knowing that Symphytum deals with ulceration and such damage from chemical toxins, I gave him Symphytum 10MM. End of story - remarkable healing set in.

Bryan and I had both taken Symphytum MM in 1993, as mentioned in Chapter 1, with the effect of white tongue and chalky tooth surfaces for a day, and white powdery elimination through the soles of the feet.

In 1997, Bryan took MM again. He developed pain in the inferior right sacro-iliac joint and the fifth lumbar-sacrum joint, with a little pain in the left SI joint as well. He also had pain in the spinal muscles at thoracic vertebrae 9-11, worse on the left. His ability to move his arms backward (from the normal hanging position) was impaired and he had constriction in the anus and bleeding haemorrhoids, an old problem. You will remember that he had been injured in the pelvic area (three bone breaks) at age fifteen, when the Hydrastis injury was incurred (Chapter 1).

The chalky teeth and white tongue did not recur, and the joint pains subsided in time, only to be reactivated when he took another dose of Symphytum, CM this time, in June 2002. This time, the pain in the inferior aspect of the right SI joint and hip rotator muscles became a real problem, causing constant pain that would, on occasion, grab suddenly and severely and take a while to wear off. Most of the time, the pain was minimal while sitting or standing, absent after relaxing in bed and noticeably worse for walking. There was also a return of the old bleeding from the bowel. The pain never stopped him from working, but no treatments we tried, whether of physical or medicinal nature, gave any relief or cure. Nothing worked.

Finally, after two months, the problem had not altered. On the basis that a chronic complaint must be re-activated into an acute one in order to be healed, I reasoned that if this remedy is activating an old injury it must be the remedy to heal the condition, and all that was required was to use more of the same remedy. We tried Symphytum 50M next, as it is second to none on healing old bone complaints. It seemed to me that there was perhaps an old infection in the bone from the failure to heal properly of the old injury. We also tried Symphytum in very low potency for several weeks. No benefit.

Finally, X-rays and an MRI were taken and indicated no bone damage in the pelvis, but revealed arthritic overgrowth of bone in the lower lumbar vertebral facets, showing that Symphytum in high potencies had not helped these bones, which would have been traumatised when the spondylolisthesis developed.

Many homeopaths have a lot of insecurity over giving high and very high potency remedies where organs or tissues are degenerating. They have a desire to use only very low potencies of drainage and reconstruction remedies in such situations. They usually get good results, over the long term.

The megapotencies of remedies restore normality to the organs at the etheric or electro-magnetic energy level, which causes instant necessity for the tissues to reconstruct themselves in compliance with the repaired and reactivated blueprint. Cells have no choice but to alter towards normal. How can this be dangerous?

When a remedy is poorly selected, if its vibrational pattern is not a match for the person's condition, generally it simply fails to affect it, no benefit is achieved and nothing is gained, nor lost, except perhaps, a little time searching for the right remedy. Bryan's bone surfaces at the once damaged facets of L4 and L5 were now arthritically rough and enlarged, impinging on nerves. We now had to reverse this process, and the remedy to do this was the remedy that had been used so long ago for the spondylolisthesis, the mighty Hydrastis, the 'I did it to myself' guilt remedy that works so well on bone.

The big lesson we had to learn from this volunteered experiment of Bryan's was that Symphytum, in its infinite wisdom, enlivened a problem that had gone into a decline that was unsignalled. His brain had not been getting the message, for years, that he had an arthritic problem developing in the lower spine. We also used Silica to reduce the arthritis.

***

Clawing your way back from debilitating or destructive disease conditions is rather like opening up a clear road through the wilderness. You are trying to create order out of disorganisation, and it can be hard work. Even though the remedies begin instantly to set you on the right track, there is always much clearing of the track to be done, and once cleared, it must be kept that way.

The body's cells have memory that conditions their responses, for good or for bad. This memory needs to be retrained into healthful responses by retraining your subconscious mind to your new understandings. Be on the lookout for lapses into old habits of thought, for they can kill. Always remember that your subconscious believes everything you tell it, and if you find yourself falling back into outdated beliefs, pick yourself up and use affirmations to re-instill the new truths on which your body is to create itself.

Remember that what these remedies are dealing with are beliefs and attitudes that have been thousands of years in the developing, and changes need reinforcement if they are to set in. Switch the points, whenever your train of thought diverts back to the old track, by visualisation. Replace any old thinking with images that fit your new understandings, and soon the brain will stop trying to slip back into the old ways. Repeat doses of your healing remedies may be needed from time to time, for years, to assist this process.

CHAPTER 17

Deal gently with people and be not harsh; cheer them and do not condemn them.
- Sufi saying.

RACISM RELEASE

Racism - the lack of a sense of brotherhood between the races of man - is widespread throughout the world, though not a feature of all cultures. It stems from fear of the unknown, distrust of others less familiar, guilt of harm done to others, fear for life or property, anger over misunderstandings, inability to forgive, intolerance, judgemental attitudes, arrogance of 'superiority' of knowledge or accomplishments, greed for the lands or possessions of others, defensiveness over your own, and probably, many other considerations.

Australia still carries a great guilt over racism. Australia's original inhabitants were localised tribes who, for the most part, kept to their own territories. On the coastal strips, food was plentiful and hunting grounds were relatively small. Inland, provisions were much more sparse, and tribes were often obliged to be nomadic to survive.

Hunger was a primary cause of battles between tribes, and against the white invaders. As white settlers came and claimed the land, they unthinkingly deprived the indigenous inhabitants of their hunting grounds, often forcing these people to hunt in the territories traditionally belonging to other tribes, or to steal from the settlers to survive.

Battles resulted in significant loss of life and the further impoverishment of communities. As white settlement encroached further, the remaining natives were eventually forced to become reliant for their survival on white missions and pastoralists.

The two hundred years of white settlement in Australia has been a period of massive guilts, heaping one upon another. The British brought their rigid class system with them - a place for everyone and everyone in his place - and the natives were, by virtue of their lack of an equivalent civilization, placed at the bottom of the hierarchy. Every attempt to fight back and reclaim their land was regarded as outright murder, never declared war, and they had no chance against the rifles and pistols of the whites.

Killing a black was no different from killing a rat, in the minds of many whites; they were regarded as vermin. Yet it was white 'civilization' that had forced these people to steal food from their stores, like rats in the night.

Australian journalist, radio and TV broadcaster Stan Grant says in his family's biography,[96] 'We'd survived isolation for tens of thousands of years, but we could not survive discovery. We had no agriculture, no domestic animals, no money, no factories, cities or towns; we had nothing the whites could call civilization. The whites came here with the microscope, telescope, barometer, clock and steam engine; yet for all their technology they would soon show they lacked the basic unit of humanity: empathy. They could not look - they would not allow themselves to look - into our eyes and see themselves.

'The whites preached from their Bible; they told us the way to civilization was through their Christian God. But they read their scripture selectively. They broke their own commandments: "Thou shalt not steal"; "Thou shalt not murder"; "Thou shalt not commit adultery"; then they told us we must have no other gods before theirs. In spite of it all, we believed them.'

As I described in Chapter 15, the predominant British attitude is the complex mindset of Staphisagria, which said to the indigenous people:

- One rule for me and another for you
- Stick to our rules and you will not get into trouble with us
- Know your place and stay in it and you will keep the peace; if not,...
- Never try to rise above your 'station' in life - you will never be one of us - know your 'betters' - it is presumptuous of you to want to better yourself
- I know what is good for you
- Let us decide whether you are better off with your families or where we send you
- These heathens need to be taught Christian values
- Training as a white man's servant is the only way you are going to become acceptable to us
- This country would be better off if all the aboriginals were assimilated by intermarriage so that the race ceased to exist
- You do not offend me and get away with it; justice must be done

Many well-meaning people with this kind of thinking felt that they were 'doing the right thing' by taking individuals, like cattle, from one mission to another, hundreds of miles away, separating them from their families and even husband from wife; and even worse, by taking aboriginal children from their families and known environment and culture and thrusting them, under lock and key, into institutions where they were taught to be household slaves and farm labourers and roustabouts.

No thought was given to the cruelty of such an act. No-one ever considered that the cruelty of removing children from their mothers and families who loved them left them bereft, grief-stricken, isolated, confused and benumbed, many of them never to see their families again.

The Staphisagria mind had closed its heart, subjugated love in the name of right and wrong, good and bad, to the point of total denial of humanitarian feeling. For some, Ledum fears of not keeping control also were strong. Many still carry powerful Ledum grievance towards aborigines generally.

Now, guilt has caught up with white Australia. Guilt causes denial, so many are still denying any responsibility for the past or for setting things right. Guilts of many kinds have caused grave damage to the native population, with the result that the cleanup now requires the use of most of the remedies in this book, both for the black and the white population.

One of our biggest problems within aboriginal society is the abuse of alcohol and alcohol addiction. This is a direct result of white men bringing syphilis to Australia and passing it on to the black girls they seduced and raped. There was no syphilis in Australia before this. Syphilis changes genes and allows a tendency to self-destruction, alcohol craving and suicidal depression to enter succeeding generations.

In homeopathy, we use Aurum metallicum, gold, a brilliant anti-syphilitic remedy, to restore self esteem and put the sunshine back into such people's lives while removing cravings for alcohol. In the megapotencies, Hydrastis removes the guilt of having been over-run by whites and the guilt of bad behaviour under alcohol and as it does so, restores liver integrity. Staphisagria helps those who drink because they believe they are small and helpless in the scheme of things, that they are never listened to by others. It lifts the helpless frustration and indignation at the offenses being perpetrated against them, individually and collectively, and gives courage to stand and be heard, without alcohol. Hypericum helps those who simply do not know when enough drink is enough and do not care, they feel worthless anyway so what does it matter? Aconite helps those who lack the confidence to go for their dream, who feel that Dutch courage is needed before they can face a new situation, particularly of an intellectual kind. It is also needed for fear and expectation of punishment or harsh treatment. Ledum (can't let go of grudges) and Conium (dependency) are also often needed.

The syphilitic inheritance resulted, in addition, to apathy to life, low self esteem, destructive eye diseases, deaths in custody by suicide and high infant mortality. Fear is a major aspect of the syphilitic miasm.

In addition, gonorrhoea took a strong hold and was passed between whites and blacks freely. The results of this were the suppression of their instinctual knowledge, massive guilt from conforming to regimentation and allowing the injustice of the Staphisagrian lawmakers and do-gooders to control their lives; petty thieving, vindictiveness, out-of-control anger and destruction and the guilt of brutality to their wives. Staphisagria and Hydrastis help these issues greatly.

To add further insult to injury, mass inoculation of the children is creating intensification of their already low self value, adding lack of respect for their elders, loss of respect for property or possessions, disregard for safety and loss of self-preservation instincts, hyperactive behaviour and rebelliousness, all these giving their parents and teachers a lot of heartache. (Read Hypericum and Staphisagria again.) The great thing is, there is very little of Ledum's heartless cruelty in our aboriginal people.

While we think of the period of the 'Stolen Generation' as having been between 1912 and 1938, children and families were dispersed, rounded up and transported into mission stations from 1880 onwards, and the practice went on, for white and black children alike, to the present day. Government do-gooders vested with a little importance, who think they know best, are still removing children from 'bad' homes, 'for their own good'. The short-sightedness of such appalling arrogance and ignorance is beyond my belief. All these bossy types need to do is treat the parents with these remedies and within a matter of months, they have cleaned up their act and are coping with their responsibilities.

What homeopathy can offer to the aboriginal population of Australia, through these remedies in megapotencies, is the creation of harmony and contentment in their lives, without drugs; respect for others and themselves; respect for property, theirs or others'; resolution of addiction, domestic and social violence, fear and aggression, and reduction of crime. While this is happening, they are also receiving resolution of the physical aspects of their health, which begins to come good as soon as the emotional issues are released.

It is their great Staphisagria helplessness that allowed them to get where they are today, lagging decades behind other indigenous populations in their integration into our multicultural society. (Strange, but only a peaceable, harmless Staphisagria people could bring out the worst in their Staphisagria oppressors.)

It is time for those of aboriginal origins to regain their own personal sovereignty. This does not require giving them land or houses, but rebuilding their self-esteem and love of life, repairing the damage done to their forebears and still being done to them today. Many are unable, without help, to rise above the past and take a strong stand for their own personal growth, to regain their individual and collective uniqueness and quality. Many now need Conium, to lift them out of financial dependency, something they knew nothing about a couple of centuries ago.

It is time to bring these people back to self-worth and confidence. They are being destroyed by the depraved behaviour (from the belief of low self value) of their young. Grief amongst parents and elders is immense, they are helpless and despairing for the futures of their kids. Homeopathy is the only answer to their problems.

I encourage all homeopaths in every state of Australia to try these mighty remedies and get familiar with seeing the miracles they can perform. Let it be known to social workers, aboriginal medical centres, prison counsellors and doctors, welfare organisations, government care departments and all who have any opportunity to influence change for the better.

A case could be made for funding for a trial to be undertaken, and I am sure the money would be forthcoming.

In the words of Sharyn Buchanan, a young aboriginal girl in my district, 'What are your hopes for your children? To attend university, obtain a good job, and have a happy family. Well, our hopes are that our children don't get hooked on drugs or alcohol, and that they don't die young, and also do not get pregnant by 13 years of age. As you can see, our hopes are similar to yours, but our children will find it harder to get a full-time job.

'Once we were a strong race of people. We took care of ourselves, we had our own tribal laws and traditions. We knew what our children were doing, we knew where they were. Our people did not have to rely on machines or shops to find food; we were self-sufficient and cared for ourselves. We had our own way of dealing with theft and crime, which was much more severe, and was feared as well as being respected by the aboriginal people and youth of the community. The youth of today just laugh at the European system of justice. Our people did not need to rely on welfare or handouts from the government, before colonisation took place.'

A race that could survive for tens of thousands of years without the need for materialism, mechanisation and industrialisation has a lot to re-discover about itself, and a lot to teach the rest of us.

CHAPTER 18

The history of human growth and development is at the same time the history of the terrible struggle of every new idea heralding the approach of a brighter dawn.
- Emma Goldman

TOWARDS A BRIGHTER DAWN

Whoever you are, wherever you live, if you are honest with yourself, having read this far, you will have found at least one remedy in this book that fits you. Individuals of all ages, in whatever line of activity, can gain something from releasing the accumulated guilts, fears, griefs and angers of lifetimes.

I would like to see these remedies understood, and even used, by teachers, counsellors of any type, psychoanalysts, community health workers, palliative care workers, aged and child welfare departments, special schools and homes for disabled and learning impaired people, aboriginal or other native welfare departments and organisations, missions, nurses in any types of work, doctors of all kinds, drug and alcohol detox units, alternative and complementary practitioners of all kinds, ambulance crews and other paramedics, police, prison doctors, psychiatrists and psychologists, diplomats and politicians, defense force leaders and medicos, work force medical officers and safety officers, homeopaths of every school, and last but not least, parents, who have better knowledge than anyone else of their children's nature and personality, history of traumas and the ways these traumas have changed their children.

Many homeopaths will not like my saying this. They also need remedies to clear their fears and guilts, few people are exempt. But as long as the principle of not repeating a remedy unless it is needed again is applied, it will be very rarely that any harm would come from use by non-homeopaths. I have proven over the years, with the enthusiastic co-operation of numerous friends and patients, that the right remedy works dramatically well, while the wrong choice rarely has any effect at all. It simply does not hit the spot and nothing happens, or if it does, it is a very temporary discomfort. If I had a dollar for every time I had taken a remedy that was not the right remedy for the problem, I'd be a millionaire by now, yet my own health has improved, little by little, over the years and I am now healthier than I have been since I was twenty. Those to whom I have given vials of the very high potency remedies, with the knowledge of when to use them, have found themselves able to make big changes for themselves and their families without having to pay me a visit. On occasions they may phone for confirmation of their choice, but often this is not needed. Any intelligent person can learn the ins and outs of one or several of these remedies, as apply to their family or those in their care, and use them successfully.

The world is in a mess and getting messier. At the same time, it is polarising, the forces for good are getting greater and greater, while the forces against good, for evil, if you like, seem to be getting greater accordingly. Yet evil is only the absence of good-consciousness, as dark is the absence of light. All we need do to ensure that destructive thought and action ceases is to switch on the light for all those in the dark.

Sounds easy, and the only reason it has been so hard, to date, is because so few people are conscious that hate, greed, anger, vindictiveness, revenge, jealousy and envy, every form of malevolence, are as easy to eliminate as I have found them to be, and that once eliminated by the great light and insights given by these remedies, there is no going back. Although some remedies bear repetition occasionally, over a few years, the enlightened sufferer never goes back to thinking the way he had before the remedies. Persistence wins out even with the most intractible criminals.

The potential for planetary healing is, therefore, quite immense.

Religion has played its part in bringing us to where we are today. For many centuries BC, spiritual wisdom, or gnosis, was gained through meditation and insights were passed on, taught in the 'mystery schools' of many parts of the world, including Sumeria, Egypt, Persia, Palestine, Britain and parts of Europe. 'Gnosis was a way of knowing that brought its initiates into intimate contact with divine reality, to the very feet of God. It was not just taught, but imparted through initiation, a form of revelation culminating in the profound and secret knowledge of the divine mysteries. The life of the newly enlightened gnostic, his beliefs, associations and comportment, were totally transformed as his new spiritual insight became a vehicle for change, creating an outward lifestyle that was truly in harmony with nature and in tune with the divine. He was aware that he was empowered to do, feel and know that which was impossible with his own unaided strength and resources. He had not only been granted the sublime gift of sacred knowledge but a new state of consciousness and being. As a result, he was set upon a path of constant endeavour and service to both the temporal and the spiritual world.'[97]

Once Saul, a Mithraian from Tarsus, while travelling to Damascus, hit upon the belief that Jesus was a reincarnation of the ancient god, Mithra, he began to create a magical God out of the gnostic initiate Jeshua, and lesser gods of his gnostic parents, brothers, sisters and friends, a distorted truth began to be promulgated. In order to perpetuate the new religion, which gave the Romans much greater power over the Palestinians, all previous cults and doctrines had to be changed into Christian ones, and eventually, 'the Church ruled its flock by credulous fear and the deliberate inculcation of guilt, so the poor sinner was engaged in a lifelong struggle to gain absolution for his sins, and ultimately, his personal, eternal salvation. What constituted a sin was, of course, defined by the Church, who was also the self-appointed lawmaker, judge, jury and executioner.

'Gnosis, on the other hand, did not require belief in dogma or even in God. The gnostic knew the vibrant spiritual reality of truth and recognised the fallacies and distortions that are an integral part of any dogmatic belief system. His primary purpose was to use his spiritual knowledge for the benefit of the community; the illusion of mere personal salvation was not his concern.'

How far away from spiritual consciousness have we drifted!

And all the while, science in the field of quantum physics and in psycho-neuroimmunology is finding more and more confirmation that we and the universe are not merely physical, visible-to-the-naked-eye matter.

Did you know that the doctrine of Immaculate Conception in the Roman Catholic Church only became official in 1862? Only two years later, Pope Pius IX officially denounced progress, liberalism and modern civilization, along with rationalism, secret societies (except his own), Bible societies and freedom of choice in religion. In 1870, he promulgated the doctrine of Papal Infallibility and, with the backing of the Inquisition of the Holy Office, bullied and menaced the First Vatican Council into voting him infallible in his own right.[98]

From that time on, 'papal infallibility' has been used to protect the heavily flawed Church of Rome from the advances of science and knowledge.

Since losing its lands and temporal power in Europe, and the freedom to burn or otherwise execute, the work of the Inquisitors focused on ex-communication, an almost as powerful tool of menace, and on controlling the literature read or written by the Catholic flock.

Only as recently as 1966 was the Index of Prohibited Books abolished by Pope Paul VI - but not before the Holy Office had contrived to control and censor the translations of the Dead Sea Scrolls[99], which threatened to enlighten us about the Teacher of Righteousness and his true identity and teachings, and about the Liar (Paul?), who twisted the (gnostic) teachings to create what later became the Roman Church. For 45 years, access to the scrolls was denied true researchers and translators, for fear that it might undermine the official dogma and doctrine of Christianity, as written in 321AD and altered by the Church itself, many times since. Did you know that it was only because of Papal policy of suppression of information that the whole of Europe entered a

700 year period of Dark Ages? It was only when travellers to the East in the eleventh century began to bring back knowledge of the wonderful architecture, artworks, mathematics, literature and medicines of Islam that Europeans began to awaken out of their long sleep - at considerable risk of being burned at the stake.

Feminism is showing Catholicism to be closely aligned with its traditional arch-enemy, Islamic fundamentalism. Today, they act in concert on such issues as birth control, abortion and feminine sexuality generally, effectively denying women to be human entities in their own right, seeking to inhibit the United Nations' efforts at population limitation and cripple the spread of western enlightenment. Look into Arnica, Hydrastis, Hypericum, Ledum and Staphisagria to reduce this mysoginistic behaviour, man's inhumanity to women, that has dominated Europe and the Middle East since before the flood. It is time to get back to normal, decent human respect - not only for women but for all people.

We were, in 2001 and 2002, offended by the savage terrorist attacks being made against the USA and its allies. Does anyone wonder why the US Administration is so hated by more than a few of the world's population?

Gonjesil told me, 'Feelings are that the US Administration is the most evil terrorist organisation ever known. Great guilts of this great nation have lost it the respect of most of the world. Guilty loss of love for this country is the reason for the suicide bombings of the trade centre and Washington. Many Americans have lost faith in the Administration now, yet feel helpless to effect any turnaround. This is a Staphisagria helplessness. Given this remedy, confidence to take a stand for the ideals on which the country was founded would return. The heartbroken embarrassment felt by millions of Americans could be turned into determination to make reparation.

'A new generation will draw the line.'

Many Americans feel that anti-terrorism need not be equated with war and aggression, which always affects many innocents. Professor Noam Chomsky, a world renowned political activist, writer and professor of linguistics at Massachusetts Institute of Technology, says[100] that the US is the only country that was condemned for international terrorism by the World Court and ordered to make reparation; that the US rejected a Security Council resolution calling on all states to observe International Law and instantly terminate the crime of international terrorism, responding by immediately escalating its attack against Nicaragua.

Chomsky points out that 'during the past several hundred years, the US annihilated the indigenous population (millions of people), conquered half of Mexico (in fact, the territories of indigenous peoples, but that is another matter), intervened violently in the surrounding region, conquered Hawaii and the Philippines (killing hundreds of thousands of Filipinos), and in the past half century particularly, extended its resort to force throughout much of the world. The number of victims is colossal. For the first time, the guns have been directed the other way. That is a dramatic change.'

Chomsky quotes the bishop of the southern Mexican city of San Cristobal de las Casas, who has seen his share of misery and oppression, when he urges North Americans to 'reflect on why they are so hated' after the US 'has generated so much violence to protect its economic interests.'

Speaking out against responding to violence with violence, Chomsky hopes that 'an aroused public within the more free and democratic societies can direct policies towards a much more humane and honourable course.'

And since first writing this chapter, the US has invaded Iraq, once again on the pretext of freeing an oppressed people, which they would not have done had they not also been protecting their own oil interests. The Big Brother never puts his energy out where there is no potential for future profit, as many suffering nations can testify.

All over the world, people with personal problems and nations with large ones could see themselves on the road to greater health and prosperity, moving towards the ideals of liberty, equality and harmlessness, and effective procedures for planetary cleanup, at a much faster rate if these mighty remedies could be employed on a general scale. Guilt release remedies free us up to create our greatest dreams, lifting us out of dreaming for revenge and destruction and enabling us to convert our enemies into brothers. They help us to rise out of helpless frustration, out of feeling a victim of others or of circumstances not of our making, and out of the perception that others are more powerful than we are.

Guilt release remedies shift our awareness out of the belief that we are powerless against the power hungry, helpless against the war machine, the controllers, the law makers and against aggression and destruction. Powerlessness, weakness, helplessness and frustration are the retreats of those who know that there are good and happy ways of being and doing, but know not how to create the reality of these ways into their lives.

When we shrug our shoulders helplessly, raise our eyebrows in mystified, despairing wonder at the state of the world, knowing instinctively how things should be but not knowing how to create them that way; when fear of anger, dissent and war paralyse, that is the time to gain inspiration and courage from Staphisagria.

When we have wonderful ideals that could be implemented if only we had the confidence to get going without fear of failure and punishment; when we feel that the forces of Evil are outstripping the power of Good in the world, that is the time to take Aconite.

When we have lost faith in our ability to survive well and happily create all we need in a world free of materialism and money; when we feel helplessly panicky and dependent in this money-oriented era, that is when we need Conium.

When life's shocks have left us devastated, unbalanced and unable to function calmly, when panic makes us rash, when we are loaded with distrust and fear of other people and it is pointless to take life seriously, that is the time we need Hypericum.

When we feel too soft at heart in a world that demands that you must be tough to survive; when this causes us to toughen our hearts against the blows of life; when life is leaving us battered and bruised from every encounter and we are losing the heart to fight the hard battle; when we must teach the young that life is tough and you might as well get used to it early; that is when we need Arnica.

When we feel that life depends on discipline and control and without these all we have is frightening chaos; when discipline and control must be applied forcefully or with threat in order to retain order; when we have lost control in some way and cannot forgive those who are not compliant with our ideas, who have not conformed to our perception of the rules of life, who have hurt us or our family or nation, that is when we need the freedom from tensions that Ledum brings.

When unforseen or unplanned circumstances throw us off our expected path in life, when we love to have plans and know what is in store for us and cannot adapt well to having those ideals and dreams shattered, this is the time to heal the past and gain fresh insights for the future from Ignatia.

When we feel it is all up to us, that we are the strong and capable who must, at any cost, support the weak and solve their problems for them; when we feel responsible for having harmed or handicapped another person or society; and when we have harmed, even without intent, through our irresponsibility, that is the time to gain new concepts of self-forgiveness and self-responsibility from Hydrastis.

And when it seems that all ceases to work, when disintegration sets in and our world begins to decay, cell by cell, unit by unit, and nothing tried is working to heal; when the body and the very framework of family life and society is eroded; that is when Symphytum can regain structural integrity and convert the breakdown into a brand new creation. Symphytum builds the matrix upon which our New Millennium, like Phoenix rising from the ashes, will be created - created by each one of us, healed and energised, playing our creative part on the world stage. The buck stops here, with every individual one of us.

The great thing is, very lovely things are already beginning to happen to allow this great cleanup to get underway. Lots of people are devoting their lives to this effort. All involved in planetary restoration must give themselves the opportunity of profiting from these great, energising remedies.

'They say the human race is falling on its face, and hasn't very far to fall', sang Mary Martin in *South Pacific*, sixty years ago. Like Mary's character in the musical, I'm another such cock-eyed optimist. 'I'm stuck like a dope with this thing called Hope, and I can't get it out of my heart.'

Inspiration

Elizabeth Fry (1780-1846), Quaker heroine[101]*, the first English woman of modern times to fight for women's rights, has been a source of inspiration to me for many years. Coming from a wealthy banking family with good social contacts, she campaigned endlessly, through family, friends in Parliament and even through royalty, writing, travelling and speaking throughout Britain and Europe for the welfare of thousands of the oppressed and the miserable.*

'Treat prisoners as though they were redeemable; treat lunatics as far as possible as if they were sane; teach children, but do not overwork them or treat them harshly - these, in various contexts and applications, were the tenets of Elizabeth Fry's gospel. And it had weight: it produced effects. In Russia, in Germany, in Denmark, in Holland, in France, in Scotland and Ireland and England, chains were removed, old cruelties were stopped, men gaolers were taken away from the control of women prisoners, lunatics were allowed books and occupations and sunshine, and to sit at table for their meals, instead of being fed like beasts, at the word of Elizabeth Fry.'

She worked personally for education and better conditions for women in Newgate prison, rallying many of her friends to help in sending the convicts off to Australia with training in sewing and outfitted with needles, pins and thread to enable them to begin earning a living; she was influential in the abolition of convict deportation; campaigned and received funds to set up libraries in all British lighthouses for the education and relief from boredom of isolated lighthouse keepers and their families; and set up the first nurses' training school, at which Florence Nightingale was a student.

In addition to all this, Elizabeth Fry was always the first to come to the aid of any member of her very large family (eleven brothers and sisters, many neices and nephews, eleven children of her own, and many grandchildren) whenever there was a health crisis. She was told in her youth, by a clairvoyant, that she would be 'a light to the blind, speech to the dumb and feet to the lame.'

I'd like to think this book could be such a Telopea, a waratah beacon to light the way.

REFERENCES

The Author apologises if any of the following web references are no longer current.

Chapter 2

1. Polonius' advice to his son, Laertes, in *Hamlet*, by William Shakespeare
2. Fred Alan Wolf, Ph.D. *Parallel Universes. The Search for Other Worlds.* Simon and Schuster, 1988. p98.
3. Swami Kripananda. *The Sacred Power.* SYDA Foundation.1995 p26
4. Candace B.Pert, PhD. *Molecules of Emotion.* Scribner, N.Y. 1997. p.187
5. Bruce H. Lipton, PhD. *The Biology of Belief.* 2001. This is a must-see videotape available from www.brucelipton.com
6. Ainslie Meares MD, DPM. *Relief Without Drugs. How to Conquer Tension, Pain and Anxiety.* Fontana. 1970
7. Jonathan Margolis. *Uri Geller, Magician or Mystic?* Orion. 1998
8. George Vithoulkas. *Talks on Classical Homeopathy - Materia Medica.* B. Jain Publ. Ltd, 1980

Chapter 3

9. Horst Poehlmann, PhD, MBBS. Pleomorphism of Germs. Similia, JAFH, Vol. 7, No. 3
10. Antoine Bechamp. *The Blood and its Third Anatomical Element.* Veritas Press, 1988
11. Aust. Quarantine and Inspection Service, ACT
12. Christopher Bird. *The Persecution and Trial of Gaston Naessens. The True Story of the Efforts to Suppress an Alternative Treatment for Cancer, AIDS and other Immunologically based Diseases.* H.J. Kramer Inc., 1991
13. Prof. G. E. R. Lloyd, Ed., *Hippocratic Writings.* 1950. Penguin Books repr, 1986. (The Oath, p67)
14. Great Books of the Western World, 10: *Hippocrates, Galen.* Encyclopaedia Brittanica, Inc. 1952
15. Dr Dorothy Shepherd, *A Physician's Posy.* Health Science Press, UK. 1981
16. Infection and Immunity, Vol. 70 No. 7, July 2002
17. April 2002, published on-line at www.cdc.gov/nchs/releases/02news/ attendefic.htm
18. Gerri Willesee. The Angry Medico - and his fight for infant lives. (Australian) Woman's Day, 1/12/1974
19. www.foundation for health choice.com
20. www.korenpublications.com. My thanks to Tedd Koren for his invaluable free newsletter to chiropractors.
21. James J. Rybacki, Pharm. D., and James W. Long, M.D. *The Essential Guide to Prescription Drugs. Everything You Need to Know for Safe Use.* Harper Perennial, 1997 Edition
22. Journal of Bone and Mineral Research, May 2002
23. Powell, Dr. A., Inspiration and Persecution: Messages from Self and Beyond. Network - the Scientific and Medical Network Review, No. 77, Dec.2001, pp17-21
24. as 21.
25. Trevor Turner. Trust Me, I'm a Doctor. New Internationalist 331. Jan-Feb 2001, p33. trevor.turner@chcst.nthames.nhs.uk
26. Science News, 2001; 160:309
27. Guardian 5 Oct 2000
28. Patrick Quillan. *The Diabetes Improvement Program.* The Leader Co. Inc., North Canton, Ohio USA; in which he quotes Sancetta SM et al, Ann.Int.Med., Vol35, p1028, 1951
29. Maebashi M et al, J.Clin.Biochem. Nutr., vol 14, p211, 1993
30. Guy Murchie. *The Seven Mysteries of Life: an Exploration of Science and Philosophy.* Houghton Mifflin, 1999

Chapter 4

31. J. Ellis Barker, *New Lives for Old - How to Cure the Incurable*. Health Science Press.1949
32. Viera Scheibner. *Vaccination - The Medical Assault on the Immune System*. 1993.
33. George Vithoulkas. *Homeopathy - Medicine for the New Man*. Arco, 1979
34. Dr Dorothy Shepherd. *The Magic of the Minimum Dose*. Health Science Press.
35. George Dimitriadis, Ed. *The Bonninghausen Repertory*, Hahnemann Institute, Sydney. 2000
36. Magneto-Geometric Applications, of 45 Dowanhill Road, Catford, London, SE6 1SX UK would be happy to receive your enquiry and will send you details and price lists of their instruments and remedy cards. They were the original producers of magneto-geometric instruments, have been in business for over 40 years and are a steady and reliable source.
37. A factual report on the study and other related publications are available from Isaac Golden at P.O. Box 155, Daylesford, Victoria, 3460, Australia, or via i_golden@netconnect.com.au. Further information can be gained from the Australian Vaccination Network, P.O. Box 177 Bangalow NSW 2479, e-mail info@avn.org.au, www.avn.org.au and by subscribing to their Informed Voice magazine; see www.informedvoice.com.au.
38. Harris L. Coulter. *Divided Legacy. The Conflict between Homœopathy and the American Medical Association*. North Atlantic Books, 1982. A detailed history of American homeopathy and allopathic medicine in the 19th century.
38b. Norman Doidge, MD, *The Brain That Changes Itself*, Revised Edition, 2010, p107. Scribe Publications.
39. Valerie V. Hunt. *Infinite Mind. The Science of Human Vibrations*. Malibu Publishing Co., Malibu, California 90265. 1985. pp109-110.
40. Samuel Hahnemann. *Organon of Medicine* (Fifth Edition + additions and alterations from 6th Edition, 1833, transl. by Boericke and Krauss, 1921.) with Preface to 6th Edition, Transl. by R.E. Dudgeon. Indian Books and Periodicals. Reprint.
41. As 5.
42. Nature 409:816, 2001
43. Nature 333.787, 1988
44. As 4.

Chapter 5

45. Pulford. *Homeopathic Materia Medica of Graphic Drug Pictures*. B.Jain Publishers, New Delhi
46. Dr Desmond Morris. *Manwatching*. Triad/Panther,1980
47. Ashley Montagu. *Touching - The Human Significance of the Skin*. Harper & Row, 1971
48. Burton Goldberg, Fight Fibroids Naturally. Nature & Health, June-July 2000
49. Diegeler A, Hirsch R., Schneider F, et al, Neuromonitoring and neurocognitive outcome in off-pump versus conventional coronary bypass operation. Ann.Thoracic Surg. 2000;69:1162-1166

Chapter 7

50. Mrs M. Grieve, FRHS. *A Modern Herbal* (1931). Tiger Books, 1992
51. Finley Ellingwood, MD. *American Materia Medica, Therapeutics and Pharmacognosy, Vol II, Botanical* (1919). Eclectic Medical Publications, 1994
52. Robert Lomas. *The Invisible College*. Headline Book Publ., London 2002
53. John Henry Clarke, MD. *A Dictionary of Practical Materia Medica*. IBPS, New Delhi.
54 Samuel Hahnemann. *The Chronic Diseases, Their Peculiar Nature and Their Homœopathic Cure*. Jain Publishing Co. New Delhi.
55. As 15.
56. Simon Winchester. *The Surgeon of Crowthorne* Penguin Books, 1999. Also on CD
57. As 53.
58. William Boericke, MD. *Materia Medica with Repertory*. B. Jain Publ. India
59. Kay Rasool. *My Journey Behind the Veil. Conversations with Muslim Women* Lothian Books, Melbourne. 2002
60. V. Sackville-West, *Saint Joan of Arc* (1936). Penguin Books, 1955.
61. Fred Alan Wolf. *Parallel Universes. The Search for Other Worlds*. Simon and Schuster. 1988

Chapter 8

62. Max Wichtl. *Herbal Drugs and Phytopharmaceuticals*. Medpharm Scientific Publishers, Stuttgart,1994
63. As 15, 55.
64. Jeffrey SL, Belcher HJ. Use of Arnica to relieve pain after carpal tunnel release surgery. Alternative Therapies in Health and Medicine 2002;8(2):66-68
65. Holsinger, Tracey et al., Head injury in early adulthood and the lifetime risk of depression. Archives of General Psychiatry (2002); 59:17-22
66. US National Institute on Aging and Duke University. Head Injury and Alzheimer's Disease - 50 Year follow-up to head injury! Neurology, Oct. 24, 2000

Chapter 9

67. Matthew Wood. *The Book of Herbal Wisdom*. North Atlantic Books, 1997
68. Dr N.M. Choudhuri, *A Study on Materia Medica*. 1929. B. Jain Publishers, New Delhi
69. George Vithoulkas. *Talks on Classical Homeopathy - Materia Medica*. B. Jain Publ. Ltd, 1980

Chapter 10

70. Dr W Strehlow and Gottfried Hertzka MD. *Hildegard of Bingen's Medicine*. Bear & Co., New Mexico. 1988

Chapter 11.

71. SMH, Sept.21-22, 2002, p48
72. Jack Welch. *Jack*. Hodder Headline. 2001
73. Chris Moon. *One Step Beyond*. Macmillan 1999
74. (withdrawn)
75. WorldNetDaily.com
76. Michael Lewis. *The New, New Thing*. Hodder & Stoughton,1999
77. Simon Andreae. *Secrets of Love and Lust*.

Chapter 12

78. Peter Evans. *Peter Sellers, the Mask Behind the Mask*. NEL Ltd. p41

Chapter 13

79. M. L. Tyler, MD. *Homoeopathic Drug Pictures* (1942) Health Science Press, 1975 et al.

Chapter 14

80. Dorothy Hall. *Dorothy Hall's Herbal Medicine*. Lothian Press, 1988
81. Andrew Jennings. *The Lords of the Rings* (1992), *The New Lords of the Rings* (1996), *The Great Olympic Swindle* (2000). Simon and Shuster

Chapter 15

82. The Australian, June 11, 2002, p1, 'At the sharp end of a medical mystery.'
83. William Shakespeare, *Julius Caesar*.
84. A. J. Cronin. *The Stars Look Down*, p9. NEL Ltd, 1975
85. ibid, p18.
86. ibid, p594
87. A. J. Cronin. *Beyond This Place*, NEL Ltd, 1975
88. Advice to Sister Anne in the film, *The Singing Nun*.
89. Peter O. Erbe. *God I Am - From Tragic to Magic*. Triad Publishers, Australia.

Chapter 16

90. Hirono, I. et al. Journal of the National Cancer Institute (USA) 1978. 61:865
90b. Grube B, Grunwald J, Krug L and Staiger C, Efficacy of a comfrey root (Symphyt offic. radix) extract ointment in the treatment of patients with painful osteoarthritis of the knee: Results of a double-blind, randomised, bicenter, placebo-controlled trial. 1016/j.phymed.2006.11.006
91. The Age, Melbourne, March 15, 1978, 'Scientists say Herb is a Killer'
92. Andrew Hughes, 1978.
93. Michael Calstleman. *The Healing Herbs.* Bookman Press, 1991
94. Dr. J. Hayman, Dept. of Physiology, Repatriation General Hospital, University of Melbourne, Australia. Out of Africa: Observations on the histopathology of *mycobacterium ulcerans* infection. Clin. Path. 1993;**46**:5-9
95. '7.30 Report', ABC-TV, 20.6.2000

Chapter 17

96. Stan Grant. *The Tears of Strangers.* Harper Collins Publishers, 2002

Chapter 18

97. Tim Wallace-Murphy and Marilyn Hopkins. *Rosslyn, Guardian of the Secrets of the Holy Grail.* Element Books. 2001
98. Michael Baigent and Richard Leigh. *The Inquisition.* Penguin Books, 2000
99. Geza Vermes. *The Complete Dead Sea Scrolls in English.* Penguin Books, 1998
100. Noam Chomsky. *September 11.* Seven Stories Press (US), Allen & Unwin (Australia). 2001.
101. Janet Whitney. *Elizabeth Fry, Quaker Heroine.* George G. Harrap & Co. Ltd,1938 Chapter 16
90. Hirono, I. et al. Journal of the National Cancer Institute (USA) 1978. 61:865
90b. Grube B, Grunwald J, Krug L and Staiger C, Efficacy of a comfrey root (Symphyti offic. radix) extract ointment in the treatment of patients with painful osteoarthritis of the knee: Results of a double-blind, randomised, bicenter, placebo-controlled trial. 1016/j.phymed.2006.11.006
91. The Age, Melbourne, March 15, 1978, 'Scientists say Herb is a Killer'
92. Andrew Hughes, 1978.
93.' Michael Calstleman. *The Healing Herbs.* Bookman Press, 1991
94. Dr. J. Hayman, Dept. of Physiology, Repatriation General Hospital, University of Melbourne, Australia. Out of Africa: Observations on the histopathology of *mycobacterium ulcerans* infection. Clin. Path. 1993; 46:5-9
95. '7.30 Report', ABC-TV, 20.6.2000

INDEX

CPSIA information can be obtained
at www.ICGtesting.com
Printed in the USA
LVHW061645060222
710360LV00044B/1290/J